"I've been in the music industry for more than 40 years. Since meeting Dr. Jay, he has provided me with the information I needed to maintain a level of health that made it possible to continue performing the world over. I recommend his work highly to anyone who wishes to remain healthy and active for as long as they wish."
– Bobby Kimball, Lead Singer for TOTO

"I have been in practice for almost 20 years and have always conveyed the importance of proper exercise, posture, rest and nutrition to my patients. This book consolidates all of these ideas and makes them easy to follow and understand. Everyone needs to read this book if they want to avoid back or neck pain while living a healthier lifestyle."
– Dr. Phil Dontino, DC, DAAPM, DACNB, FABDA, CICE

"Being a professional drummer and doing a lot of session work and travel was wreaking havoc on my body. Under Dr. Jay's care and listening to his advice, I am keeping up with my hectic schedule. Dr. Jay, YOU ROCK!"
– Dave Northrup, drummer for Travis Tritt and Nashville sessions musician

"A lot of books promise a miracle cure or tell you fluff when it comes to your health. This book is different. It delivers information you need, in a format anyone can understand, backed by solid research. This is the last book you will ever need regarding your complete health."
– Dr. Richard F. Gennaro, Jr., DC, CSCS, CFT, MUA.
Founding Member and Vice President of the ICA Council on Fitness and Sports Health Science

Back
At Your
Best

Balancing the Demands of Life With the Needs of Your Body

Dr. Jay M. Lipoff, C.F.T.

Back At Your Best provides of information that is practical, reliable, as well as easy to understand issues relating to diet, exercise, sleep, spinal health, posture and ergonomics. This information comes from many research studies, scientific facts and over 20 years' of experience treating patients. This book is intended to be a source of information to help you achieve better health through informed decisions, and a better understanding of how your body works with what it needs.

Always consult your personal doctors before attempting anything new when it comes to your diet or exercise, because your doctors know your clinical case best. Dr. Lipoff does not receive any endorsements from any company or products contained herein.

First Edition 2011
Second Edition 2013

Copyright © 2013 Dr. Jay M. Lipoff, C.F.T.
Photographs & Drawings © 2013 Dr. Jay M. Lipoff, C.F.T.
Design & Layout by Mark Boyce @ www.558studio.com
Editing by Alexandra Mueller-Blysak at www.articulate-LLC.com

contact: www.BAYBBook.com at drjay@backatyourbest.com

ISBN-13: 978-0-9836147-7-7

> *"The person who makes a success of living is the one who sees his goal steadily and aims for it unswervingly. That is dedication."* – **Cecil B. DeMille**

Dedication

This book is dedicated to my patients whom I have had the pleasure to treat and get to know over the years. You are like family to me. May these words find you in good health and the ideas remind you of all the times I nagged you to: sleep like this, get the wallet out of your back pocket, stop doing that, and to stretch, stretch, stretch. Remember, it is only because I care about you and your health.

To my family, friends and colleagues, thank you for your years of guidance, friendship, encouragement, support and love. Without you, I would be nowhere.

To my wife Julie, there is no life within me, without your love around me. I love you from the top of my heart to the bottom of my soul. Our sons are without a doubt our greatest accomplishment.

> *"The best and safest thing is to keep a balance in your life, acknowledge the great powers around us and in us. If you can do that, and live that way, you are really a wise man."*
> **- Euripides**

Acknowledgements

The list is long but I will limit it to the people who have influenced my education. My friends know who they are and they are really special to me.

Mrs. Van Wie was the best 3rd grade teacher who really captivated my attention. She made learning fun and when she retired the world lost a phenomenal advocate for learning. Mr. Jim Vittorio was my 6th grade teacher and the father of one of my best friends. So I was pushed and encouraged a little more because he wanted me to succeed. He knew I could always do better. They are still friends of mine to this day.

The instructors who enhanced my education and passion for natural health the most are Drs. Phil Dontino, Vinny Loia, and Dino Patriarco. Your guidance will always be appreciated.

Next are my study buddies with whom I spent many long hours hammering out information into the early morning. Granted, some of that time was wasted during breaks of basketball and Madden Football on the projection screen. They have been a constant source of inspiration, friendship, laughter and ever-lasting support. I am fortunate to have you as my friends. Thank you Drs. Art Atkinson, John Barnes, Mark Fronczak, Richard Gennaro, and Gary Kane.

My friend Dr. Jack Barnathan who has unmatched energy and enthusiasm for educating his colleagues and the public on how to become more physically fit and healthier. Thank you for your motivation and commitment to your work.

Special thanks go to my brother-in-law Greg and my wife Julie. These dedicated souls sacrificed their time for me to take a ridiculous amount of photos to visually demonstrate the proper ways to exercise and stretch. They were really good sports about it.

Mark Boyce has the patience of a saint. He never yelled out in frustration where I could hear it, to endure all of my questions and pickiness to get this book formatted.

Alexandra Mueller-Blysak. Thank you for all of your hard work. I truly appreciate it! You make me look like I have a frim grasp of the English language and the grammar rules. Which apparently I don't. Thanks for making me look good kid!

Thanks guys.

> *"The doctor of the future will give no medicine, but will interest her or his patients in the care of the human frame, in a proper diet, and in the cause and prevention of disease."*
> **– Thomas A. Edison**

Foreword

There are two reasons why I wrote a book about back health, posture and many of the things that may affect them. I have treated patients for more than 15 years and love what I do. I always create a friendly environment in which I explain what their problems are and how they can help themselves. That is how I want to be treated, so why should it be any different for my patients.

My goal as a doctor is to treat my patients as if they are my family and to do whatever is needed, whether that was in my office or somebody else's, so they could get relief and get back to enjoying life. I don't mind who gets the credit for helping someone get well or feel better, as long as they do.

One day in my office I was reading yet another patient the health riot act so she could help herself. I then realized it was time to help a larger pool of people. After years of explaining things about the body, the benefits of a healthy diet, proper exercise and correct posture, I decided to write this book.

My goal for this book is to explain difficult subjects so anyone can understand them and implement these ideas, without all the medical mumbo jumbo. Sure I may use some big words, but I will define them and use analogies that readers can relate to in their life. The book should be non-intimidating, educational and fun while offering practical solutions and applications enabling people from any background to benefit.

This book gives you an opportunity to learn how your body works to make you more responsible for your own health. When you understand how you can change the way you perform simple everyday tasks, you have a wonderful chance to regain, maintain and preserve your health.

Admittedly, there may be some dry spots due to the research studies I have included, but I will attempt to make their findings thought provoking and meaningful. I hope to do this in a light-hearted way, because learning is easier if it's fun.

All people have interesting stories. My job is to listen and learn about your habits and lifestyle demands so I can develop an effective approach when I help you. The question is will you listen to my ideas about how you can help yourself?

If someone explains to me that he is a workout nut, like Tony, then my program for him has to be aggressive. He isn't going to sit around. If I tell him not to do something physical or not train, he isn't going to listen to me. As an athlete, I can relate. I want to compete too.

When Dennis had a captain and crew golf tournament his low back hurt. I told him, if he was playing, to initially let the other guys drive the ball and limit his swinging. As he got closer to finishing his day, then go ahead and swing more. That way he can participate the entire day, instead of trying to hit yards further then his team on the second hole and ruining himself for the day.

Day after day people are hindered by pain. It keeps them from things like work, family, hobbies and sleep. Many patients have come in complaining of headaches, neck pain, sciatica, or low back pain. In most cases, they have contributed or created the major source of their pain. Sometimes it is from one specific event, but many times it is from making simple repetitive movements during every component of life. This is one of the health concerns I want to address and help you correct.

People don't realize weak muscles, unhealthy diet, lack of exercise, skeletal imbalances and stress can influence their health. Likewise these can all be affected by work, play, sleep, working out and your everyday lifestyle. So learning how to better care for your body could make a huge difference in every member of your family's lives.

Each day we make simple mistakes that will lead to problems down the road, or we ignore the importance of caring for our bodies. I have seen many patients overlook caring for their health monetarily so they were able to get their vehicle fixed, get a special haircut or have enough money for their dinner plans. What they failed to recognize is that good health is invaluable!

The human body is too often not cared for properly, and only receives the attention it deserves, when it's too late and you can't get out of bed or turn your head. Now the repairs are a priority and will cost more to fix. Patients come in when they are *"dying in pain"* or can't move. Now everything on the home front is on standby. Wouldn't it be great to not let things get to that point?

So I treat them and give plenty of instructions on things they can do at home and in everyday life to help them get well and prevent injuring themselves again. Stretching, using ice or heat, lifting properly and listening to their body are just a few of the many ideas I give patients, to facilitate the healing process. Some patients listen. Some get too busy, forget or start to feel better and stop doing anything.

The more they did to help themselves with these *"free"* activities, the greater the chance that they would have a speedy recovery. It would help me help them. It's a win-win. Otherwise I have threatened to follow them around all day to keep an eye on them because theoretically I only see them for 15 – 30 minutes in my office.

After that they are on their own. Usually back to doing the same things and probably doing them the same way, which led them to needing some form of care in the first place. We are creatures of habit, to a fault. You have to take some responsibility for your healing.

I have had patients tell me the treatment wasn't working because their backs still hurt. In one instance, I asked a patient what she had been doing when she proclaimed her back pain was getting worse, after she had just improved tremendously. She responded, *"I was feeling good so I tried to catch-up on cleaning my house and slipped in the tub, landing on my backside."* That might have something to do with her resurgence of back pain. She is not alone.

It is no treat to have a patient come in time after time complaining. If I wanted to hear complaining, I can go home for that. Haha. Some people listen and play an active role in regaining their health. Some let the doctor do all the work, and then there are those who have decided they know what is best for their health and don't use any recommendations. Which type of patient are you?

When a patient does get better, inevitably they forget everything that helped them get well, or stop doing the stretches once the pain is gone. Regaining your health is great. Maintaining your health is even more difficult because it is a constant battle but has greater rewards. I have to remind myself to do my stretches too.

Easy changes in our posture, nutrition, exercise and eliminating bad habits that directly affect your body could help you stay healthy and enjoy life to its fullest. It is never too late to make a change for the better.

My personal motivation for writing this book is I have experienced many of the same spinal problems as my patients. I give new meaning to the saying *"doctor heal thyself."* I have made mistakes. I slept on my stomach. I lifted with my back. I ate candy without a wrapper. I ran with scissors. I did it all, Baby. I lived on the edge. You can learn from these mistakes and stay well, as I have. Who better to learn from than someone who has experienced debilitating pain first hand?

For instance, when I was 27, I was completing my doctorate program. I had always been strong but lifted too much by myself or worked out improperly when I was younger. One day I bent correctly, or so I thought, and lifted our three-legged dog Cody to put him on the couch. He was battling an aggressive type of cancer called Osteosarcoma and lost his leg.

I felt a pop with pain like nothing I had experienced before and I went to my knees. Years of lifting, throwing my body around in sports, motorcycle wipeouts, etc., I had stressed my back enough that this was the final performance that finally caused my first disc bulge.

Whether it was lifting the dog or not, I had put such a large amount of stress on my spine over the years that this was the straw that broke my camel's back.

I could barely raise my leg in bed every morning. For three months I crawled after getting out of bed in an attempt to stand upright and then went to school to treat my patients. If I sat for five minutes I would have to crawl on the clinic floor to get back upright. Not pleasant.

I can't tell you how many patients have come in doubled over complaining that they went to pick up a pen and their backs just went out. This is what happens when we ignore all the factors that affect our health, like sitting incorrectly, ignoring muscle spasms or staying flexible. Pain may come and go away initially, but eventually it will debilitate us. Been there. Done that.

No one is perfect. Especially not me. If you ask my wife she'll be glad to tell you. In fact, she could probably write another chapter in this book about the subject.

I do many of the same things you do, and I don't always do things correctly. Stuff always has to get done one way or another. I just try to limit the damage I may be causing by being careful and using some common sense. I'm a big believer in if you want something done, and done right, you have to do it yourself.

However if I can use my expertise and years of knowledge as a way to help you, or prevent you from experiencing pain, then it is well worth the time I invested to write this information down for you. Every little bit can help you decrease the amount of stress you put on your body and keep you pain free.

Unfortunately, no one gives us a handbook on how to care for our bodies. It would be great to turn to page 38 for instructions on what to do for headaches, why you get them and how you could help prevent them. The best instructions I received growing up were *"sit up straight," "keep your head up when you walk"* and *"don't do that or your face will freeze in that position."* Okay, not the last one, but it is a classic.

In this book, I cover the basics first. Feel free to skip around if you already understand certain areas, but each section complements the next one. In some cases you may see a similar study or comment. That isn't because it was real late while I was typing, but because I felt the information was worth repeating to reiterate the point.

The first section of the book is titled *"Message In Your Body."* It is focused on helping you understand your body, how it develops, its framework and how it works, by starting at the beginning.

Once we have this foundation I will discuss many of the factors in life like common health conditions you will come across, proper nutrition, relieving stress, proper rest, smoking, understanding posture's importance and much more, because everything affects your health.

With more improved knowledge, healthy ideas, appreciation and respect for your body, you can prevent health problems. Now let's be honest here. Part of this section will be a little dry due to the anatomy, science and research. I can assure you it couldn't be me.

The information will be useful in helping you understand many of the common skeletal or muscle ailments you hear about from doctors. So after your doctor tells you that you have blah, blah, blah and it will blah, blah, blah, and you have no idea what they said, you can look it up in this book. I explained most common ailments in terms you can understand.

This is followed up by section two, *"In Search Of The Healthy Grail."* I discuss proper eating and dieting strategies, uncover the truth about some of the fad diets, and help you save some money you won't waste on gimmicks and empty TV promises. This is followed up by descriptions and visual examples of ways you can workout at home, at a gym or in your office. Afterwards we cover stretching, its importance and include examples for each muscle group.

Last is section three entitled, *"You Can Teach An Old Back New Tricks."* This takes an in depth look at all of the things we do every day and why we can be the cause of many of our health problems. I will discuss correct and alternative ways to perform many common tasks from sunrise to sunset, so you can limit the amount of damage to your body over the years. Topics to be discussed include: ergonomics, sleeping positions, pillows, office chairs, computer workstations, laundry and more.

I won't ask you to change or re-evaluate anything that I haven't done for my own family, or myself. What good is knowledge if you can't share it with someone to help enrich their life with the gift of better health? You are now my extended family. What time is dinner?

TABLE OF CONTENTS

SECTION I – MESSAGE IN A BODY

SECTION II – IN SEARCH OF THE HEALTHY GRAIL

SECTION III – YOU CAN TEACH AN OLD BACK NEW TRICKS

The Morning Ritual......308
– The best ways to wake up and get your day started without pain.

Travel......318
– Practice good posture when traveling to guarantee a great time.

Work and Chores......325
– How to do both correctly, using good posture to protect your spine.

Play Time......349
– Concerns about your spine with certain activities.

Children......357
– How to raise them, without aches and pains.

Activities I Don't Like......367
– Things that make you go *"hmmm."* There's got to be a better way.

Final Thoughts......371
– Unloading every last thought I have in my melon. May take a while.

Reference Words......375
– If I didn't tell you, or you forgot, here's a brief recap to bookmark.

References......379
– I'm not just making this stuff up.

Recommended Reading......389
– Some good literature to help you and your family stay well.

Index......391
– Tracking down the topics that are important to you.

Section I

Message In A Body

> *"Our body is a machine for living. It is organized for that, it is its nature. Let life go on in it unhindered and let it defend itself, it will do more than if you paralyze it by encumbering it with remedies."* — **Leo Tolstoy**

You've Got A Great Body

Your body is a marvelously complex machine. The magic started when an egg and a sperm got together, liked each other, and became what is known as a zygote. It split and became two cells, then repeatedly until there were an amazing trillion of stem cells. These cells have the remarkable ability to multiply almost endlessly or become more specialized into cells like a brain or liver cell.

They continued to multiply, divide and each choose their own destiny. Some became skin cells, some liver cells, some cartilage and the rest as they say, is history. The most amazing creation is born without any intervention from us.

This body of yours will try to keep you alive at all costs. If you have a cut, the body will stop the bleeding and repair the skin. A broken bone will also heal any way it can to keep you going. Throughout your life your body will replace the cells that make up your skin, your blood, even your bones to keep you in tiptop shape.

Sneezing is your body's way of getting rid of bad germs, so don't hold them Did you know the air is expelled at 100 mph? That's why you cover your mouth. You could lose your teeth. No. You expel a tremendous amount of germs into the air.

Ever notice that when winter starts, 40 degrees feels cold, but by the end of winter 40 feels like a heat wave. That's how efficiently your body adapts to its surroundings, whether it is presented with a physical, emotional, nutritional, biomechanical, environmental or chemical changes.

I remember my dog Cody who had Cancer. His leg was amputated to try to save his life at age five. It later metastasized, traveling into his front leg. Believe it or not, that dog would still run on two legs, find his green five-gallon bucket lid *"Frisbee,"* and bring it to me to throw. His body adapted for the sake of his survival in any way it could.

Using just the front right and the back left leg he was able to shift his balance in order to still get around. Unavoidably the stress on two legs wore down his body faster than normal. The same thing happens to us when we alter our movements due to pain or structural changes.

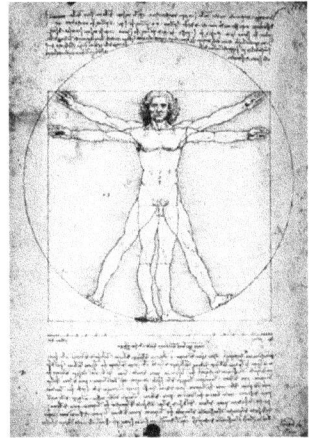

When I broke my right hand after wiping out on my bicycle, I learned to write with my left hand. My body also adapted; enabling me to peddle and chew gum at the same time.

When we are first born, our spines are still pliable. The cartilage that makes up our spines at birth are not the rigid bone that we develop later; and, the birthing process isn't easy on the frame of our bodies. Our spines have to develop so our bodies can absorb the stress of life. I want to explain this area that few people truly understand because posture is mostly about your spine.

> *"...the brain of man was God's drugstore and it had all liquid, drugs, lubricating oils, opiates, acids and anti-acids, and every quality of drugs that the wisdom of God thought necessary for human happiness and health."* – **Andrew T. Still, D.O.**

ANATOMY 101

When you are born you have 270 soft bones in your body. After childhood when growth is complete, many of them fuse together and you are left with only 206. Most of these affected are in your hands and feet.

The skull wasn't formed so we could wear neat hats. We have our skulls to protect our brains. It protects the brain for a reason. The spine, which is comprised of multiple moveable segments called vertebrae, protect our spinal cord. Our ribs protect our internal organs.

The brain is like the fuse box to your house. The wires coming off of the fuse box go to every room and outlet in your house and provide electrical information. The brain is the control center that receives and sends out information to control what the body is doing at all times. It controls everything your body does in a split second; whether you are relaying messages like when to swing at a good fastball, or simply digesting food. It needs to be protected.

Human Skeleton

A. Humerus. **B.** Clavicle.
C. Skull. **D.** Sternum
E. Ribs. **F.** Radius. **G.** Ulna.
H. Metacarpals. **I.** Carpals.
J. Phalanges. **K.** Metatarsals.
L. Phalanges. **M.** Tibia.
N. Fibula. **O.** Patella or Kneecap.
P. Femur. **Q.** Ilium.

The spinal cord is like a conduit of wiring that travels safely within the spine and exits to provide vital information to organs, muscles, etc. Your body does all of this while allowing you to swing a golf club, spin your dance partner around or sit down to have dinner with the family. It is truly an engineering masterpiece.

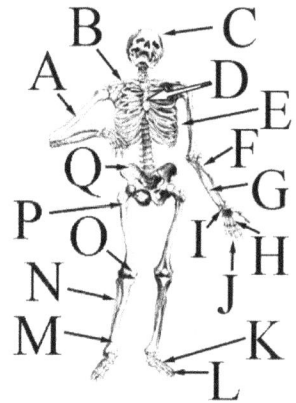

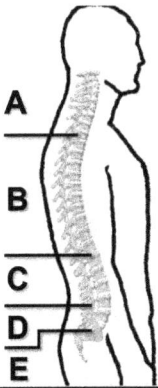

Spine Identification
(side view)
A. Cervical Spine.
B. Thoracic Spine.
C. Lumbar Spine.
D. Sacrum. E. Coccyx.

The bones of your spine are designed to fit together in an S-shaped column of curves. They are balanced so your bodyweight is evenly distributed throughout your spine, allowing you to stand upright and see forward. If these curves are out of alignment and balance, they can cause stress to the muscles, spine and discs, and eventually cause pain.

When we are born we already have the primary curves in our midback, or thoracic region, and our sacrum, which is below the belt line. As we lift our head up with crawling we develop our cervical, or neck curve. When we eventually start walking our lumbar, or low back curve develops.

These curves play an important role in the way your body handles everyday stress. When something changes these curves such as gaining weight, an accident causing alignment problems or micro trauma from repetitive motion, your posture is compromised.

The anatomist Raymond Dart made two profound statements regarding the topic of posture. One was *"Lack of poise, i.e., fixity of positioning and its terminal result, faulty posture. Unfortunately it is the most prevalent condition of the human body."* The other *"concomitant with.... the intensification of civilized life during the last century is the pandemic condition of malposture amongst urbanized mankind."*

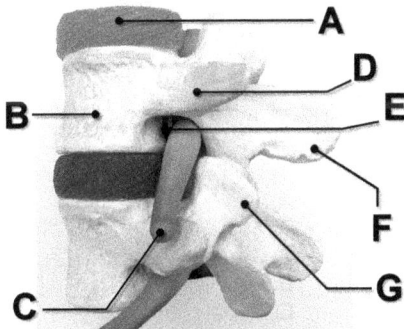

Healthy Vertebra

(left side view)
A. Disc. B. Body.
C. Spinal Nerve.
D. Pedicle.
E. IVF or Intervertebral Foramen.
F. Spinous Process.
G. Facet Joint.

The spine is made up of 24 individual bones, called vertebrae, not including the sacrum and the coccyx. The front part of a vertebra is called the body (B) and is a square shaped structure that rests on the discs. A disc (A) is a shock absorbing spacer, above and below each vertebra and is a common cause of back pain as we get older. Behind each vertebrae and disc is the spinal canal, which houses the spinal cord.

On the side of each vertebra is a space called the IVF or intervertebral foramen (E). The foramen is created by the pedicles (D) above and below, the back of the vertebral body, the disc (A) and the facets (G). This opening allows the nerve (C) corresponding to that spinal level to pass through it and relay information back and forth from the brain to the area it supplies, so it knows what to do.

When the laminas **(F)** meet they join in the center where the spinous process **(C)** is located. These are the bumps up and down the spine you see on someone's back. Many muscles attach to the lamina and spinous process.

A condition called Spina Bifida may be present when the laminas don't join and form a spinous process. There is nothing blocking the spinal cord and nerves from protruding backward and may result in neurological problems.

Lateral, or to the side of the facets are transverse processes **(F)** that stick out an inch or so and these too are a common attachment for muscles.

The spinal canal is made up of the: rear portion of the body; the pedicles **(D)**, which are bridges to the back portion of the vertebra; the facets **(G)**, which are articulating surfaces that form joints with the bones above and below; and the lamina, which joins both sides between the facets together.

So these vertebrae are a set of blocks stacked one on top of another to create a very precious building known as your spine. They work together with the bones above and below them. If a vertebra is not in its correct position, your *"building's"* balance becomes disrupted and less stable. This can lead to problems down the road.

If you were building your dream house and found out there was a problem with its foundation, would you keep moving forward with construction? Or would you try to resolve the issues concerning the base of your house so nothing else would go wrong in the future?

Now that we have explained your anatomy, let's learn more about why it is important and learn how to stay well with a topic we affectionately call correct posture.

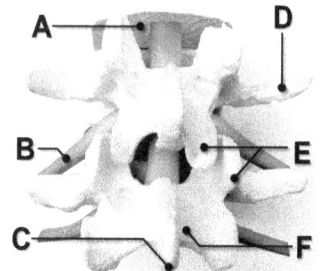

Healthy Vertebra
(posterior view)
A. Disc.
B. Spinal Nerve.
C. Spinous Process.
D. Transverse Process.
E. Facet Joint.
F. Lamina.

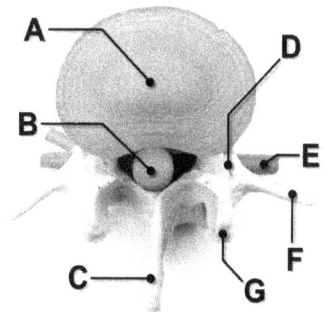

Healthy Vertebra
(top view)
A. Disc.
B. Spinal Cord.
C. Spinous Process.
D. Pedicle.
E. Spinal Nerve.
F. Transverse Process.
G. Facet.

"Sit up straight!" – **every Mom in America**

Is Your Posture Out To Pasture?

According to Merriam-Webster's Dictionary, posture means the position or bearing of the body, whether characteristic or assumed for a special purpose. In other words, how you normally position your body when doing a certain task.

Our posture is important for many reasons. It is the position of balance and alignment your body adapts and always returns to throughout our life. Over time it changes depending on our activities, lifestyles, and the demands we place on our bodies. Posture is how our spine relates to the muscles attached to it, during movement or rest.

Much of life has our bodies sitting at a computer, a desk, in front of a TV, and can ruin the good intentions of Mother Nature who designed our spines to allow us to walk upright, be active and survive.

During our lifetimes, some people may stand tall and have good posture, while others may slouch and have less than desirable posture. This can be a direct reflection of our occupation, sports we play, lives we lead and even how we are perceived by society.

Good posture enables our bodies to move around and breathe easier. Circulation is improved, we have greater visual acuity and fields of vision and our hearing acuity is sharper[1,2].

Maintaining proper posture, you can attain a higher level of competitiveness in sports with a body that is more efficient. Posture distributes stress and forces throughout the body to limit the likeliness of injury, and the amount of damage your body sustains over years of use.

The bones and muscles of your body all function together to create movement. A *"musculoskeletal problem"* is a term used to describe conditions involving both the muscles of our body and the associated bones of the skeletal system. Every time we move to pick up a pencil, lift our children, hit a baseball or roll over in bed, we are depending on our musculoskeletal system to allow for these desired motions.

Poor posture alters the redistribution of weight forces throughout the body. It is inefficient and can lead to damage. Even bending over once and lifting with your back, without regard for maintaining stability in the abdominal region by curving of the lower back, is all it takes to sideline you for a while.

As far as what position causes the least amount of stress on your back, standing upright causes 100 pounds of pressure per square inch on the low back.[3,4] Leaning forward to brush your teeth, wash dishes or to bend and pick

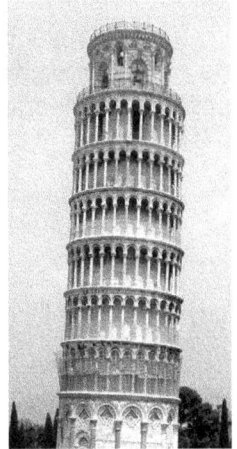

something up, causes 200 pounds of pressure.

When you lift a 30 lb. laundry basket or cute little Alex, multiply the actual weight by 10 – 15 times[5,6] to figure out the amount of compression force impacting your lower back. This number will vary depending on how far the weight is from your body, how high you are going to raise it and how tall you are.

That is an additional 300 – 450 pounds of pressure on your spine to lift the weight. Now add that to your forward body weight of 200 pounds and you have lifted 500 – 650 pounds of disc crunching and degenerative changing force to your back. Each time we lift, these forces get distributed to the discs, muscles, ligaments and supporting structures but there is damage nonetheless. Now, will you bend your knees when you lift?

Similarly, when we sit the knees should be slightly higher than the hips. This position exerts 100 pounds of pressure. When we slouch in school it creates 150 pounds of pressure and when we hunch over the desk it creates 200 pounds of pressure.[3,4] This clearly shows why posture is so important to our overall health.

Posture is affected by muscle tone, flexibility, weight, alignment, genetics, work habits, stress, hobbies, sleep positions and habits of the body all day long. Likewise, posture can have a negative effect on your sleep, healing abilities,[7] athletic performance, singing and overall quality of life. Having a strong, flexible and well-balanced spine has a dramatic impact on your posture.

This is why it is so important for everyone to understand that everything you do affects your health today, tomorrow and well into the future. Knowledge is power. Knowledge is health!

"By three methods we may learn wisdom: First, by reflection, which is noblest; Second, by imitation, which is easiest; and third by experience, which is the bitterest." – **Confucius**

WHAT AM I LOOKING AT HERE

You can watch and see bad posture everywhere. Some people have rounded shoulders. Others have their heads forward with their ears in front of their shoulders. Their midbacks have an increased curve and they walk with a limp. Some are arching backward at their waist; and their backsides may cross the finish line a full second later due to an increased low back curve. Or the whole body could be leaning forward in front of their feet.

When looking at your body straight on in a mirror, your head should be straight with your nose in line with the buttons of a shirt. Standing with your arms at your sides with your fingers an even distance from the ground, your

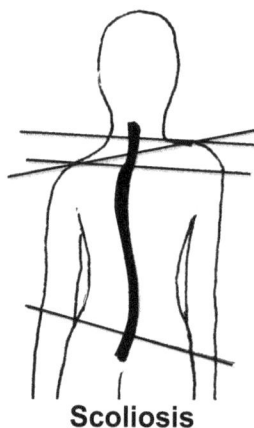

Scoliosis

shoulders should be level to the ground.

Your waist should also be parallel to the ground, with legs straight and feet pointed directly ahead. If you really pay attention you can learn a lot about a person's posture when they are in the standing phase.[8]

Vertical lines of your shirt being pulled to one side, pants rotating so the zipper or a seam is off center, or a cuff hanging lower on one side, are all visible signs of postural distortion. Any variation could be a hint that a person is not enjoying a positively, perfect, posturing physique.

From the side, you should be able to draw a straight line down from your ears intersecting your shoulders, hips, knees and ankles. Shoulders are back, chest out and stomach in, like standing at military attention. In fact, remember the military position and hit that pose to correct your slouching.

Remember that your body was designed to be in this position, so try to do all of your activities while respecting this design.

If you can modify your behaviors to minimize the stress you put on your body, it will last longer and thank you in the end.

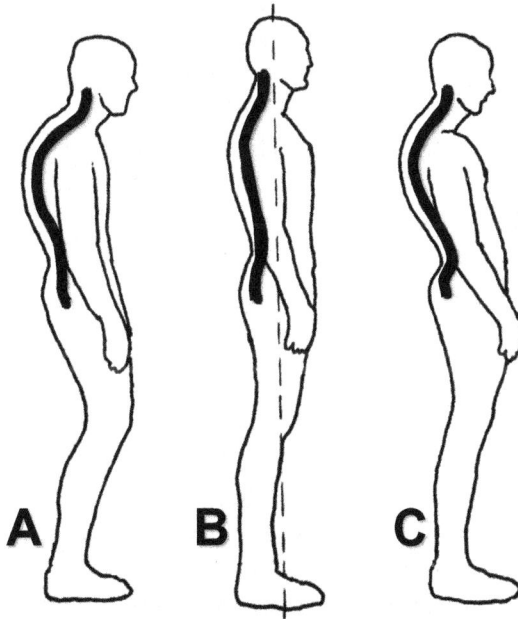

Posture Examples

A. Increased Kyphosis in Mid Back.

B. Proper Posture.

C. Sway Back,
Increased Low Back Lordosis
and Mid Back Kyphosis.

"The best lightning rod for your protection is your own spine." – **Ralph Waldo Emerson**

Cervical Spine

The neck typically has seven segments, with the upper section providing much of the rotation to turn your head. It has a lordotic curve in which the middle of the neck curves inward toward the front of your body, otherwise called the anterior. Your ears should be in line with your shoulders when viewed from the side. Many muscles attach to the neck to create movement and protect it. Some of the more common muscles are the Trapezius, Sternocleidomastoid (SCM), Scalenes, Suboccipitals and Levator Scapula.

Common Cervical Problems

ARTHRITIS

As we age everyone experiences changes in their body. Some sooner, due to abuse their bodies withstood over their lifetimes, others because of genetics. Arthritis is a condition that can seriously limit the movement of people of any age as they become older. The healthy joints that we are born with become worn; a condition known as degeneration. This can lead to abnormal motion and eventually instability of the area.

Your body will try to stabilize a troubled spot by depositing bone where there is too much stress or uneven wear. Bone can grow on our vertebra and is called osteophyte formation **(A)**. Such growths can interfere with your motion affecting space for the spinal cord and its nerves.

Arthritic Vertebra Changes
(left side view)
A. Osteophytes on vertebra.
B. Disc Degeneration.
C. Spinal Nerve Pressure.

Arthritis is a slow process that decreases the range of motion in our necks. With less space between our joints and an inability to move our bones like we once did, our muscles corresponding to these regions will also shorten and become tight. Many elderly people will notice less motion and flexibility in their entire spines as they age.

This is an adaptation to the change in ranges of motion due to arthritis. The more we repeat an activity, the more the affected area will be under stress and break down over time.

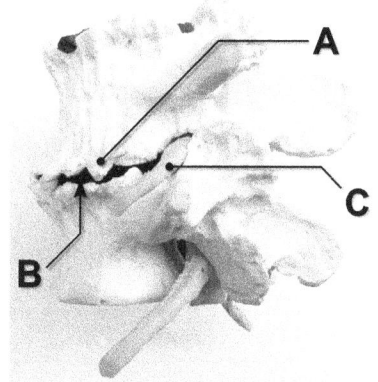

The most common type of arthritis, Osteoarthritis, commonly forms after degenerative changes occur over time, after an injury or an infection.

Two other types of arthritis are Rheumatoid and Psoriatic. In these cases the body actually attacks itself, destroying the joint space, leading to deformation of the joints involved. Grandparents whose fingers become splayed away from the thumb or have large swollen joints, probably have one of these conditions.

I know they call them the *"Golden Years,"* but I have yet to have one patient confirm this proclamation. Everyone always tells me, *"It gets worse after 40,"* *"Doc, wait until you hit 50,"* *"After 60 it's all downhill,"* etc. So in light of these patients' statements I've decided to never grow old. I think this time called the *"Golden Years"* was named by because doctors who see patients more and more during the natural aging process. It is *"golden"* for the doctors in terms of money.

Specific dietary changes and supplementation with glucosamine sulfate and chondroitin sulfate may prove beneficial for some patients. There will be more information about these sulfates in the Vitamin and Mineral Section.

DISC INJURIES

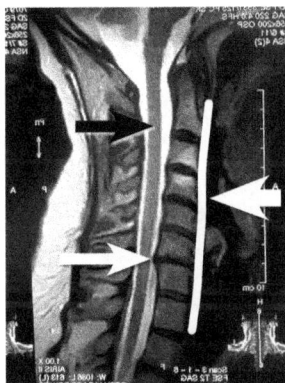

Cervical Disc Bulge

(right side view)
Large White Arrow & Line.
Showing no curve.
Black Arrow.
Spinal Cord.
Smaller White Arrow.
Cervical Disc Bulge from increased stress to region.

Each cervical disc is like a shock absorber between each of our neck bones. Overuse or injuries lead to excessive wear and stress to the disc causing abnormal function. Stress can cause it to bulge. Think of it like a jelly donut. When you press down at an angle on the jelly donut, the jelly is forced to the far edge and may bulge. A disc will typically bulge straight back, or to the left or right.

The problem with a cervical disc injury is that it affects the flow of information below the neck traveling back up to the brain. The spinal cord is larger in the neck because of the amount of nerves it contains. The lower in the spine you go the smaller the number of nerves existing in the canal and the narrower the cord.

When a disc is bulging, it may press against the spinal cord or a nerve. Either of these scenarios can cause shooting pain that radiates into your midback, or into your arms and fingers. You may notice a change in sensation, reflexes or have muscle weakness in your arms or hands.

FORWARD HEAD CARRIAGE

This is a condition in which the head is sticking out forward more than it should be. It may develop from a sudden impact or a fall that jerks the neck violently, changing it permanently.

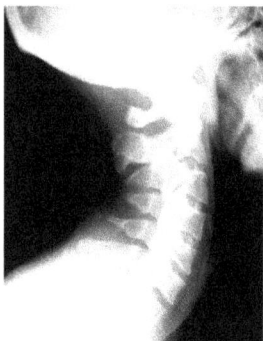

**Normal
Cervical Curve**

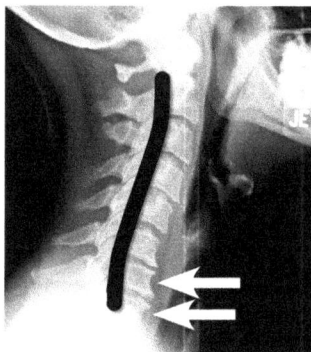

Cervical Curve Reversed
(right side view)
Black Line.
Showing a straight and slightly reversed neck curve.
White Arrows.
Arthritic Changes called Osteophytes

Inventions to increase productivity or enjoy recreation time have also negatively affected this region. With TV, computers, computer games and driving many people hold their heads too far forward.

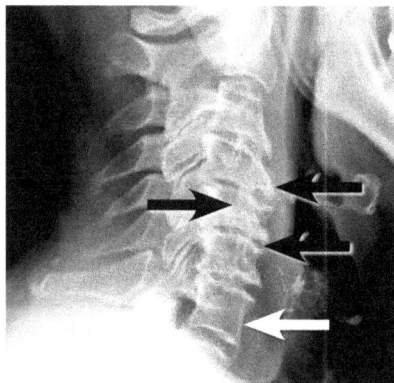

Cervical Arthritis
(right side view)
Black Arrows.
Large arthritic changes or Osteophytes.
White Arrow.
Normal shape of a vertebra.

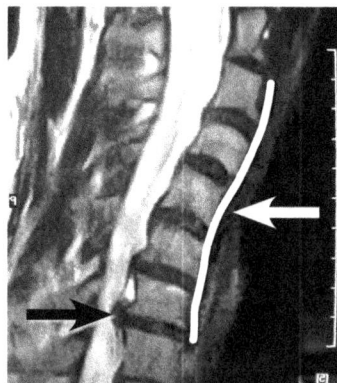

Cervical Disc Bulge
(right side view)
White Line.
Showing reversed curve.
Black Arrow.
Disc Bulge caused by stress of reversed curve.

Over time, the head and neck will actually permanently move to that position. This will change the amount of stress placed on the neck bones and the discs when we use our necks. Altered mechanics and movement, such as forward head carriage, may lead to long-term muscle strain, early arthritis of the joint space, or cause serious injury to the discs and nerves.[9]

For every inch your head is forward in relation to your shoulders, it causes a compressive force to the neck that is increased by the additional weight of your head.[9] So if your head is forward just one inch, the resulting stress would be twice the weight of the head on your neck. That can spell trouble not to mention pain.

With two inches of forward head carriage you would have to endure two times the weight of your head, plus the weight of the head that a normal neck would support. That is a total of three times the weight of the head on the neck. Now you can see how important it is to have your head in a proper position in relation to your overall posture and body's mechanics. So please, no more leaning forward when you work at a computer.

HEADACHES

Almost no one is immune to a headache. In your lifetime at least 95 percent of all women and 90 percent of men will experience one.[10] Great news, huh? About 20 million Americans will suffer from some type of headache this year, accounting for approximately 156 million workdays lost.[11] This will result in a loss of productivity totaling $13 billion.[12]

Besides impacting work, headaches can be debilitating and ruin plans. In fact almost 50 percent of people also noted they had decreased effectiveness if they went to work, stayed home or were at school.[13, 14]

There are two main classifications of headaches. The first type is a primary headache, which includes: migraine, tension, cervicogenic (headache caused by problems in the neck or cervical spine), and cluster headaches. These headache types are the most common, comprising 90 percent of all headaches and have no associated medical condition. A secondary headache can result from tumors, infections, etc., and account for less than 10 percent of all headaches.

Some common symptoms associated with the majority of headaches are: sharp, throbbing pain in different regions of the head; constant ache, localized neck or occipital (base of skull) pain precipitated by abnormal movements. The range of motion in the neck will be decreased and your posture may be altered due to hypertonic (tight) muscles, which may also be tender.

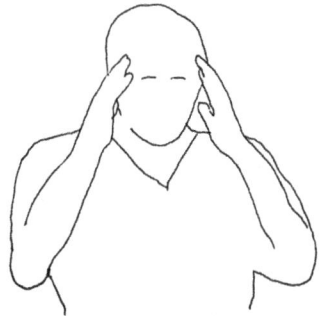

After seeing a doctor, and provided there is no history of a major problem causing your headaches, you may benefit from some easy ergonomic tips, exercises and stretches. This simple approach may help you prevent, reduce and eliminate future headaches altogether.

Relatives used to tease us about sitting up straight and keeping our heads up. Research shows they were right. In fact, proper body posture and ergonomics play a major role in a lot of the things we do on a daily basis. Placing your neck or head in an unnatural or vulnerable position while exercising, driving or at home, are things that can lead to a headache.

Dr. Peter Rothbart, MD, FRCPC, President of the North American Cervicogenic Headache Society, proclaimed in the Toronto Star, *"We've been able to put together a scientific explanation for how neck structure causes headaches- not all headaches, but a significant number of them."*

In addition, noted Researcher Nikolai Bogduk, MD, PhD, Professor of Anatomy at Newcastle, Australia, commented: *"The model for cervicogenic headache, (headache caused by the neck), is not only the best evolved of all headaches but is testable in vivo, in patients with headache complaints."*

One of the specific areas that have been linked to neck pain and headaches is the facet joint, also called the zygapophyseal joint, which is located toward the back of the vertebra on each side. It is the joint created when one facet joint articulates with another one from the vertebrae above and below it. No, I did not make up that word for your next scrabble game, but it would fetch a boatload of points. This joint has been linked to 54 – 60 percent of chronic neck pain and 58 – 88 percent of chronic headaches.[15]

These findings support the importance of proper posture and alignment of the neck. If there is an alignment problem, then the muscles and the bones of the neck will be under increased stress, and this may result in a headache.

Another overlooked source of headaches is eyestrain. When was your last eye exam? Are you supposed to be wearing glasses but you forget or don't think you look good in them? Would you rather look good, feel lousy and not know who's looking at you or feel good and see clearly?

HYPOLORDOTIC CURVE

This is a decrease in the neck's curve and can be associated with an increase in the midback curve as a way to compensate for the neck. It is sometimes referred to as a Military neck because it is straight. In some cases it is actually reversed and bends forward instead of backward.

Leaving your head forward for too long, like reading with a book in your lap, or having a case of whiplash, will force the body to change how the curve is oriented. This will affect how simply turning your head distributes pressure in the neck and will lead to the potential break down of the spine.

MUSCLE SPASM

This can be associated with one muscle or an entire group of muscles. Its onset can be a sudden involuntary contraction or associated with another condition. It may last for seconds or days, depending on the cause.

Muscle spasms cause pain and tightness, decrease your range of motion and may even affect your nerves. Muscles are used with every aspect of motion. When we move we always contract the muscles, but we rarely take enough time to relax them by stretching. If you never stretch them, you cause your muscles to build up tension and tightness and eventually they may not want to let go.

PINCHED NERVE

This condition occurs when there is some encroachment around the nerve. The most common sources to cause nerve compression are arthritic changes, muscle tightness and disc bulges. Even the slightest narrowing of the space the nerve passes through can cause pressure on it. This interferes with the nerve as it relays information back and forth between your brain and your body.

Nerves supply motor function or information for movement. Nerves also regulate sensory information and reflexes to your muscles. Think about placing your hand on a hot stove. Sensory information is sent to the brain that it's hot and a message is sent back to move your hand. In the neck, you might experience changes from your neck down to your fingertips. Each nerve supplies a different region. For example, on one arm there could be numbness in just your pinky and half of your ring finger, while the rest of your arm feels normal.

This is why doctors may examine you with a reflex hammer, perform muscle testing or use a pinwheel to check your sensory levels. Sometimes the doctor may order a nerve conduction velocity test (NCV), which can determine the exact nerve being pinched. Nerve pain can be sharp, achy or numb. It may be aggravated, or alleviated by certain neck or arm movements.

STENOSIS

Behind each vertebral body is a space that creates the spinal canal. This space contains the spinal cord and is big enough to accomodate bending within each curve of the spine. You can see an example of this in previous pictures.

When the spine deteriorates, it causes stress to other supporting joints and ligaments. As the body deposits bone for additional support, the ligaments and joints also enlarge. These changes decrease the size of the space for the spinal cord to pass. This can cause compression that irritates nerves on one or both sides of the body. Sometimes a progressive disc bulge may contribute to the decreasing size of this space. It is more prevalent in men and usually occurs during their middle ages.

STRAINS AND SPRAINS

A strain occurs when there is an overstretching of the muscles or the tendons that attach the muscles to bone, or possibly even a tear in the fibers. Reaching for an object, lifting improperly or playing sports can cause this condition. Symptoms may include pain, tightness, swelling and bruising.

Another form of this is a repetitive strain, which can happen when you do the same thing for an extended period of time and keep the same muscles contracted. Playing guitar, washing dishes, painting, or lifting trash cans are examples of this.

Sprains involve a ligament, which attaches bone to bone. A common example is an ankle injury. This is mostly associated with the mechanism of overstretching but can include tearing or rupturing of the structure.

We all suffer from occasional aching or stiff necks that usually go away in a day or two. When pain persists longer, our necks are telling us that they need help. Some of the common causes of neck strain are joint dysfunction or improper movement of the neck bones, weak muscles, bad posture, working too long without moving the neck around, tension and degenerative conditions that affect the joints and discs.

TORTICOLLIS

This is a severe spasm of the muscles in the neck. Sometimes referred to as wryneck in children, patients are born with Congenital Torticollis. It can be associated with a trauma at birth that leads to a contracted and eventually shortened SCM muscle. It can also be caused by spinal or spinal cord abnormalities. When this muscle tightens the head is rotated to the opposite side and may be laterally flexed.

In adults with acquired torticollis, a sudden contraction can occur and be very painful. The range of motion is non-existent to one side and limited on the other. This isn't fun. I once walked around like Frankenstein for four days. My problem was I had the fan blowing air directly on me during a hot summer day. My neck muscles cooled and when I tried to move they went into spasm.

Don't do this. Point the fan away and circulate the air in the room. Trust me on this. I have had several patients show up in tears due to the intensity of this type of spasm.

WHIPLASH

Whiplash is a sudden forward and/or backward movement of the head after an accident or a fall. This can cause postural abnormalities and joint dysfunction. Too often patients admit to being in a car accident but believe it wasn't too bad. I ask, *"How bad was the car?"* They reply, *"Oh it was totaled!!!"*

Now how is it a 3,000-pound chunk of steel is damaged but the 150-pound soft tissue body strapped in, except for the head that bounces around, is okay? The exterior of the car doesn't magically correct itself. Neither does the spinal damage to your entire body.

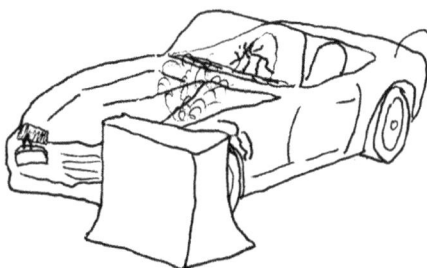

Many patients have problems today because they ignored their own health. Sadly they believed that the damage to their bodies had to be seen or felt, or they are okay after a fall or a car accident because they feel fine. WRONG! I guarantee they had their car fixed before they used it again because it was *"unsafe"* whether they could *"see the damage"* or not.

If you broke a tooth you would have it fixed immediately because you can see it. If there was a gelatinous cover over your car and you looked at its exterior after an accident, it would look fine. But would you still have it fixed? Yes, because you understand that the vehicle damage doesn't have to be seen to be present.

Current studies have shown the damage to the neck and back from a blow to the head, a motor vehicle accident (MVA) or a fall may be felt immediately, not for hours, or sometimes even years.[16]

The impact to the driver is 2.5 times greater than the force to the vehicle itself.[17] So whatever damage you see to the vehicle, realize the force to your body was 2.5 times greater. Changes of speed of only 2.5 miles an hour during crash tests caused occupants symptoms of soft tissue injuries; whereas damage to a vehicle may not be seen until 8.7 mph.[18]

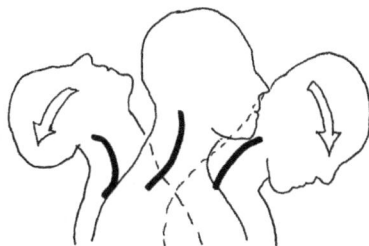

A study conducted by The George Institute (University of Sidney in Australia) found that accident victims recover rapidly during the first three months after an accident. Beyond that, recovery is slow and limited, further supporting the fact treatment should be sought immediately.

If left untreated or uncorrected, resultant adaptive changes will occur in the architecture of the spine. The soft tissue and bones of the neck will cause pain, muscles will become fibrotic or less pliable, scarring will develop in the tendons and ligaments and there will be degenerative changes in the spine.[19] A 1996 *Injury* article reported that chiropractic adjustments significantly helped reduce pain in 93 percent of chronic whiplash patients after medical and physical therapy did not.

When the ligaments heal, they will develop a cross linkage or net-like mesh of their fibers that create inferior strength in the tissue. Unless these scars and adhesions are disrupted by mobilization or adjustments,[20] the result will be the tissues involved will now fail at only 40 percent of the original strength.

Your neck has a wide range of motion, so you put greater bending, twisting and turning demands on it than you do on the rest of your spine. The seatbelt protects your torso making the neck the most vulnerable part of your spine, especially during an auto accident.

Even minor whipping of the cervical vertebrae of the neck can cause severe trauma to the neck muscles, ligaments and soft tissues. A hit during a football game or slipping and falling may have the same result.

A 2003 article in *The Spine Journal* about Whiplash research found being un-aware of the impending impact will lead to much worse damage than if you were braced for it. With forward and backward head motion of a surprised accident victim, amplitudes were 180 and 25 times worse, respectively.

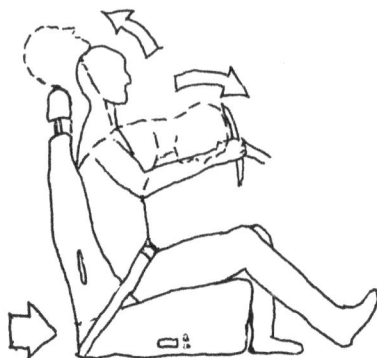

In a rear-end collision your neck is forced to move into extension starting with the lower vertebrae first. This motion is completely different from the normal motion of the spine during extension and can be a source for understanding how the neck is injured in an accident.[21]

It is a common example of a strain injury and sometimes a sprain if ligaments are involved. Although overlooked by many people, including health-care professionals, whiplash occurs more than they realize. Most people escape severe injury like fractures. The damage to the spine can go undetected and lead to biomechanical stress, which later results in chronic pain.[22] In fact, 20 – 40 percent of accident sufferers will have symptoms that persist for years.[23] This is called late whiplash syndrome.

The Spine Journal reported in 1994 that the average amount of time to reach maximal improvement after whiplash is seven months, one week, while some whiplash-injured patients could take two years to stabilize.

Neck position at the time of the accident also plays a role in the amount of damage that occurs. Over 55 percent of people who were complaining of persis-tent symptoms for more than two years after their whiplash injury, reported they had their head rotated at the time of impact.[24]

In a sudden rear-end collision of only 20 mph, a force of 12 Gs is placed upon the neck during the extension phase of whiplash (head moves backward) and 16 Gs of force on the flexion recoil of the neck[25] (head moves forward).

The term G forces means at 4Gs your body weighs four times the force of gravity. So at 12 Gs your head weighs about 120 pounds. A patient, who is a pilot, told me the F-15 fails at 10 Gs!!

The normal curve of your neck is C-shaped. Whiplash produces an S-shaped curve[26] during the initial stages of an accident, with hyperextension occurring at the lower cervical levels. The damaging hyperextension happens in 75 milliseconds (ms) after impact, while it takes 200 ms for the body's muscles to develop enough force to brace the spine.[27]

Essentially there isn't enough time for the brain to send a message to the muscles that prevent the overstretching from happening. By the time the muscles contract, it is too late. Your body has no chance to fully protect your neck from injury during an accident. When the muscles do contract, they are supporting a damaged spine.

The hyperextension of the neck is the cause of facet joint pain and demonstrates the biomechanical process of whiplash.[28] That muscle tightness or pain you feel the next day is your body's incredible recuperative attempt to stabilize itself during and after such a collision.

Left untreated the muscles will remain tight and adapt to this new position. This will alter your Range of Motion (ROM), the spine will wear unevenly and lead to degeneration due to the atypical stress. These are the people who have symptoms years after an auto accident and don't grasp the connection.

One study followed whiplash victims over a period of time and compared their spinal health to an age similar control group. They found the whiplash subjects to have 39 percent more disc degeneration than the control group that had only six percent degenerative changes.[29]

When you fail to give your neck proper attention immediately following an injury, pain and stiffness can develop and lead to limited motion, changes in your posture, headaches and muscle tension. These problems can lead to disc bulges, nerve pain, hypolordosis, arthritis and instability as shown below.

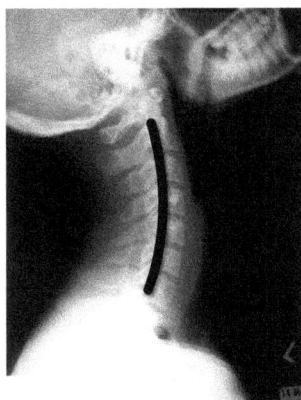

Cervical Extension Position (side view)

Black Line. Neck has continuous curve as if there are no problems.

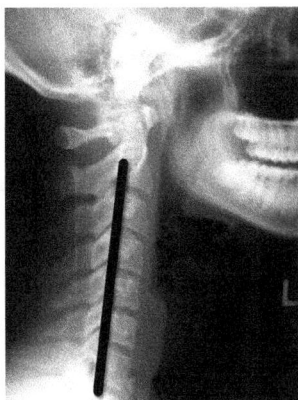

Cervical Neutral Position (side view)

Black Line. Showing a straight spine or military neck. Should have a curve. (Hypolordotic)

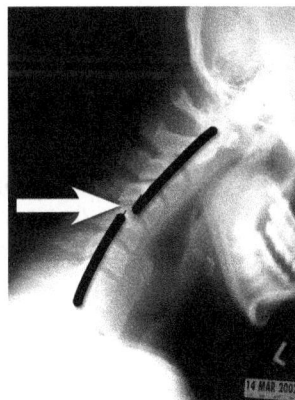

Cervical Flexion Position (side view)

White Arrow. Instability.
Black Line. Break in normal alignment.

"Rigid, the skeleton of habit alone upholds the human frame." – **Virginia Woolf**

Thoracic Spine

Below the neck is the thoracic curve, which has 12 segments or vertebrae. There is less motion here in part due to the stability created by the ribs, which are connected on both sides of the spine. This area has a reversed curve when compared to the neck and the low back, called a kyphosis.

The middle of this part of your spine curves more toward the back of your body or your posterior. Some of the common muscles attached to this area of the spine are the Trapezius, Rhomboids and Erector Spinae.

Common Thoracic Problems

ARTHRITIS AND HYPERKYPHOSIS

Like the previous arthritis section, it results from too much wear and tear in an area. Nobody wants that big dowager's hump like Aunt Betsy, which makes her look hunched over and frail looking.

I have had several patients with that problem because of what they did in life. One example is Carl the crane operator who sat all day hunched forward to look out his front windshield to see the boom of his machine. That habitual forward bending posture curved his midback over into what is called a hyperkyphosis, or an excessive kyphotic curve. Reading can do the same thing.

Another reason why this forward curve has a tendency to increase is because of the shape of the bones in the thoracic spine are shorter in front and higher in back. As the discs between them degenerate and shrink, this allows the curve to increase. To some degree it can be part of the normal aging process.

DISC INJURIES

Discs may also be injured in the midback by a fall or car accident, violent coughing or sneezing, or aging. The thoracic spine is more resistant to disc problems. This is partly because of the stability created by our ribs as they come off of these thoracic vertebrae and connect to the sternum, the *"breast bone"* between our chest. In addition most of our bending occurs in the neck and low back.

It can be tough to take a deep breath when a thoracic disc is irritated due to the expansion of the rib cage when your lungs fill with air. You may also feel a pain that wraps around your side and ends somewhere in the front of your chest or stomach. This occurs if one of the nerves become irritated as it runs along the inside of the ribs.

FRACTURED RIBS

The ribs were created to protect our inner organs including the heart, lungs and pancreas. We normally have 12 total pairs. The first seven pairs attach by cartilage to our breastbone or sternum, and the spine. They are called *"true ribs."* The remaining five pairs are called *"false ribs"* because the first three attach indirectly to the sternum with long cartilage attachments and the lower two shorter ribs are floating, because they don't attach to anything in the front.

Feel your ribs rise and expand to allow the lungs to fill with air, and lower as they return to normal and air is expelled out of our lungs.

Getting hit hard in the side, coughing, being struck by an object, even reaching for something can break a rib. The other scenario is that the cartilage between the ribs can be overstretched inhibiting breathing and movement.

I remember getting ready for a football game against another dorm at Syracuse University. My friend Matt held in a sneeze just before the game. He immediately had pain and couldn't take a deep breath. Time Out! Off to the emergency room we went. He had strained his cartilage between the ribs.

Don't hold in a sneeze. Remember your body is trying to get something out of it. Cartilage takes longer to heal because it has a poor blood supply and it takes a while for nutrients to get where they are needed for healing.

OSTEOPOROSIS

As men and women age, we BOTH lose levels of calcium, phosphorus and other important minerals from our bones. It can be due to poor diet, lack of exercise, genetics, metabolic problems, smoking, alcohol, long-standing usage of steroids and hormone changes to name a few culprits.

The bone density changes as fewer nutrients remain in the spinal bone's composition. It's like removing some of the walls and studs from your house and expecting it to withstand wind, rain or snow.

As we age and continue to put stress on our body there is less support. We come home for Thanksgiving and can't wait to see our nieces, nephews our grandkids. We eagerly bend over and pick up little Johnny, who is now 32 pounds, placing that lifting load on our spine.

With severe osteoporosis, the vertebrae or spinal bone can collapse due to such an amount of force. Also, when we lift we compress the discs as Newton's Third Law states, *"For every action force there is an equal and opposite reaction."*

So the disc pushes back toward the spinal canal, or above and below, into the surface of the vertebra it is contacting, called the end plates. If their integrity is weakened, the disc can push right through.

Until we are around 30 years of age, our body stores calcium in our bones like a bank. After that, we make withdrawals from our savings account. Continued exercise and proper nutrition are a few ways to limit how many withdrawals you make from your bank. Due to hormones in our food supply causing early development, some researchers believe today's kids only have until their early 20s to store their calcium.

Research shows that astronauts lose muscle tone and mass, and develop osteoporosis during space travel because they are not weight-bearing. Without the strain of gravity on our bodies they start to wither and weaken. That is no different than when we're sitting on our bottoms. That confirms the move it or lose it theory. Bus driver, *"Move…that…BUTT!"*

PINCHED NERVE

This is the pain I described before that wraps around your ribs. It will feel like a sharp, shooting, stabbing pain that could last for a few seconds or for a while. The disc bulging, degenerative changes of arthritis and even muscle spasms commonly cause it.

SCOLIOSIS OF THE THORACIC REGION

Everyone has heard this word. This is an abnormal lateral, or side to side, curve in the spine. It can be caused by abnormal variations in your vertebra, postural distortions, disease processes and genetics.

Some people have a genetic predisposition for having some type of scoliosis in their back. This is known as Idiopathic Scoliosis. Growing teenage females have a higher tendency to develop scoliosis than teenage males. The only reason I could find for this was either due to a mother who had scoliosis, or from magnesium deficiency, which could be associated with menstruation.

Low levels of magnesium can lead to muscle contraction and possibly curvature of the spine. Vitamin K may also reduce the amount of blood loss. To cover your bases make sure your teenager takes a good multivitamin daily.

Being a right handed person can cause you to develop increased muscle strength on that side side of your spine and pull the bones to the bones to the right.

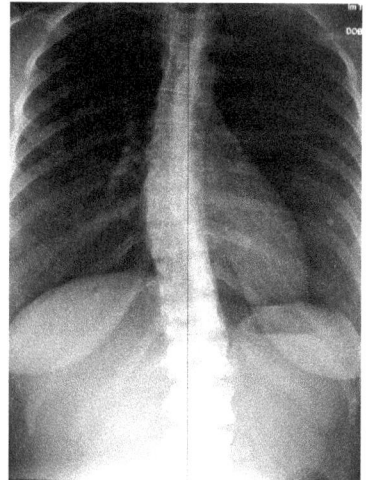

Scoliosis (back view)

This would be considered more of a deviation but more severe cases where the spine curves laterally to the right would be classified as a Dextroscoliosis. If the spine curves to the left it is called a Levoscoliosis.

If you don't sit up straight and always lean to one side you can develop a curve because your body will adapt to what you do. Just like if you lift weights you will get bigger and stronger, provided that you are eating a nutritionally balanced diet. Your body's main concern is self-preservation, so it adjusts.

Another variation is when one leg is longer than the other causing the top of the pelvis and sacrum to become tipped. The lumbar spine starts off at an angle toward the low side; only to over correct itself and head in the other direction, and thereby affecting the thoracic spine.

Sometimes exercises, massage, yoga and realignment of the spine can help. Other times a lift may also be needed for the shoe on the shorter leg side, to raise the low side up. In extreme cases of scoliosis, a rod is inserted into the spine when the curve becomes too great and poses a threat to the internal organs and breathing.

Signs of a scoliosis postural defect would be a bra strap that always falls down, tilted shoulders, a prominent shoulder blade, rib humping when the person bends forward, uneven shirt sleeves, or buttons or lines of a shirt that seem crooked.

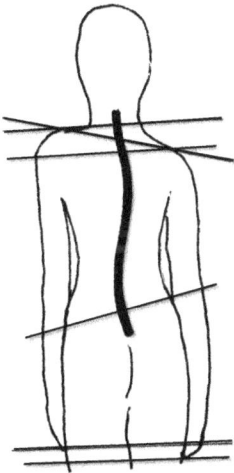

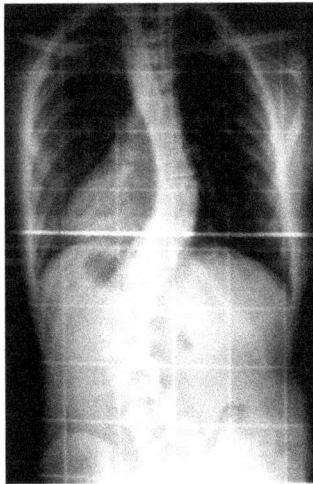

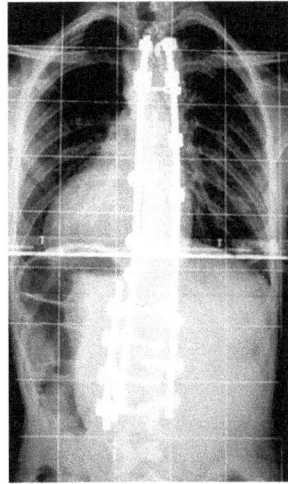

Left Picture Picture of a person with Scoliosis.
Middle Picture How severe it is on an x-ray.
Right Picture Their only solution was to have rods surgically implanted to prevent progression and future compromise of their internal organs.

THORACIC OUTLET SYNDROME (TOS)

This is a condition in which muscles along the side of your neck disrupt the nerves and blood supply traveling through your shoulder and down to your fingers.

The nerves that leave your neck and travel to your arm make up the brachial (meaning arm) plexus. This large group of nerves is similar to the group of nerves in your low back that form the sciatic nerve to your legs. Pain can be sharp, achy, throbbing or numb; or manifest as changes in sensation, reflexes or muscle weakness in your arm.

The subclavian artery, vein and vertebral artery are the vessels that can become compressed in this region. Symptoms are typically coldness and pain in the hands and fingers, or a tired out feeling when working overhead due to poor circulation.

The muscles involved in this condition are called the scalenes. When they get tight they can pinch off any of these structures mentioned. The clavicle, or collarbone, and an occasional extra rib in the lower neck can also obstruct or occlude the vessels and nerves.

> *"If you cannot get rid of the family skeleton, you may as well make it dance."*
> **– George Bernard Shaw**

Lumbar Spine

The lumbar spine is made up of five segments with a lordotic curve similar to the neck region. This area is usually under a lot of stress because most of us lift improperly creating a fulcrum at the lowest part of the lumbar region, like a seesaw. Repetitive bending movements at the waistline can suddenly create a problem or occur overtime.

Some sources will tell you back pain will resolve on its own. This is proof of the body's amazing recuperative abilities to stop pain, but does it solve the problem is the real question. Most episodes of back pain return with increasing severity as time passes. The same holds true for the rest of your body.

About 80 percent of the population at some point will suffer from Low Back Pain (LBP). Some common muscles attached to this area are the Erector Spinae, Quadratus Lumborum and Psoas Minor.

Common Lumbar Problems

ARTHRITIS

The longer you are alive, the greater your chances are of developing arthritis. I'd rather take that chance then consider my alternatives. When we bend and lift to do everyday chores or work, most of us bend at the waist instead of keeping our backs straight and lifting with our legs. Over time this causes excessive wear and tear, like a hinge on a door, and that can lead to deterioration.

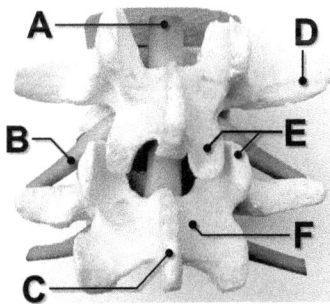

Healthy Vertebra (back view)
A. Spinal Cord.
B. Nerve.
C. Spinous Process.
D. Transverse Process.
E. Facet Joint.
F. Lamina.

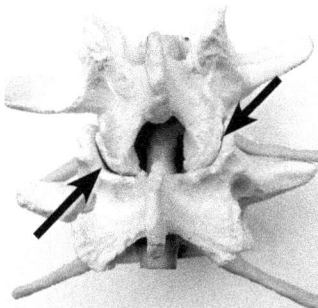

Degeneration of Vertebra (back view)
Black Arrows.
Facet Degeneration.

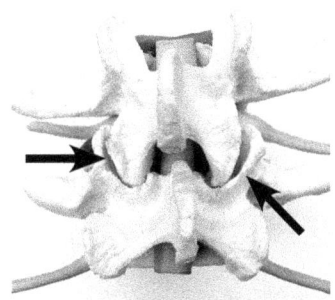

Arthritic Vertebra Changes (back view)
Black Arrows.
Facet Degeneration.

As the discs wear down, the space or height between the vertebrae decreases too. This means there is less space for the nerves to exit this region along the side of these vertebrae. This is often called Degenerative Disc Disease, Degenerative Joint Disease or Spondylosis.

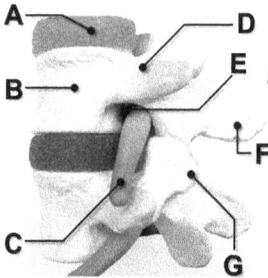

Healthy Vertebra
(left side view)
A. Disc.
B. Body.
C. Spinal Nerve.
D. Pedicle.
E. IVF or Intervertebral Foramen.
F. Spinous Process.
G. Facet Joint.

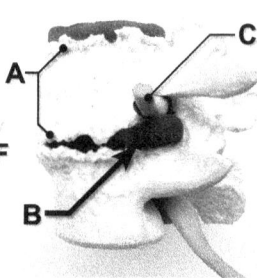

Degeneration of Vertebra
(left side view)
A. Osteophytes forming as the vertebra degenerates.
B. Bulging Disc.
C. Spinal Nerve Encroachment.

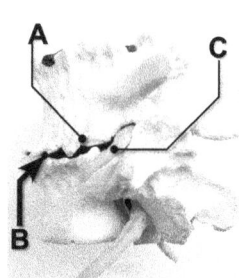

Arthritic Vertebra Changes
(left side view)
A. Osteophytes on vertebra.
B. Disc Degeneration.
C. Spinal Nerve Impingement.

A minimal decrease in disc height results in more stress on the surrounding segments of the vertebra and has been shown to cause degeneration in the facets.[30,31,32,33] With closer proximity of moving parts there is increased resistance. This will cause abnormal movement of the spine and worsening arthritis. A 2007 study by Eubanks et al. found at age 60, 100 percent of their subjects had arthritic facets. The kicker? Arthritic facets can cause chronic pain.

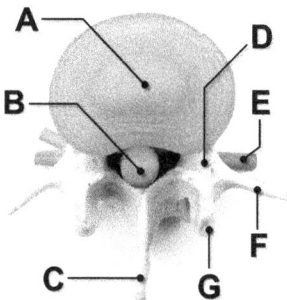

Healthy Vertebra
(top view)
A. Disc.
B. Spinal Cord.
C. Spinous Process.
D. Pedicle.
E. Spinal Nerve.
F. Transverse Process.
G. Facet.

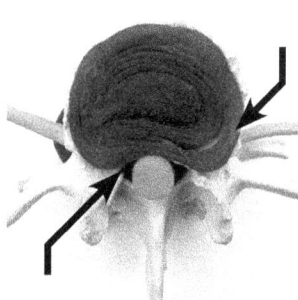

Degeneration of Vertebra (top view)
Upper Black Arrow. Disc degeneration. Notice disc is black.
Lower Black Arrow. Decreasing width around spinal cord.

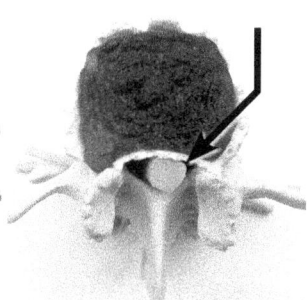

Arthritic Vertebra Changes (top view)
Black Arrow. Spinal Stenosis.

With more and more stress, the discs will continue to change size and the body will respond and adapt. Calcium will be deposited to stabilize the area as a direct counter measure to the continued stress.

These new growths are called Osteophytes, or spurs, and will grow anywhere necessary to secure the spine. If spurs grow in the foramen, or opening where the nerves exit the spine, there may be too little space and the nerves can become painful either at the site of restriction or down into the leg.

Arthritis is closely associated with genetics, the time and amount of stress placed on the spine, posture, weight, alignment and flexibility.

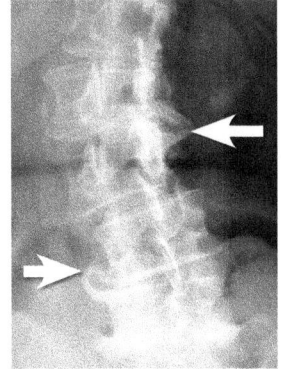

Lumbar Spine
(back view)
White Arrows.
Major arthritic changes and bone spurs being designed to limit motion of tipped vertebrae.

DISC INJURIES

Discs can only handle so much stress. The longer we stress them and the harder we work them, the more likely they are to wear down. These shock-absorbing cushions can bulge or herniate and lead to nerve problems.

Several factors can contribute to how healthy your discs are over the years. The most common are stress to the area, the workload, posture, nutrition and exercise, as well as smoking. The normal aging of a disc will cause it to potentially dehydrate, shrink, harden and develop faulty biomechanics for lifting. When posture, ergonomics and all the other abuse is added to the equation it only further compounds the problem.

Restricted movement of the joints and supporting tissue will occur from less space between the vertebrae and will alter the normal rotation of the joints,[34,35] causing pain,[36] and leading to arthritis.

Poor posture can double low back pressure when lifting incorrectly. If you raise an item higher than your waist you are only increasing the stress on your spine when you lift. This could result in a 10 – 15 fold increase in pounds of pressure per square inch of the disc depending how much you lift, how you bend to grab it and where the object is in relation to your body.[4,38]

Want to try it for yourself? Hold a gallon of milk close to your body and then far away. It feels a lot heavier the further it is from your body.

Factoring the 10 – 15 times the weight when lifting improperly in front of the body formula into everyday life, lifting a 10-pound can of paint out of a car trunk would be up to 150 pounds of pressure on the low back. So in my case, bendng to pick up a 60-pound dog would be an even 900 pounds of pressure per square inch on my back. That's what dropped me.

The most common area to be affected by a disc problem is the lower lumbar spine, in the middle of your back at the level where your belt would be. The 4th Lumbar disc, also known as L4, and L5, the next one below it, are the two discs typically involved in more than 95 percent of back pain. They take most of the abuse from lifting heavy loads, bad posture or repetitive movements.

Each disc's mechanical behavior is dependent on its location[39], like at the belt line where it is a fulcrum for lifting. Higher in the lumbar spine would require less bending for lifting than required by the lower spine. The loading and history of loading from constant lifting can affect the integrity of the disc's health.[37] L4 and L5 are commonly injured because they are used with constant bending, as well as lifting.

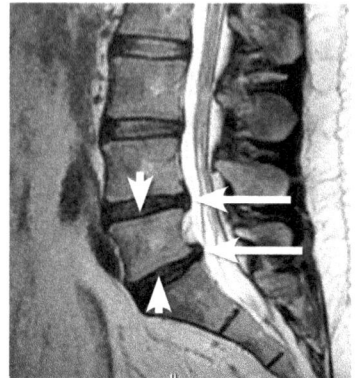

Lumbar Disc Bulges
(side view)
White Arrows.
Two discs bulging back into the spinal canal.
White Arrow Heads.
Both discs are darker because of increased degenerative changes.

A permanent decrease in the thickness of a disc from abnormal loading or repetitive movement is a source of pain in the lower back.[40] There is also a change in its axes of rotation,[36] which means the spine turns less efficiently.

Every time each disc is compressed, it forces water and metabolic waste out. When you sit or lay down the disc is relaxed and replenishes itself with nutrients and fluids. This pumping mechanism to move fluids in and out of the disc allows the disc to stay healthy by maintaining its nutritional and mechanical requirements.[41]

Making one mistake lifting a heavy object, a light weight, stumbling or even a single fall can result in damage to a disc.[42] When someone double dared you to lift something ridiculously heavy, and you did, or you carried your big brother on your back when he outweighed you by 40 pounds; these are classic examples of how we injured our backs long before we even knew it. When we lift a laundry basket of wet clothes and turn to put it on the counter we are loading the disc and compressing it down under pressure.

The lumbar disc is especially vulnerable to something known as fatigue failure because it has a poor blood supply.[40] While it is loaded it has fluids being pushed out of it and no new nutrients can make it in. That's like trying to blow air into a balloon while someone is squeezing it. Air coming out is greater than the air you are trying to inflate the balloon with; so it never inflates or gets new air inside the balloon.

As the disc is under increased pressure it influences disc cell metabolism and may accelerate the degeneration of the disc.[43] This explains why constant lifting or stress can increase the likelihood of experiencing disc degeneration as we age. The pressure doesn't allow cells to function properly and no new nutrients ever make it into the disc during this stress to replenish themselves.

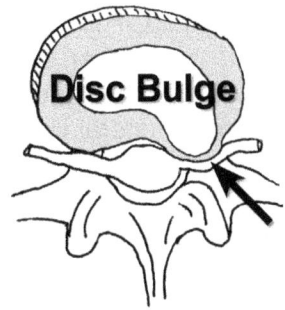

Disc Bulge
(top view)
Black Arrow. Pinched Nerve.

It's like doing yard work for a long period of time with no new workers with energized muscles and hydrated discs to help. The ones that you are still working become increasingly less effective, exhausted and are more susceptible to injury.

An example of how the body brings nutrients to help repair the damage is seen when numerous blood vessels develop in response to a herniated disc[44] and as degeneration occurs.[45] This increased blood flow is directed toward the annular fibers of the disc that is degenerating; not into the vertebral end plate,[46] which is the part of each vertebral bone that makes the roof and floor as it contacts each disc. As the disc continues to degenerate, more blood vessels are seen.

Many people mention a slipped disc. There is no such thing. The disc is securely fastened in between the vertebra by its annular fibers. There are additional supporting structures that further make it impossible. It is not like squeezing a fresh pumpkin seed and having it pop out between your fingers.

A disc can however expand outward in either direction and form a lump or bulge. As fluid is lost due to continuous compressive forces, more weight is directed to the outer annular layer of the disc.[47]

Under this stress, this layer will become predisposed to lateral instability and degenerative changes.[48] It may become hardened, crack and even split, as in a tear. Notably these changes do not have to be the result of a specific injury, but may be caused by the accumulation of minor events that stress the spine.[49] That is why repeating movements that negatively affect your posture can have a long lasting result, and a painful one at that.

If a disc bulges or pushes backward toward the spinal canal and spinal cord, it can press against them or the nerves that exit the spine and then cause pain. These nerves in the lumbar region provide vital information to your lower body.

Pressure against either the cord or the nerves can cause mild to severe pain that is local or radiates down either leg. If you've never had it, don't judge someone who is in pain or cranky due to this type of injury. Once you've had back pain, you will develop new respect for anyone who does.

HYPERLORDOTIC CURVE

If the lumbar curve increases too much, then stress loads are unevenly distributed on the body. In a side, or lateral view of the lower back, the center of this curve will be well in front of the sacrum, where it should be, causing stress to the posterior portion of the back's lower vertebra.

This is why healthcare professionals stress the importance of core training to strengthen the mid section and stabilize the spine. Along with strength; flexibility, alignment and posture are extremely important too.

The foundation for how our spine handles many of the stresses we place upon it daily is a strong mid section. It comprises the abdominals and obliques, the erector spine muscles of the back, the quadriceps in the front of the upper legs and the hamstrings on the back of your upper legs.

Unfortunately too many of us suffer from weak abdominals and tight hamstrings, which are perfect for accommodating a hyperlordotic spine. This condition is visible when a person's backside is sticking out, or someone has a protruding stomach.

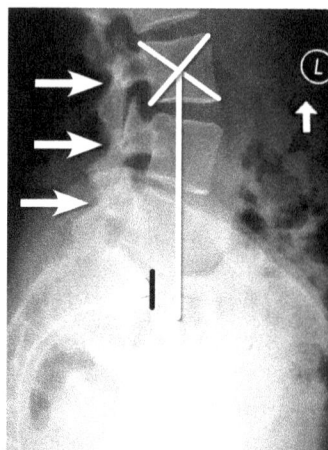

Lumbar Forward Stress
(right side view)
White "X". Center of 3rd Lumbar vertebra or L3.
Large White Line. Gravity line or showing where stress is with relation to the spine.
Black Line. In a normal spine the large white line should be behind the black line intersecting the sacrum.
White Arrows. Areas where stress will be increased in spine, not including discs.

PINCHED NERVE / SCIATICA

The sciatic nerve is made up of two lumbar nerves and three nerves from the triangular-shaped sacrum, which is below the lumbar spine. As they combine, they become the largest nerve in the body and travel down both legs, also referred to as, the lower extremities. Sciatica is when the nerves roots exiting the spine are compromised and cause pain down one or both legs. This is also known as radiculopathy.

The nerves supply the necessary information to your legs so you can go about your daily life. When the slightest pressure disrupts the sciatic nerve it can cause an increase or decrease in information relayed to your body. You might feel less on one side, have weakness in some of the muscles or have a change in your reflexes. In an effort to reduce the pressure on the nerves, a person will lean away from the side of pain, known as antalgia.

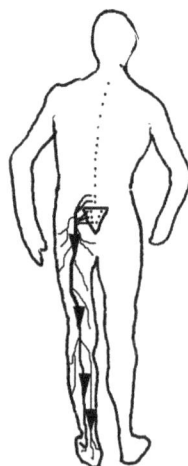

When there is a lot of pressure against the spinal cord and its lower portion, you could lose control of your bowel and bladder. This is called Cauda Equina Syndrome and usually requires a surgical repair.

Dr. Kirkaldy-Willis, MD reported in a 1985 *Canadian Family Physician* study that chiropractic spinal adjusting basically fixed leg and low back pain in 81 percent of disabled patients when other treatments couldn't help them

Sciatic pain does not have to involve a disc injury. Degenerative changes, arthritic changes to the spine, pregnancy, weight, posture, alignment and even tight muscles can also contribute to cause it.

SACROILIAC PAIN

Also known as SI pain, this is the area where your right and left iliac bones of the pelvis meet the base of your spine and the sacrum. These two bones form a bump, or a dimple, called the Sacroiliac joint. It is located just above your buttocks, around belt height and about three inches from the center of your back.

Sometimes the muscles attached to this region can tighten and limit the SI joint movement. These joints move when you walk, run or cross your legs. Pain can be localized or may even refer pain down into the upper leg.

If one SI joint isn't moving well, the other side may start to move more to compensate for the lack of motion on the other side, creating hypermobility and discomfort.

SCOLIOSIS OF THE LUMBAR REGION

This is when the spine curves to one side or the other, when it should be straight when viewed from behind. If the spine looks like a " (", the vertebrae will be tipped to the right and create a concavity on the right side of the spine.

Physical demands on the spine and vertebrae will produce more stress to the inside of the curve because it carries more weight. This can lead to deterioration of the disc and lead to arthritic changes in the bones. It may cause more problems than just structural strains from wear and tear.

The result is the openings for the nerves to exit become smaller on the right and provide conditions favorable for pinching a nerve. To demonstrate, put one fist on top of the other; tip the upper hand to the right and you will see the hands get closer together on the right, but further apart on the left.

Scoliosis is not just the lateral bending of the spine. It can be more complicated and involve rotation of the vertebra as well. As the spine bends the vertebrae may rotate to one side or the other. Muscles will change and you may feel more musculature and tightness on one side of the lower back.

SPASMS & STRAINS

Two examples. One is the person who overdoes it by raking the lawn most of the day. Muscles used over a long period of time remain constantly contracted forces. When you continue to tighten the muscles, they might not relax when you want them to and may go into a spasm. They could also tighten as you become less active and the muscles cool down later in the day.

Spasms will limit your motion and can be very uncomfortable. The longer the muscles stay tight the harder it will be to get them back to normal.

The other example is the person who tries to lift the mower to get under the deck, and even worse, attempts to do so after sitting or being inactive. Not only do the discs fill with fluid after inactivity, but the muscles of the back will also tighten up from remaining motionless.

Lifting something heavy, whether the person is in good shape or not, may just require too much from the body at that instant, creating muscle strain or spasms. Both can cause restricted ranges of motion and pain that could last days to weeks.

SPONDYLOLISTHESIS

This means that one of the vertebrae became unstable and slid either forward or backward from its normal position. There are two types of spondylolisthesis. One is acquired and the other is degenerative.

An acquired Spondylolisthesis can occur when we are born, from a serious fall, an injury when we are young, an accident later in life, or from our normal genetic development. Teenagers more involved with sports have a higher degree of probability of acquiring this condition.

The defect occurs when there is discontinuity from the attachment of the vertebral body, either on one side or both, to the rear portion of the vertebra via the pedicle. Most people don't have any symptoms or pain until later in life, after wear and tear have over worked that area.

There are strong ligaments and muscles still supporting this region but with continued stress, arthritis will develop and vertebral movement can occur.

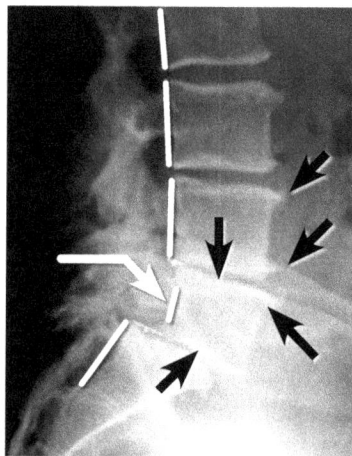

Spondylolisthesis
(right side view)
White Arrow.
Movement of the vertebra forward.
White Lines.
Back of vertebra, which should be a straight line.
Black Arrows.
Degenerative changes.

The more common Anterior Spondylolisthesis is forward movement of the body; whereas Posterior Spondylolisthesis is backward movement. Degenerative spondylolisthesis develops as the disc and articulating facets degenerate. Vertebrae move closer together, have a little more play or looseness, so the body responds by depositing calcium to strengthen and stabilize the region. This increased arthritic calcification can lead to stenosis (see below) as the spinal canal becomes smaller.

Surgery may eventually be needed if the progression becomes too great or unstable in either case. The procedure will fuse or brace the bones to prevent further motion and halt arthritic changes. The problem with fusions in the spine is now two segments move as one.

As the body requires more support from surrounding vertebrae to pick up the slack to allow motion, it will place more stress than normal on those bones and cause them to degenerate. It can become a cycle of degeneration and then surgery over the years. Better posture, biomechanics and ergonomics are just a few things to try to limit your back's stress and potential surgeries

STENOSIS

Behind each vertebral body is a space that creates the spinal canal. This space contains the spinal cord and is big enough for it to permit bending within the curves of the spine. You can see an example of this in previous pictures.

When the spine deteriorates, it causes stress to other supporting joints and ligaments. As the body deposits bone for additional support, the ligaments and joints also enlarge. These changes close down the space for the spinal cord to pass. This can cause compression and irritation of nerves on both side of the body. Sometimes a progressive disc bulge may contribute to the decreasing size of this space. It is more prevalent in men and usually occurs during their middle ages. Bending or flexing your spine forward typically offers some temporary relief.

Less Common But Worth Mentioning
ABDOMINAL AORTIC ANEURYSM (AAA)

As we get older, calcium deposits can form in our blood vessels. The aorta runs from our heart down to behind our lower stomach, before it divides and travels down our legs. If too much calcium gets deposited in the aorta the outer rim can become rigid, like a bagel that has been left out too long. It loses its flexibility. Now as blood pressure increases inside of it there is a greater chance of causing a problem.

An aneurysm is an area in a blood vessel that expands. As it does, the side that balloons out becomes vulnerable to rupturing. If that happens you've got big trouble as it is commonly fatal. Most aneurysms occur from the stomach region down toward the feet.

The problem with an AAA is that it mimics low back pain. Patients think their pain is just normal low back pain and ignore receiving proper attention or having x-rays taken. Pain can be deep and steady yet relieved by changing your position. You could also notice a pulsation that is prominent in your abdomen. If there is extreme low back and abdominal pain and you have an aneurysm, you must get to the hospital immediately.

Surgery can be done and is more successful if the aneurysm is small, around four to six cm. The replacement is done with a synthetic graft. There is a higher prevalence of this with smokers, anyone with hypertension or heart problems, a family history of them and the elderly.

LIPOMA

This is a benign, or non-cancerous, tumor made up of a slow-growing lump of fat cells that forms between your skin and the muscle layer beneath it. They will feel like doughy, palpable masses in your lower back along the level of your belt and a few inches from the center of your back. However they can be anywhere on the body. Genetics and possibly a minor injury may have a role in why these fat cells form in the body. Being overweight is not a factor.

A lipoma mimics many ailments of the lower back like sacroiliac pain or sciatica, and can cause intense pain. Some medical and alternative treatments can be beneficial. I had one on my shoulder blade that if pressed wrong, felt like a knife in my back. I had it removed and the problem was resolved. It is a relatively easy procedure. Doctors will remove it if you can't resolve the pain, a large lump forms and it bothers you cosmetically, or you need to do a biopsy on it for further evaluation.

"Walking is man's best medicine." – **Hippocrates**

Sacrum

The sacrum is made up of five segments that eventually fuse in our younger years and resemble an upside down triangular shape at the base of the spine. It rests between our iliac crests, which are the bones you feel if you push in from the sides at your waist. It has a kyphotic curve to counteract and absorb the shock of the lumbar spine.

Common Sacral Problems

PIRIFORMIS SYNDROME

A common muscle that can irritate the sciatic nerve is called the Piriformis muscle, which is located diagonally in the buttock. It is connected to the outer hip and the sacrum. The sciatic nerve can run above, through or below the muscle. If this muscle becomes enlarged, tight or inflamed, it can press on the nerve. If you look at the diagram for sciatica from the previous section, you can see how a muscle running across that nerve could cause a problem.

Women may experience sciatic pain and piriformis syndrome when they get pregnant. From my experience and understanding of the human body's biomechanics, I believe that pressure from inside the womb is not the only reason this occurs.

As women reach later trimesters they gain weight. Sometimes it is a little and sometimes a lot. As the inner thigh becomes thicker women lose the ability for their normal walking pattern and swing of their legs, because one thigh touches the other thigh. They are forced to externally rotate the legs and swing them outward when walking to make an adjustment for this change. This is affectionately referred to as waddling.

This motion can contract the piriformis muscle and irritate it or make it bigger. When this happens there is a good chance the sciatic nerve can be pinched. I've seen many patients with this condition in my office over the years. Darn kids.

SHORT LEG SYNDROME

Sometimes the sacrum is tipped and causes the spine to curve sideways. Much like a house with a crooked foundation. If it has a slope, then when you build the next floor, it too will tilt.

Many cases of Scoliosis and Low Back Pain have a short leg syndrome associated with them, in which both legs are not the same height. Sometimes the upper leg bone, the femur, may be shorter or the lower bone, the tibia, may be the problem. This is as common as people not having the same size feet. It's true. None of us are perfect. Sorry to be the bearer of bad news.

Many patients wonder why they have problems with short leg syndrome now if they've had this condition their entire lives. Well I could lift a 25-pound can every day with my left hand and a 50-pound can with my right without a problem. If I had to do it for years it would become cumbersome and eventually wear the right side down. The same thing happens when your body carries your bodyweight unevenly. It will support you for awhile but eventually the body will get tired and cause symptoms.

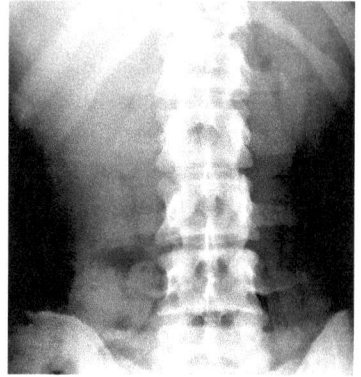

Lumbar Spine
(back view)
Normal

If you look in the mirror you may notice one side of your pants is higher than the other with one pant leg hanging longer on one foot. You might even notice uneven wear of the heels of your shoes. For example, try poking your side above the waist with your thumbs and slide down until you feel a bone. That is the iliac crest. If you keep your fingers there and look into the mirror, does one finger appear higher?

To visualize the movement, take your left hand's pointer finger and the middle finger, and try to press down on just the tips of those fingers like the fingers walking for the yellow pages ad. You will notice the easiest way to do this is to bend your middle finger.

A classic sign of this is when you stand. Do you feel stable? Is it more natural to stick one leg out? That is because it would be uncomfortable to stand on the longer leg, or middle finger. The shorter one would be floating.

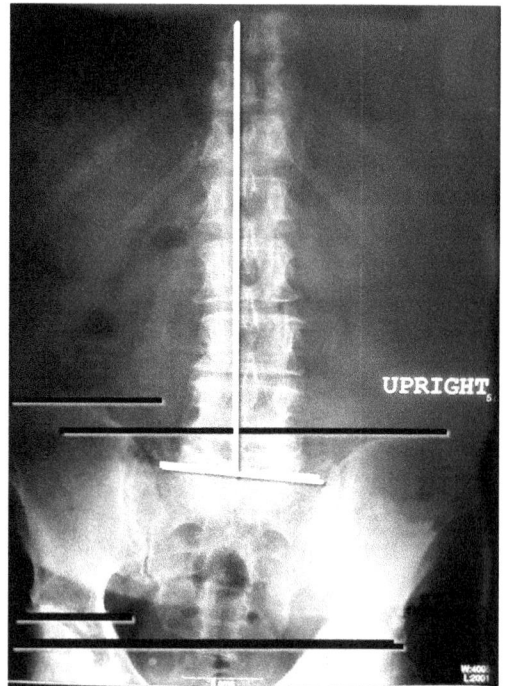

Short Leg Syndrome
(back view)
Black Lines. Upper line shows a lower right waist and the lower black line shows a lower right hip.
White Line. Shows a tip of sacrum or base of spine.
Vertical Thin White Line. Where the center of the spine should be.

Using your left hand, try to move the fingers and simulate walking. You will notice when the middle finger tip is making contact, the pointer finger is up in the air and moves freely. When you place the pointer finger down, the middle finger hits the surface before it can swing unless you tip your hand to the short side and swing the middle finger outward.

In relation to your anatomy, when you stand on the long leg, the short one can swing fine as you take a step. As you drop to the lower side, the longer leg will hit the ground and start to wear the heel down. You then compensate by externally rotating your hip, or toeing outward, to create more room for the long leg while tipping more of your weight onto the shorter side. This overworks the piriformis muscle.

The other problem with having a short leg means that one side of your body is carrying more weight than the other. So in addition to having the lumbar spine curve toward the low side, your unequal distribution of weight causes uneven wear on the hips. Notice in the previous picture there is increased whitening above and below the lower black line on the right. That is calcium being deposited to strengthen that area due to increased stress.

One hip socket will have a joint space that degenerates and becomes smaller due to the stress over the years. Sometimes patients will note a clumsy feeling when they walk or that they constantly catch one of their heels on the ground as though they are stumbling.

A functional short leg is when the leg appears shorter due to ankle pronation, flat feet, a tipped and rotated pelvis or a difference in knee angle when compared to the other side. Anatomical short leg could be due to a healed fracture, joint replacement, misalignment, tight muscles or from normal development. Whatever the source, correction is needed before the curve develops or becomes irreversible and leads to more serious problems.

A common way to evaluate this is to lie on your back, bend your knees as though you were about to do a sit-up and have your feet together. If you looked at the knees from the side you might notice one knee sticks forward more or is higher than the other.

Some healthcare practitioners measure from certain reference spots in the pelvic region. These include the belly button or the front of your hip bone on the side, down to the inside of your ankle while lying down, or to the floor when evaluating you while standing.

Another evaluation technique is to shoot an x-ray with the patient standing, so the patient is weight-bearing, and the film will show you what the body is doing inside. Lying down films will allow hypertonic, or tight, muscles to distort the pelvis on the film. It will make it look the opposite of what is really happening when you are weight-bearing. I have several sets of films that were taken supine, or lying on the back, and then again standing. The difference is amazing.

> *"Get knowledge of the spine, for this is the requisite for many diseases."*
> **– Hippocrates**

Coccyx

This is a small section below the sacrum that is comprised of three to five fused segments, also known as the tailbone.

Common Coccyx Problems

COCCYDYNIA

This area can be fractured or injured from slipping on ice and falling on your buttocks or during childbirth. It causes pain and some people require a donut-shaped cushion or padding so sitting does not aggravate the area. Over the counter meds may help relieve any inflammation or dull pain associated with the injury.

> *"The art of medicine consists in amusing the patient while nature cures the disease."*
> **– Voltaire**

The Disc

Between each vertebra is a disc. It is like a fresh jelly donut. Not to make you hungry, but the inside of the disc is jelly-like and referred to as the nucleus pulposous. The outer surface is tough and is called the annulus fibrosus. The disc's purpose is to allow for motion between vertebral segments, act like a hydraulic shock absorber, and to distribute forces throughout the spine.

The inner layer is about 80 percent water when we are younger but loses hydration and nutrients as we age. Between degeneration and decreased water content, people can lose about three inches of height due to these changes. This is why our parents and grandparents appear to shrink as they get older. Their discs resemble old, stale and dried up donuts that aren't very pliable.

This outer fibrous layer has interlocking fibers that withstand pressure from the disc within and support the disc when weight is applied to it. These fibers also prevent excessive motion of the joints when we move.

If you press straight down on a donut the jelly spreads out evenly. When you compress the front edge of the donut continuously over the years, it forces the jelly to the other side of the donut. This is essentially what happens to our discs.

When the outer edge is under too much stress, it causes a bulge or protrusion in the outer fibers. The bulging can occur on any side of the disc. This malformed disc can put pressure on nerves or the spinal cord, and cause local or radiating pain.

An annular tear is when there is so much stress to the disc that the outer layer weakens and splits. Material from the nucleus can start to ooze out. It takes about 300 pounds of pressure to tear these fibers. A tear that involves leakage of the nucleus pulposous can also be referred to as prolapsed disc.

In more severe cases the jelly will tear the outside layer and may even seep out into the spinal canal. If the material fragments, it can float through the spinal canal fluid and is called an extrusion. This piece could then get lodged anywhere in the canal and the patient becomes an immediate surgical candidate.

A sequestered disc is when the piece that floats gets lodged against a nerve, or the spinal canal, causing serious pain. Surgery is usually needed to relieve the pain by removing the fragment.

The Stages of a Disc Herniation

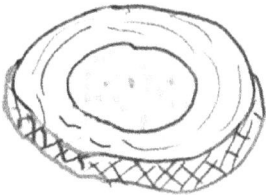

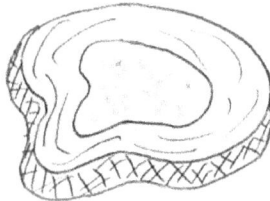

Normal	Protusion or Bulge	Prolapse

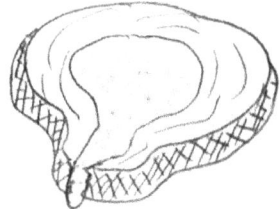

Disc degeneration and sciatic pain can be associated with posterior disc bulges that are causing low back pain. A disc problem can occur suddenly or be felt as a pain that gets worse over time. There may be pain shooting out sideways from the level involved or it may irritate a nerve and send sharp or numbing sensations into your arms or legs.

Your range of motion can be drastically reduced. You might think a bone or joint in a different area is causing the problem due to referring pains from the disc. Visually look for a severe tilt to one side (antalgia), trouble standing up, or the ever popular bodily shift that looks like illusionist Chris Angel cut you in half and shifted your upper body three inches to one side of your waist.

Coughing, sneezing and using the toilet can make things worse because they all make the disc enlarge. If you sneeze and the disc enlarges it will tap the nerves close by and you will feel it. Leaning forward and placing you hands on your knees may help reduce the sharpness of the cough or sneeze by increasing the space between your vertebrae, the discs and the nerves.

Some 80 million Americans have back pain each year. I don't want you to be one of them.

"The important thing is not to stop questioning. Curiosity has its own reason for existing. One cannot help but be in awe when he contemplates the mysteries of eternity, of life, of the marvelous structure of reality. It is enough if one tries merely to comprehend a little of this mystery every day. Never lose a holy curiosity." – **Albert Einstein**

Fibromyalgia

One of the biggest mysteries in health conditions that encompass many of the topics covered so far is Fibromyalgia. Currently more than 12 million Americans have been diagnosed with it. Interestingly, women are ten times more likely to get this disease and it usually starts between the ages of 25 and 50, but these numbers can vary. A lot of controversy exists within the medical community on whether the diagnosis is even real. There is no one specific test for it. Many times the diagnosis is found by ruling out other conditions like Arthritis, Hypothyroidism and Lyme Disease because of the similarity and overlap of symptoms.

People with this condition will tell you it is painful and exhausting. They experience long-term and wide-spread areas of painful points, or trigger points, and tightness all over their bodies; like in the joints, tendons, muscles and more. These points are commonly found in the shoulders, neck, chest, shins, knees, hips, elbows, buttocks and lower back. This disease may also be associated with fatigue, moodiness, headaches, abdominal complaints, stiffness after immobility, inability to exercise, depression and sleep problems.

The cause of this condition is the mystery. It often involves physical or emotional trauma or genetics; and sometimes an illness triggers symptoms. In practice I have often seen it in patients who have experienced multiple accidents in a short period of time.

After the body is damaged from a car accident and the muscles and tendons are healing, another accident occurs to the same area and these tissues become injured again. The repetition of trauma causes the muscle fibers to lose more and more of their elasticity, which once allowed them to stretch and move freely, causing a chronic rigidity in the joints and scar formation in the muscle and tendon fibers.

This disease is more prevalent in women. I have also seen many patients who have been in abusive relations, both physically and mentally, at some point of their life. A physical relationship can result in the same stress to your body as being involved in multiple car accidents. Constant stress or damage to the body will cause the muscles to get tight and never let go.

There are several options for relief and these vary widely for each person. One of them is diet and nutrition. Most experts agree people should avoid: Aspartame, sugar, fructose and other simple carbohydrates; MSG and nitrites in your foods; caffeine from soda, chocolate, coffee and tea; yeast and gluten; dairy; and the nightshade plants like tomatoes, potatoes, eggplant and chili or bell peppers.

You can see how your body responds after you eiminate any of these to see if they are a factor for you. Other options for some relief would be medications, chiropractic, therapy, massage, acupuncture, yoga and medical marijuana.

> *"Thoughts, like fleas, jump from man to man, but they don't bite everybody"*
> **– Stanislaw J. Lec**

Lyme Disease

Deer ticks that are able to transmit Lyme disease carry a bacterium called Borrelia burgdorferi. These little monsters sit perched on the edge of a plant with their front legs extended so they can latch onto anything that has blood that walks by. Then they look for a nice place to set up camp on their new host.

For every case reported about seven to 12 are not according to the CDC, and overall the reported cases are definitely rising. Part of that is because we are more aware of it now.

There is also a Lone Star tick, which has a white spot resembling a star (it's not a Cowboys fan). These guys rarely transmit Lyme disease but can carry a bunch of other diseases. Memo to self, all ticks are bad.

Prevention Ideas:
- Dress in light clothing so you can spot the ticks.
- Duck tape your pant legs to your shoes or tuck them into your socks.
- Apply bug spray with deet or permethrin on your clothing to repel (permethrin is formed from a derivative of a chrysanthemum plant, however both may have dangerous side-effects when used repeatedly and directly on the skin)
- Permethrin is hands down the best repellent and used by the military.
- Drop your drawers before going inside and put the clothes in the washer immediately.
- Have somebody thoroughly check you from head to toe when you come in from outdoors; especially on the back of knees, genital areas, waist line, arm pits and head.
- Place a gravel or wood chip barrier between your lawn and the weeds or woods as ticks like shade and moist environments.

If you do find a tick the best way to remove one is with a pair of tweezers. Grab the head, grip it and rip it. No I'm kidding. Work that little bug out and try not to squeeze the body as that will push bacteria into your body, increasing the chance of infecting you. Also according to the CDC a tick usually needs to be attached for 36 – 48 hours to transmit something to you.

If possible, put the offending tick into a zip lock bag in case you need it to be tested or brought in for identification. It isn't as rewarding as squishing it, but it will die a slow death in there eventually. Slap it on the fridge with a magnet or tape it to the inside of a cabinet door. You could also use a jar to hold your alleged criminal.

When I captured a tick I tried out various repellents and here are my findings. The natural germanium oil, lavender, garlic and citrus don't hold a candle to the chemicals. I think the tick was doing the back stroke and working on his complexion in the natural concoction; but boy did he turn, run and then curl up after getting near the permethrin. Winner!

Permethrin has the potential to kill every bug ever to roam your backyard. I did threaten to wipe out our lawn of all life forms. However, Rambo did also read it can harm cats, dogs and of course our kids, so I will spray our clothes instead. Besides I like spiders. Essential oils can also harm other wild animals so always use caution with them too.

So if you are bitten, seek medical attention immediately so you can start a course of antibiotics to reduce the chance of infection. If you see a red rash, redness and swelling or the classic bulls eye appearance where the bite occurred you need to see your doctor.

Early symptoms of Lyme disease include:
• Redness
• Swollen lymph nodes
• Headache
• Joint and muscle stiffness
• Fatigue

Later symptoms:
• Bell's palsy or facial paralysis
• Nerve problems in the hands or legs
• Inflammation of heart muscle, which can lead to abnormal heart patterns or heart failure
• Arthritis like symptoms, joint stiffness and pain

Many patients seek relief from professions like medical, chiropractic or massage treatment to alleviate the pain and stiffness they have in their joints. Often the symptoms make the patient believe it is arthritic pains, Lupus, Chronic Fatigue Syndrome or Fibromyalgia.

Blood work can be done to see if there is a specific arthritis causing the problems to better determine a solution. Sometimes the blood work will be negative. In that case a Western Blot test or Elisha blood test may be ordered to try to diagnose the condition as Lyme related.

Different types of antibiotics are used to fight the symptoms of Lyme disease depending on how long the patient has presented with symptoms. The sooner you start antibiotics once you have determined it is Lyme disease the greater your chance of reducing the symptoms.

I have friends in their 40's who complain how painful it is to get out of bed, how they feel like they're 90 and that their joints bother them constantly.

Ticks vary in size too. They can be as small as a "period mark" of a sentence or 1mm to the size of an apple seed. Usually the most harmful ones are about 1-2mm. That is why you want help checking for ticks when you come back indoors.

That means hunters, landscapers, construction workers, Public Utility employees, apple pickers and fall lovers should be careful. Although most bites occur during the spring and summer, a tick will bite you whenever it has a chance. Always be prepared.

> *"Somewhere on this globe, every ten seconds, there is a woman giving birth to a child. She must be found and stopped."* – **Sam Levenson**

Pregnancy

Pregnancy is similar to an elite athlete training and stressing their skeletal system, as well as their muscles, tendons and ligaments. A lot of changes occur over the next nine months, which can cause pain for the expecting mother.

The only bonus of nine months of pregnancy is that your body has time to strengthen in accordance with the growth of your child. That's why it's not fair to just slap the 30-pound sympathy belly contraption on us guys so we feel your pain. We get it. Each extra pound pulls forward and compresses the low back at a 10:1 ratio. So a 25 pound stomach is 250 pounds of additional low back pressure.

Some common problems associated with pregnancy are low back pain, Sacroiliac joint pain, Piriformis Syndrome and Sciatica. Low back pain can be caused by the unborn child pressing against the spine, but as pregnancy results in the stomach increasing in size there is also more stress to the low back.

A 2012 study in Chiropractic & Manual Therapies found chiropractic very helpful for low back pain related to pregnancy, as did *The Journal of Midwifery & Women's Health*.

Sciatica we discussed earlier. This is pain into either leg caused by pinching the nerves in the back or by a muscle in the buttock region, known as the piriformis.

The Sacroiliac joint or SI joint is also another common source of LBP for women. These are the two bumps you can feel just below your belt line and about two fingers from the midline on both sides. *The Journal of Family Practice Research* reported 91% of test subjects reported relief from SI pain after receiving manipulation.

Another common pain during pregnancy is headaches. It could be from changes in your body, hormones, everyday chores becoming more difficult, the fact that *"there's a baby coming,"* stress and even your disturbed sleep pattern.

Among the multitudes of headache studies that show chiropractic manipulation helps headache sufferers, a 2009 study in Complementary Therapies in Clinical Practice specifically found headaches in the pregnant patient also responded well to chiropractic.

Lastly, Carpal Tunnel Syndrome (CTS) is another common ailment of pregnancy. It involves less space in the wrist for nerves and blood vessels. Symptoms will usually diminish after childbirth, although chiropractic and physical therapy can help temporarily decrease symptoms.

> *"The reason we have two ears and only one mouth, is that we may hear more and speak less."*
> – **Zeno**

The Temporal Mandibular Joint (TMJ)

This is the joint on the outside of your cheeks in front of your ears. It is a delicate joint that allows your mouth to glide when it opens and closes. It can be injured by getting popped in the chin, a car accident, clenching your teeth, or chewing gum. To nip this quick, stop chewing gum if you have a TMJ problem.

Many of us want our shoulders rubbed but who asks to have their jaw massaged? The fact of the matter is many of us ignore this region, yet we use it constantly. For instance, you use your jaw for talking and eating. Some of us do one of these too much anyway.

I see many patients, including myself once, who have popping noises when they chew. An imbalance can occur in the muscles of mastication, or the chewing muscles: the buccinator, masseter, lateral and medial pterygoids.

When these get tight you need to stretch them too. Don't worry you won't have to bite on a dumbbell or anything. A bite guard can help protect your teeth but it won't solve why you might be clenching your teeth or why the muscles are tight. Stress is probably the cause.

Put two fingers in the bottom of your mouth over your teeth. Pull down and stretch your mouth open. Theoretically we are supposed to be able to fit three middle knuckles from our fingers into our mouths. Some people can fit their foot in their mouths, so for them this shouldn't be too difficult of a stretch.

Likewise you can glide your palms, or the meaty part below your thumb region, along the side of your jaw as you open your mouth. This massages the muscles when you open the jaw. Don't worry about looking silly doing these exercises; I have a worse one yet.

Take the palm and place it on the side of your chin. Gently push the lower jaw to one side, hold it there for a second or two and let go. Do this for both sides. This will stretch the little pterygoid muscles that open and close the mouth. Take your time doing these in the privacy of your home, while driving or during TV commercials. They may do the trick.

> *"A slip of the foot you may soon recover, but a slip of the tongue you may never get over."*
> **– Benjamin Franklin**

Your Feet

We walk, stand, run and pound our feet day after day. Those poor aching feet. There are 26 bones and 58 joints forming a pedestal for us to move on. They take the impact of our bodyweight, which can be as much as 3.5 times your bodyweight. So if you are 200 pounds your feet are withstanding 700 pounds of pressure with every step.

That can add up to around four to six million pounds of pressure each day. That's why a good foot massage feels really great. Share one with your someone special or get a mechanical massager. Give the hooves a break.

Your feet play a vital role in balance of the body and are critical in maintaining spinal posture. If your feet have a problem it will be transferred to the knees and hips, and eventually the rest of your body.

Knee or hip pain can alter your gait and create spinal distortion or back problems. Make sure your feet are not the culprit causing these aches and pains of yours.

Your feet are the gravitational connetion between your spine and every step you take. Like an architectural suspension bridge, each foot maintains an arch and has fat pads to withstand the force of the ground and our bodies.

When we take a step the heel strikes the ground first. The arch lowers as the foot makes contact and turns outward slightly pronating. As we raise the heel the arch rises and the foot turns slightly inward, known as supination, and supports the foot as we push off.

Many people have fallen arches or have flat feet because their arches are somewhat pronated or are less than the optimal arch for their bodies. Pronation can lead to conditions like short leg syndrome because of a tilted pelvis, bunions or plantar fasciitis, which is pain on the bottom of the foot. Supination can lead to chronic ankle sprains.

Orthotics can be a way to support and preserve the arch if there is a problem. When they are casted make sure your ankle is in a proper alignment and your arch is corrected. There is no reason to just step into a mold and cast a foot with bad arches. You haven't done anything supportive.

Other options that may provide support and relief include over the counter brands of supports and orthotics but they are not specific to your foot. I just want to make sure you get the support you need and can get off on the right foot.

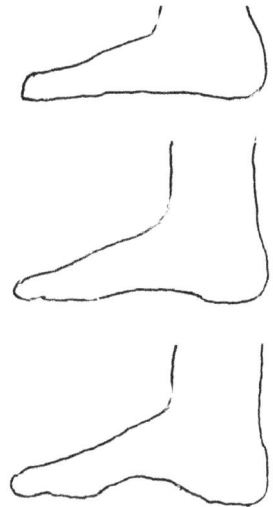

Common Foot Problems
BUNIONS AND CALLUSES

A person may put a foot in his or her mouth. Somebody else might move like they have two left feet. Some folks try to walk in other people's shoes. Then there are those who put the shoe on the other foot.

I want to talk about shoes for a moment. Look at your foot. Does it have a point where the toes are? No. Traditionally the anatomical relationship of your toes is that they are an extension of your feet and splay outward. They shouldn't look like you've been squeezing five pounds of potatoes into a two pound sack.

When you wear shoes that don't fit properly, aren't comfortable (especially if it is in the name of fashion), are too worn in the heel, provide little support in either direction, or take a lot of abuse while you are exercising, you may develop growths or structural changes in your feet.

When you buy shoes, make sure they fit well, don't squeeze your toes together and hurt your feet. You need these puppies to last say, 85 years or so. Calluses form because there is too much pressure against your foot and your body is trying to compensate by creating a protective pad. If your toe angles in, you may have redesigned the anatomy of your toe and this could be accompanied by a growth known as a bunion.

You might look hot, but how hot are you going to look hobbling around like Quasimodo because of your blisters and bunions. Not to mention the attempt to make a pad with Band-Aids and gauze. I have friends who have had their bunions surgically removed and it is painful and takes awhile to heal. Find shoes that fit your feet and are comfortable. I never win the discussion of heels with women, especially if they are vertically challenged or want to look five pounds thinner. I've heard all of the excuses.

I've been to parties and the ladies' first comments to my wife actually were, *"Those are great shoes."* How about nice to see you or how have you been? Society has placed a lot of expectations and self-induced stress on women to keep up with trends and beauty products so they are fashionable.

Either way, there are cushions for heel spurs, bunions, calluses and arch supports or heel cups for any situation. Podiatrists can fit you with orthotics, administer cortisone shots for the pain or do surgery if necessary to correct the problem. Or you could get better, more comfortable shoes and keep the *"little piggies"* happy.

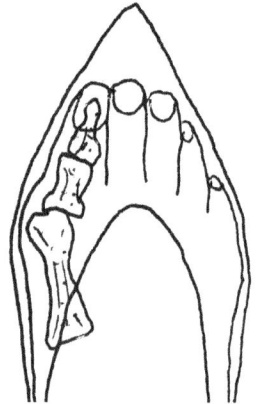

Speaking of keeping things happy, some runners are going out naked, with nothing on their feet silly. This is a family book. That's crazy you say. People have been running from lions and saber tooth tigers long before running shoes were available. The runner's stride becomes different without shoes and they are more in tune with their movements.

The foot strike comes down more toward the ball of the foot rather than the heel, as with shoes. About 75% of us run with the heavy heel strike. Is that causing our leg pains?

According to Daniel Lieberman, PhD, professor of human evolutionary biology at Harvard University, barefoot runners have an incredibly different foot strike pattern. The result is much less impact to the foot than landing on the heel first. Runners have a little extra spring in their legs. He also found that cushioned shoes may actually add to the number of foot injuries we suffer because of the force of every heel strike, but more research is needed.

These shoes look like gloves for your hands and allow more of a natural movement of your feet. Using the au naturale approach, the runner experiences a more interactive, stimulating, exhilirating feeling and an increase in speed. Research has shown barefoot running, and lighter shoes, will improve your speed. I always chose lighter spikes when I played baseball to give me every advantage and it helped.

Before you take off for a long run you should start slow. I would recommend trying a rubber track to get the hang of it or use five finger shoes to provide comfort and protection. These shoes look like gloves for your hands. They allow a more natural movement of your feet. Give your feet time to toughen up and to build strength in your calf and foot muscles.

My patient Rob tried these shoes on for the first time and then ran seven miles. He was pretty sore but he really likes them a lot. So do weightlifters.

MORTON'S NEUROMA

The nerves on the bottom of our feet are vulnerable to becoming pinched or irritated by all of the moving bones and pressure when we walk or run. Sometimes they do get pinched and usually this occurs in between the third and fourth toes. This can be caused by pressure of our bodyweight, an injury or from wearing the wrong shoes.

There is a thickening of the tissue around the nerves and this may cause burning or sharp pain in your foot. It may feel like there is something in your shoe causing a bump. It feels like you're stepping on a marble. Sometimes anti-inflammatory meds, rest, supports or even surgery may be needed to resolve the problem.

PLANTAR FASCIITIS

This is a tightening of the muscles on the bottom of your feet that run from your toes to your heel where they are attached by a tendon. Often when you wake in the morning you have to walk gingerly because there is so much pain in your feet.

As you move around, the muscles warm up and the symptoms decrease. As you become less active or wake the next day the muscle have cooled and retightened. You need to break this cycle.

Over time, due to stress, the body deposits calcium in the tendon to strengthen this region where it attaches to your heel and creates heel spurs. This can be due to: weight gain, bad arches, improper shoes, Achilles tightness or poor foot alignment.

You can try to have them broken down by ultrasound or work on loosening the muscles in this region. If they are really inhibiting you, surgery may be your only relief.

The first thing you might want to do is invest in new shoes. Take a look at your current selection. Are the heels worn down or do your feet fall sideways over the soles? Is there a hole in one of them? These are clear signs that it is time to replace them. Good shoes can be invaluable. If you are going to put pressure into them for six or eight hours a day, you want good support.

You could also try switching shoes each day or every other. Ladies, I know this is easier for you because of the small Nine West closet you have, but it is worth considering. If it is last year's style, then donate them and take the write-off.

Guys, you need to have two different pairs of work boots or several pairs of dress and comfort shoes for the other activities in your world. I have three pairs of dress shoes and rotate them throughout the week because each wears and feels differently. I work on a cement floor, which is terrible for my feet and knees, but my shoes make a difference.

Make sure you have the right shoes for the job. I recently went diving for Megalodon teeth (a prehistoric, 60 foot, great white shark from 30 million years ago) and Captain Steve, who runs the dive shop, mentioned he had foot pain. Being inquisitive and empathetic I asked him about it. He was going to go running and forgot his sneakers so he jogged in the boat shoes he had on.

The next day his feet were killing him and they never stopped being sore. I told him what to do for it and then worked on his tootsies after the dive. First I massaged and loosened the muscles and then adjusted each foot. He had some instant relief and we identified the culprit of his pain. Wrong shoes.

To relax feet muscles you can massage and work the bottom of your feet with the knuckles of your hand or your thumb. Better yet, get a massage and let a pro help, as long as you aren't ticklish.

I have a patient who is explosively ticklish. I treat this condition using a special massage unit I have at my office. Bart is a big man and is so ticklish and laughs so loudly, everyone can hear it in the entire office and it makes them all laugh. He has a great, robust laugh that probably carries over to the next street. Sounds like I'm tickling Santa.

The other option is to roll your foot on a golf ball while sitting or standing. You can also put the golf ball in a tub of warm water. The warmth of the water may help to relax the muscles, while the pressure from the golf ball works the muscles from the base of the toes to the heel. If you have a doctor confirmed heel spur, don't press the ball into that area, because it is bone and it will really hurt.

Some people freeze water in a 12-ounce plastic bottle and roll on that. It kind of works the same way to break up adhesion in the muscles, but to regain my step I prefer to use the ball or my thumb. That way I can really get in there and make something happen. Either process isn't super comfortable but both are extremely effective. The longer you let plantar fasciitis go, the worse it will get.

Something you could try to strengthen your plantar muscles is to squeeze marbles or a pencil with your toes and try to bring it toward you. You can even pull your toes in while you have shoes on. Just curl your toes and that will help recreate the arch of the foot.

"It is better to die on your feet than live on your knees." – **Emiliano Zapata**

Your Knee

The knee is a vulnerable joint that moves like a hinge. It enables us to move and is only protected by several ligaments and tendons. It is made up of three long bones. The upper thighbone, or femur, meets our two lower leg bones: the tibia, the shinbone and largest of the two lower bones; and the fibula, which is on the outside of your leg and forms the bump of your ankle.

The surfaces of the bones that come into close contact have articular cartilage on them to allow the segments to slide and move easily. Your knee may sustain such injuries like minor tears and strains that recover naturally.

Sometimes this can lead to uneven force on the knee or altered mechanics of the joint due to scar tissue.

The American Academy of Orthopaedic Surgeons estimates that more than four million people seek medical treatment for knee problems each year. Like most injuries it is difficult to prevent them in the case of an impact or fall, but for everyday activities there is a lot you can do. Make sure you are properly prepared.

You don't just walk into a meeting and you don't step up to the plate without preparing. Make sure you are warmed up. Most of us have recognized our bodies have aged more than our brains so we need time to loosen up the old bones.

I don't care if a whippersnapper challenges you. When they do, don't play one-on-one fresh from your commute home in your high heels, loafers or Timberlands. Make the shoe fit the activity and take time to loosen up your muscles.

Watch out for the weekend warrior scenario. Try to stay active and remain in good shape year round by eating right, exercising and stretching regularly. With a strong foundation, nothing can sideline you easily.

Common Knee Problems

ARTHRITIS

Time is the enemy. Often micro traumas we endure as youngsters can lead to us gimping around later. Minor injuries, repaired or not, have a tendency to weaken, create instability and change our movement.

The protective coating allowing the bones to glide over one another can deteriorate, as we grow older. Over years of consistent sports, chores and movements it will wear down further. As the stress becomes too great on any joint it will lead to degeneration and arthritis. This can cause calcium build-ups, known as spurs, to form as the body tries to stabilize the knee. We will feel pain and stiffness in the joint. Ever watch an ex pro football player walk? It is horrible. Their knees have been so badly abused they walk as if they were 95-years-old.

Another prominent reason for knee troubles at any age is our weight. As we continue to grow larger as a society, some medical professionals have recognized that being overweight by just one pound could result in around five pounds of additional stress to the knees. So being 10 pounds heavier than you would like to be could mean 50 pounds of added weight to your knees.

BAKER'S CYST

Remember the jelly donut analogy? The lubricating fluid between the knee bones are contained by a capsule or covering. Like a disc in your back, when stress is placed upon the knee unevenly it will force a bulge behind the knee.

As the force increases it pushes a pocket of fluid backward between the hamstring tendons. This is called a Baker's cyst, named for the surgeon that first described it.

The cyst can cause pain and swelling and reduced movement. It is usually worse with weight-bearing activities. Some people experience cysts in their wrists that they can whack with a heavy book to break them. It hurts and doesn't solve their problems permanently. They could have them drained or surgically corrected.

CHONDROMALACIA PATELLAE

The kneecap, or patella, is connected to the quadriceps, or the front thigh muscles, by a tendon. The lower portion of the kneecap attaches to the lower tibia bone by a tendon as well. The kneecap is known as a sesamoid bone. They form in the body when a tendon crosses a joint. The bone allows the tendon to stay taught during movement and keeps it away from the surface of the bending joint preventing friction or rubbing.

Sometimes our thigh muscles become stronger on one side of our body, pulling the kneecap to that side. This causes uneven wear of the smooth surface on the underside of the bone and makes it rough. Trauma, muscle weakness and overuse are also common causes.

You may hear popping and cracking noises when you bend your knees. There may be pain with walking down stairs or hills, or upstairs, as the knee becomes weight-bearing and the leg is straightened. Another test is pressure directly on the kneecap into your leg. Now contract your thigh while your hand applies pressure on the patella, preventing it from sliding upward as you contract. Pain with either of these two manuevers may indicate arthritis behind the kneecap. The injury is common with sports like soccer, skiing, running and cycling.

LIGAMENT DAMAGE

The collateral ligaments and cruciate ligaments protect our knees from excessive motion. There is a lateral collateral ligament (LCL) on the outside of the knee to stabilize the joint and the medial collateral ligament (MCL) on the inside of the leg to secure the inner knee.

You may have seen a football player get tackled and hit on the outside of the knee. When the knee is hit from that direction it tears the ligament on the inside of the leg because as the knee bends from the hit, the inside of the knee joint widens and separates the MCL too much. The LCL would be damaged with a hit to the inside of the knee.

The anterior cruciate ligament (ACL) is in the center of the knee and functions to limit rotation and forward movement of the tibia, the big lower leg bone. The ACL is usually damaged when an athlete plants and twists their foot. Stepping in a hole and twisting the knee will also simulate the movement for all of you non-athletes thinking you are safe.

The posterior cruciate ligament (PCL) is also in the center of the knee joint and limits backward motion of the tibia bone. If a player is hit from the front it forces the lower leg too far backward and can tear the PCL, because it is designed to limit backward motion. There is usually instant pain and a loud *"pop"* that accompany the injury.

OSGOOD - SCHLATTER'S DISEASE

Many youngsters up to their early teens may complain of knee pain in one or both legs. The disease affects mainly boys involved with sports. The tendon attaching the kneecap to the tibia is being stretched too much. In some cases it can actually tear the bone away from the tibia.

Pain is brought on by activity. There can be inflammation below the knee. Rest and ice relieve it. Limiting your vigorous sports helps the healing process while enabling some light exercise along the way. It can resolve and reappear many times. Sometimes the result will be a large bump just under the knee. Getting a child to not participate in high impact sports is difficult but will allow the body to rest and heal.

TORN MENISCUS

In between the bones of the knee are the meniscus, which are tough fibrous cushions that absorb impact and provide stability.

There is one on the inside of your leg called the medial meniscus; and another on the outside of your leg called the lateral meniscus. They are crescent shaped. When there is a tear you may notice a clicking in the knee and there may also be restricted motion. The joint may feel wobbly or like you need to shake the knee to realign it.

The meniscus is often injured by getting hit from the side and by twisting while the knee is supporting your weight. When an athlete runs and tries to avoid an opponent they have to step and twist. Once you plant and then twist, your foot stays put and much of the stress hits the knee joint. Old, tacky surfaces like Astroturf increase the likeliness of this injury exponentially. They have been replaced with natural grass or grass-like fields because grass allows the foot to move when turning and has more give. This reduces knee strain.

> *"No problem is so formidable that you can't walk away from it."* – **Charles M. Schulz**

Your Hips

The hip joint is a ball and socket joint like the shoulder. The upper leg bone, the femur, is like your fist, and its housing unit, the acetabulum, is like your other hand loosely covering the closed fist. There are a lot of muscles, tendons and ligaments trying to keep this joint stable. The surfaces of the bones are covered with a layer of articular cartilage allowing the bones to slide smoothly against one another.

Every step we take adds stress to this joint. If you are having knee or ankle pain it will definitely be transferred into the hip joint with each weight-bearing movement.

A study I think would be interesting is to evaluate how many hip and knee problems small tribes in third world countries experience considering there is no diaper pushing the thighs of a growing child outward. Just a thought. The outcome of the study would probably be messy.

Common Hip Problems
ARTHRITIS

The most common problem we encounter over the years is degeneration of the hip. This happens from increased stress and normal wear and tear. The actual joint is basically located behind your pocket. The femur comes up and the head of the femur bends at an angle toward your midline, where it meets its joint. That's why I say, *"If the pain is behind the pocket, it's the socket."*

Considering that we have two hips and they are the same age, one would expect them to wear down at the same time. This is often not the case for many reasons. If you are overweight you are forcing more stress to this joint, accelerating the loss of joint space between the bones.

Certain types of injuries from our youth, faulty pelvic alignment and lower leg problems can also cause too much weight to be carried on one side. The symptoms patients may notice include hip pain with movement, a loss of range of motion when compared from side to side, or many complain of groin pain behind their front pocket.

There are certain arthritis conditions that can deform the hip socket. This will hasten the degenerative changes that occur in the joint. It can be debilitating and make a surgical replacement the only option.

Next to the knees, the hip is the second most common replaced joint in the body. Some patients may not need a replacement but can have a newer procedure performed called resurfacing. I think of this like sanding down the rough spots and smoothing out the contacting surfaces so they glide easier. It is a simpler procedure and should be tried first if possible. Trying to keep the parts I was given, has always been a cardinal rule for me.

BURSITIS

Your body can develop a pouch of lubricating fluid called a bursa, which functions as a way to reduce friction in an area. This allows the bones, tendons, skin, etc., to slide without catching on one another. There are more than 150 bursae in the body and their locations range from the shoulder, elbow, feet and hip.

Anytime there is an inflammatory process, the suffix – *"itis"* is used. Appendicitis is inflammation of the appendix. Pancreatitis is inflammation of the pancreas, and so forth.

The typical ways to develop bursitis are overuse, injury, infection and arthritis. Activities like sports, gardening, kneeling and incorrect posture can aggravate these little sacs. They cause pain and stiffness in the joint. Loosen up, stretch, take breaks and use correct posture to decrease your chances of experiencing this discomfort. Treatment includes heat or ice, therapy, rest, support wraps and injections.

TENDONITIS

Tendonitis is inflammation in the sheath of the tendon, which attaches muscle to bone. The tendons are fibrous and strong. When your muscles contract they pull the bones they are attached to and create movement. When there is too much stress by way of overuse, the tendon can become inflamed. The sources for causing damage and forms of treatment are very similar to bursitis.

> *"It was on my fifth birthday that Papa put his hand on my shoulder and said," Remember, my son, if you ever need a helping hand, you'll find one at the end of your arm."* – **Sam Levenson**

The Arms

I am grouping some of the more common arm problems into one section because they don't affect your posture like walking with a bad knee or foot. I will discuss some of the more common ailments you may experience during your life.

Your shoulder is a ball and socket joint like the hip. Your elbow is a hinge joint like your knee, and your wrist has multiple small bones, which allow a wide range of motion, like your ankle.

Common Arm Problems

CARPAL TUNNEL SYNDROME (CTS)

Everyone has heard of this problem in the wrists. According to the U.S. Department of Labor, it affects some five million Americans and causes almost 50 percent of the workplace injuries and lost production. The wrist is very complicated in that there are eight small bones that make up a curved structure. A tendon passes over it and connects the sides like a roof. Underneath this ceiling are nerves, arteries, tendons and more, all trying to make their way through this tunnel.

Many of the jobs or hobbies we do require our hands to do a lot of bending, pulling and straining. Typical culprits are computers, either typing or mouse movement, sewing and knitting, repetitive motions like hammering, vibrations like jackhammers, but there are other causes. Chronic sprains or arthritis can lead to degenerative changes in the wrist bones and form spurs, or calcium deposits, which further limit the amount of space within the tunnel. If the tunnel changes shape, something starts pressing on the structures within, tissues become inflamed, the area becomes compressed and you may start to notice pain and other symptoms.

More common symptoms include pain or numbness in the fingers, loss of strength, a change in sensation in the hand, radiating pain up into the arm, forearm pain and swelling. Before you try surgery, seek professional care and limit the motion of the area. Stretches may loosen the muscles surrounding the wrist to alleviate stress. Also reevaluate your work place or repetitive habits to see if you can make some smart ergonomic changes. This may help solve your wrist problem and prevent others.

TRIGGER FINGER

This occurs in the tendons of any one of your fingers. Around each tendon is a sheath that protects it and is lubricated inside so it can glide when movement occurs. With repetitive motion and strain there is swelling in the tendon sheath and motion becomes restricted. Your finger may feel like it is stuck in a bent position. When you do move it, there is an audible click. For all of you computer mouse clickers, beware. Make sure you switch and stretch the fingers.

A diagnosis that is sometimes confused with trigger finger is Dupuytren's Contracture. It can occur simultaneously but is a little different scenario. It involves shortening and thickening of the tendon and can also cause the finger to bend.

On your palm you may visibly notice or palpate a bump. This is where the problem is. It is usually worse in the morning and there are few remedies you can try first after discussing the problem with your doctor. Massage the area. Rest the hand, splint the hand or soak in warm water. Medications, when combined with these remedies, may also help you avoid surgery.

GANGLION CYSTS

These are fluid filled sacs that form around a joint. These often form near the wrist, ankles and behind the knee, where they are called a Baker's cyst, and can be rather large. The fluid within the joint seeps through a tear around the joint and becomes encapsulated to form this cyst. The fluid may leak back into the joint and refill again later.

You may notice a bump limits your range of motion and causes discomfort. In general, pain is not a symptom associated with a ganglion, unless you are referring to smacking it with a dictionary. This is the old tale of whacking the bump with a large book to eliminate it. Of course it may go away on its own, you might need to have the fluid removed by a needle, known as aspiration, but then why go the easy route? Let's smack it with a heavy book.

If that doesn't cure it, smack it again. I'm just kidding. Ganglions can disappear as fast as they showed up. But if they are persistent, consult your doctor to diagnose a potential degenerative process that may be causing the ganglion cysts.

TENNIS ELBOW

Tennis elbow is tenderness on the outside, of your elbow. Pain on the inside is known as Golfer's Elbow. Either way this is tendonitis or inflammation of the tendon, where it attaches to the elbow joint. The elbow is a hinge joint, like your front door. Now imagine trying to constantly force your open door, upwards or downwards, by the doorknob. This illustrates stress forces to the door hinges and is similar to how you stress your elbow.

As a baseball player, I probably started batting practice in the cage months before the season started, had team practices where they couldn't get me out of the batter's box, played games and went to the cage many times each week of a six to eight month season. I bet I hit 2000 baseballs before the first pitch of the season. Every time you make contact, a ball is coming at you at 85 miles an hour and you are hitting it with a bat in the opposite direction. When you do that over 20 years, a lot of stress bombards the elbow joints. And if you asked my teammates, none of that practice did any good for my hitting. Haha. Anyway, I still feel it.

If you play tennis, constantly lifting things with your palms facing center, like grabbing a bucket handle or using a hammer, this will cause the pain I'm talking about. You can try braces, ice, rest, medications, gentle massage to the muscles, and creams; but, reducing the stress to the joint is the only way to get relief naturally. Otherwise you may have to try steroid injections or surgery.

ROTATOR CUFF PROBLEMS

The shoulder is very vulnerable while providing a tremendous amount of motion. The muscles that protect and provide this movement are referred to as the rotator muscles. The four muscles can be damaged from: repetitive overhead activities, overuse, trauma, and inflammation in surrounding tendons, bursa and the ever-present arthritis. Pain is most commonly located in the front of the shoulder. It may hurt to move the shoulder away from the body and you may notice limited motion in general.

Ask the reason I am not playing baseball regularly. I can tell you it feels like someone sticks a knife into my shoulder after I throw the ball too hard. Overtime you may notice weakness, pain and loss of motion. That is because tendons get torn, muscles contract and there is inflammation. Some people experience a frozen shoulder after they have protected and not fully moved the area for too long. If you allow no motion whatsoever, the entire region will freeze and become immobile.

With mild cuff injuries you could try ice, rest and medications. Eventually you may be able to incorporate a rehab routine for the muscles using just five pound weights. Any more than that and you will recruit other muscles to assist you and diminish the results you are trying to achieve. I have to say my shoulders feel a heck of a lot better if I am diligent and do these exercises. I try to do them when I watch TV but even doctors can make terrible patients.

If the problem progresses you may need cortisone shots or surgery. Once again, reevaluate your habits, job and hobbies to see if you can make ergonomic changes or change your body mechanics when participating in sports to prevent further injury and keep you in the game.

"Today's scientists have substituted mathematics for experiments, and they wander off-through equation after equation, and eventually build a structure, which has no relation to reality." – **Nikoli Tesla**

Biomechanics

Each part of our body was designed to function a certain way. If we alter the motion intended then problems can occur. Look at the demonstration of Newton's Cradle or colliding balls. Five balls, each attached to two strings, hang from a parallel bar so the balls set up in line with each other. When you pull one and let it go, it hits the next one and redistributes the force right through to the last ball.

With the proper alignment of the balls you have conservation of movement. The first ball will collide with the next ball. That force is transferred through the next few balls and the last ball will bounce outward and then return the force. This will go on for some time. It is similar to making a combo shot in the game of billiards.

If one ball is aligned just a little differently, then when you try this experiment it will end in disaster. You will have no continuation of motion and the balls will displace in every direction.

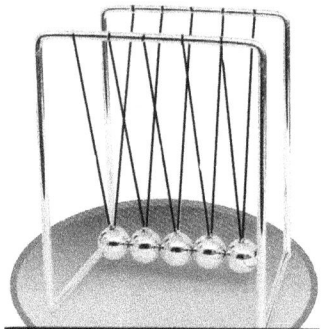

Newton's Cradle

Your body has tremendous abilities, but also has limitations if one area is unable to perform as expected. Have you ever hurt your knee or ankle and hobbled around for a few days or weeks? All of a sudden you start to have pains in different areas than your original complaint. That's because, *"your knee bone IS connected to you hip bone."*

Your body compensates for the change from normal motion and tries to provide you with your customary movement by any means possible. That could mean stressing out another perfectly normal area.

Realistically any alterations from your normal form and motion can affect other parts of the body because it is considered to be what we call a closed kinematic system. A simple knee problem like a strain, can have a profound effect on your body in terms of balance, stress, alignment, efficiency and posture.

A family member of mine was having calf spasms and knee problems. She was seen by her doctor, examined and checked for a vascular problem in that area. The tests were negative. She had knee surgery due to knee damage and went to therapy. They did exercises and some stretching. The knee improved but both calves were still having episodes of spasms. Could it be nerve pain? They tried medications and more exercises to no avail.

I talked with her and watched her. As part of her rehab, she was doing too many calf presses to strengthen the calf. She was sitting in a recliner with her toes pointed forward for hours, which keeps her calf in a shortened and contracted state. Due to the knee pain she had been walking on her toes more than the average person. I advised her about some stretches, not to walk on her toes, to sit with her feet flat on the floor and recommended moist heat and massage.

I talked to her about mechanics, posture and muscles, and she listened. In two days she noticed a huge difference and in two weeks the symptoms were gone. Sometimes we are our own worst enemies when it comes to our health.

> *"Those who do not find time for exercise will have to find time for illness."*
> **– Earl of Derby**

Muscles

There are three types of muscle tissues; cardiac, smooth and skeletal and each type has its own function.

Cardiac muscle is synchronized to push blood through the body and allow the other side to fill before being moved through the body again.

Like cardiac muscle, smooth muscle is also considered involuntary because it contracts on its own. It is present in the vascular region, digestive and intestinal system.

The type of muscles that provides motion and force is skeletal muscle. There are basically two types of skeletal muscle. They are fast and slow twitch fibers and each possesses its own traits. Muscles respond differently to training depending on which type of muscle fibers influence the muscle most. Almost all muscles have a balanced mix of slow and fast fiber types.

Your genetics play a major role in determining which type of training your muscles will respond to best. You might have realized your muscles are more geared for fast and explosive movement so you stole bases in baseball or threw the shot put. Others may have found they excelled in running long distances and ran cross-country.

Slow twitch muscles fibers (Type I) need oxygen because cells within them are extremely efficient at replenishing their energy and are considered aerobic. They are great for endurance because they fatigue slowly. A marathon runner is a good example of someone with a higher concentration of slow twitch fibers.

Some muscles are considered to be fast twitch (Type II) because the fibers that make them up are designed to generate short bursts of speed. They cannot sustain this output very long. These are anaerobic because they do not require oxygen to create more energy. A 50-yard dash sprinter has a large concentration of these muscles.

Fast twitch fibers have further been divided into Type IIa and Type IIb. Type IIa fibers are considered to be intermediate fast twitch fibers because they contain both slow and fast fibers, producing energy with or without oxygen.

Type IIb fibers are the elite of fast twitch muscle fibers. They come out of the gate like gangbusters but fail to have enough energy to make it very far because they tire quickly. Let's say your football team is down by a score with less than a minute to go. They hand the ball off to the running back. His Type IIb fibers quickly blast him through the 5-yard line, like a sprinter, as he goes toward midfield, spinning and shaking off tacklers.

As the other team's pursuit continues, the elite, fast twitch fibers start to fatigue around the 45-yard line and the Type IIa kick in. They provide a little more gitty-up and go as the runner rushes toward the end zone. As he distances himself from the competition, the slow twitch, Type I fibers can put it on cruise control, like a jogger, and allow him to casually, high step it in to the end zone from the 15-yard line. TOUCHDOWN!!

"The human body is made up of some four hundred muscles; evolved through centuries of physical activity. Unless these are used, they will deteriorate."
– Eugene Lyman Fisk

Muscle problems

Your muscles can be also be classified into two categories when referring to your posture. Some are there for support and are called postural muscles, where others are mainly for movement.

Tonic muscles are sometimes referred to as slow twitch because they don't fatigue easily and have good circulation. They are stimulated quicker and respond to faulty loading, which can be viewed as over-use, abuse or disuse of the body. They become tight and short, or hypertonic. These muscles work most of the time and help to maintain our posture.

On the other side of the track are the phasic muscles. They tend to weaken and lengthen when faced with faulty loading. These are considered a fast twitch muscle, since they develop more size and strength and are explosive in their action.

The muscles that are considered tonic and are often tight in the body, including the: low back muscles (erector spinae and quadratus lumborum), the chest (pectoralis major and minor), the neck (upper trapezius and levator scapulae), back of the leg (hamstrings), hip flexors (iliopsoas) and hip rotator (piriformis). You may notice in your own body that your neck or low back is often tight.

The phasic muscles of motion are the: midback (rhomboids, mid and lower trapezius), back of the arm (triceps), shoulder (deltoid), abdominals, the rump (glutes) and the front of the thigh (vastus lateralis and medialis of the quads).

An example would be the low back muscles, like the lumbar erector spinae and quadratus lumborum, are tonic and are often overused when lifting. They become tight while the opposing muscles, the abdominal muscles become weak because they are phasic. This is a classic example of why many people suffer from low back pain. Another would be the fact that many people have tight shoulders around the neck. The trapezius muscle may be tight from having your head forward as you drive, sit and watch TV or work on the computer. But the other possibility is that the lower trapezius muscle is weak. Strengthen that and you can balance the muscle altogether.

If someone is even slightly overweight, every extra pound of weight in the front of your stomach is an additional 10 pounds of stress in the low back. It is not rocket science that many people with large stomachs also have back problems or that pregnancy can lead to back pain.

All of the muscles in your body, especially the neck, shoulders, back, abdominals and legs either attach to the spine directly or have a close enough correlation to be considered a major player in your spine's health. If they become tight, they can pull your spine out of its normal position or proper alignment.

If your neck has a spasm, usually one side of your neck will be tighter than the other. When you turn or move your head you will have greater motion in one direction and limited in the other. For every muscle pulling on the right side of your body, there is another balancing it by pulling from the left side.

When a muscle gets stronger, say from being right-handed, the muscles become short and tight. Whereas, the other side of this tug of war battle will be stretched and weaker. When the muscles are weak and the opposing muscles are strong, it affects the alignment and the posture of the body as a whole.[50]

With whatever you are doing, if there is resistance, the job is a lot harder. When the body's movement is restricted through its normal range of motion, stress becomes a factor to many regions. Not only does it cause problems to the area of limited motion but it also causes stress to the bones and muscles that try to overcompensate and makeup for the lost motion. They do too much and become overworked so you can still accomplish what you need to do. Imagine trying to drive with one wheel that has a brake sticking so it turns harder than the others. You will still be able to drive but it will take more effort and cause damage to other areas as well.

Also, if you have muscles that are tight in your neck, they can lead to decreased movement. The longer the muscles remain tight, like after a car accident, the more apt they are to stay that way. They will become short and tight and you will lose the normal range of motion of your spine. It will take time to change the rigidity of these muscles. If left unattended, over time it will lead to degenerative changes of the joints and supporting segments.

Muscles of the Body

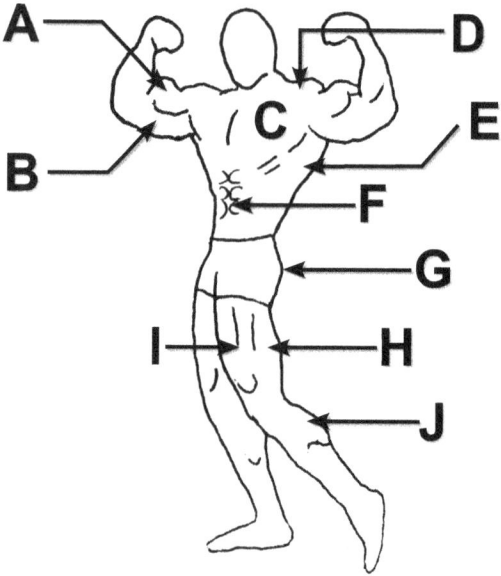

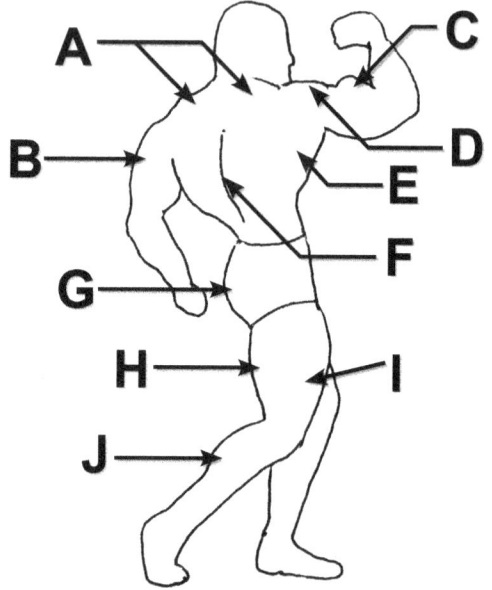

Muscles of the Body (front)
A. Biceps.　　　　**B.** Triceps.
C. Chest or Pectorals.
D. Deltoids or Shoulders.
E. Latissimus.　　　**F.** Abdominals.
G. Glutes.　　　　**H.** Hamstrings.
I. Quadriceps.　　　**J.** Calf

Muscles of the Body (back)
A. Trapezius.　　　**B.** Triceps.
C. Biceps.　　　　**D.** Deltoids.
E. Latissimus　　　**F.** Rhomboids.
G. Glutes.　　　　**H.** Hamstrings.
I. Quadriceps.　　　**J.** Calf

"Everyone has a doctor in him or her; we just have to help it in its work. The natural healing force within each one of us is the greatest force in getting well." – **Hippocrates**

Trigger Points

What is a Trigger Point (TP)? There are a total of 696 Muscles according the Basle Nomina Anatomica. We learned there are three types of muscle in the body, cardiac, smooth and skeletal. Skeletal muscle can account for 40 percent or more of a person's body weight.[51] Normal skeletal muscle does not have fibrous regions or taut bands, also called nodules, and the muscle will not cause pain upon pressure. A trigger point, is that area in the muscle that can feel like a bump or a knot and cause pain.

Any skeletal muscle can develop a syndrome known as Myofascial Trigger Points and develop either local pain, or refer pain to other areas of your body. It is a poorly understood and too often overlooked condition in the diagnosis of a patient. It is believed that 75 percent of all pain could be associated with trigger points and every pain a person feels has some trigger points involved to a certain degree.[51] For example, many headaches can be caused by trigger points in the neck muscles.

Overuse, poor posture, injuries, stress, intense training, spasm and inadequate stretching are some of the possible causes of their formation. Myalgia (myo – muscle, algia – pain) means pain emanating from muscles. Sometimes this shooting pain will imitate common conditions like sciatica, jaw pain, shoulder pain, carpal tunnel syndrome, headache or even radiating arm pain.

TPs can exist for years and then become irritated and suddenly painful. Muscles can be tight with reduced motion and decreased circulation in that area. Toxins then build up as muscle fibers join to each other, or adhere, and form these lovely knots.

There are two kinds of trigger points, active and latent. Active trigger points cause pain that is deep, achy and even radiating. The severity can be mild to debilitating. They are sore whether you are in motion or not. They don't care. They cause discomfort and they limit how much freedom you have to move.

Interestingly, the area or size of the muscle containing a trigger point does not equate to the amount of pain associated with it. So a thigh and thumb trigger point can cause the same amount of pain.

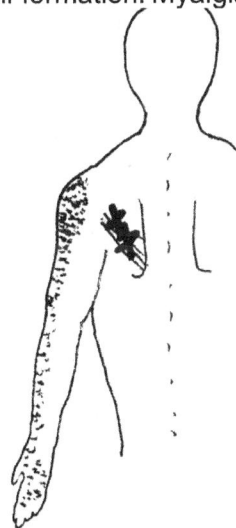

Trigger Point
Black "XX".
Trigger Point in the Muscle.
Black Dots.
Indicate where the referral is and the intensity by how dense the dots are.

Common areas involved are the postural muscles that are overworked like the shoulders, the trapezius, neck and low back, rotator cuff and hip rotators. These are active spots that may disappear on their own, become dormant, and later become latent trigger points (LTP).

LTP do not cause pain at rest but can cause weakness in a muscle and restrict your motion. They are usually only painful when pressure is applied to them.

Left untreated, they reduce the quality of life of an individual due to lingering pain and restricted range of motion of the affected region. Pain and spasm of the muscle can fluctuate for years resulting in poor posture, altered biomechanics and decreased flexibility.

> *"The goal of life is living in agreement with nature." –* **Zeno**

How does Trigger Point Therapy work?

Treatment of TPs consists of pressure in the area from a finger or a hand-held device, pressure, heat and stretching. Pressure is sustained for 10 – 20 seconds and gradually increased as the TP releases. Sometimes the body is still while work is done. Other times the patient is instructed to move their muscle through its normal range of motion while pressure is being applied to strip the muscle fibers as the muscle elongates.

The pressure on the TP is a way to increase blood flow, flush the muscle out, break adhesions in the fibers, and relax any taut bands in the muscle fiber. Muscle fibers can form a network of cross-linkages as they heal from an injury. Instead of the muscle fibers being in line with each other, they are randomly woven together. Like scar tissue, the area has less flexibility and movement. Cross friction massage helps to disrupt these fibers.

I have treated several female patients over the years who complained of severe back or shoulder pain and an inability to comb their hair. Now I know I should have called 911 because this is a crisis, however I decided to see what I could do. Every time they made the motion of brushing their hair back they were using muscles that externally rotate the shoulder to do so.

The infraspinatus and teres minor muscles are located on the back of the shoulder blade. When they get *"fired up"* they can really be limiting. They are overused in baseball and I've had my run in with them before too. Anyway, the ladies couldn't even raise their arms above their shoulders. I used some heat and some thumb pressure. After a few treatments they were back to having beautiful hair. Now, that can make my job rewarding.

There are more comfortable ways to spend an afternoon, but the outcome with TP therapy is usually tremendously helpful.

"The preservation of health is a duty. Few seem conscious that there is such a thing as physical morality." **– Herbert Spencer**

Alignment

Alignment is another important key to maintaining your spine's health. The same bones of your spine that protect your spinal cord and allow movement also get pulled one way or the other by the muscles attached to them.

These contractions happen every time you reach for something, take out the trash, throw a ball or slip and fall. Simple everyday life can cause muscle spasms and spinal misalignment. Because the muscles are attached to the spine, it is necessary to correct the alignment of the bones if you want the muscles attached to them to also relax. Otherwise it is like trying to lose weight when you are not eating sensibly. The two go hand in hand.

Good posture allows your body to function optimally. When your body is working at its best you are more productive at work, perform better at sports and can enjoy life to its fullest.

Have you ever noticed that when you are in pain or having difficulties moving, that you are completely exhausted at the end of the day, or sooner? That is because your body is working harder to allow you to function and the additional stress tires you out.

This is another reason why proper alignment and muscle balance are integral to having a healthy posture. You will have more energy as a result of your body functioning with minimal strain and greater efficiency.

If that isn't incentive enough, your brain is trying to communicate with the rest of your body via the nervous system, which exits through the spine telling every muscle, organ and cell what to do. It is also relaying information back to the brain. In fact, in a recent study discussed on Good Morning America which found that chiropractic adjustments to the upper neck can reduce blood pressure by 16 points. Usually it takes two medications to accomplish this chemically, when properly aligning the body may do it naturally.

If the body was smart enough to divide, create specialized cells and become the living, working marvel you are today, it only makes sense to ensure that the brain has that same opportunity to tell your body how to function without any interruption throughout your lifetime.

Just as your car runs best after a tune-up and wheel alignment, your body runs best when it is in proper alignment. When your tires are out of alignment, you can still drive, but the car starts to run less efficiently.

Your car will pull to one side, the steering wheel will shake and the tires will wear unevenly. You may have to replace them and eventually the brakes, rotors and calipers if you continue to stress out that area.

The same thing happens to the most complex machine you own, your body!

If it is not functioning properly, with all its parts working as they should, the spine will wear unevenly and prematurely.

Since you cannot replace your body as you can tires on your car, it is wise to keep it tuned-up and running as efficiently as possible with regular chiropractic care.

Most pro and college athletes from all sports, like football players who experience repeated collisions, have their spines checked so they can perform the way the body was intended. Guys like Michael Jordan, Tom Brady, Emmitt Smith, Evander Holyfield, Muhammed Ali, Joe Montana, Derek Jeter, Jerry Rice, Wade Boggs, Wayne Gretzky, Tiger Woods and Arnold Schwarzenegger just to name a few. So they want to keep these elite athletes from having injuries and healing fast. That would make sense for everyone.

Tire Alignment
A. Uneven wear from Misalignment.
B. Uneven wear from Bad Alignment.
C. Even wear from Good Alignment.

To correct a misalignment problem, a gentle force is applied, by hand typically, in a direction to reposition the vertebra or any joint in the body. This restores freedom of motion again and there is less stress on the bones and muscles closely affiliated with the segment needing attention. This decreases the stress on the supporting bones, discs and nerves and allows proper functioning of the spine to resume.

Mobilization is when a practitioner uses passive motion of the joint to stretch and re-establish proper movement. There is no popping noise with this procedure. It is a slow deliberate series of stretches to return proper motion to the joints.

Manipulation is a term used to describe what happens when a joint is adjusted or repositioned and an audible release can be heard. This noise is called a cavitation and occurs when the gas filled void between the joint surfaces is gapped. Nitrogen, oxygen, water vapor and carbon dioxide, which are produced by normal cell metabolism, are reabsorbed into the body after they are released. This is the same mechanism you hear when you crack your knuckles.

While I'm talking about that, nowhere in the *Annals of the Rheumatic Diseases, Western Journal of Medicine or Journal of Manipulative & Physiological Therapeutics* were there any studies proving there was joint damage that could be associated with knuckle cracking.

However, there may be soft tissue damage if the person does it too often. Some people make it a habit and pop their knuckles 10 – 20 times a day. After 20 years of this, you can have some visual changes, strength changes and swelling. In other words … stop cracking your knuckles all the time.

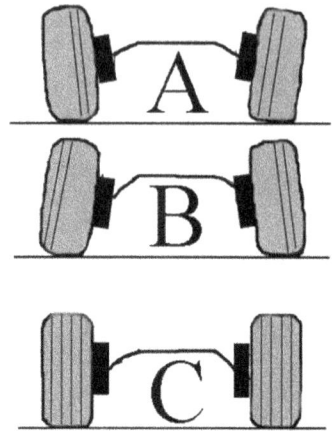

> *"Despite the tendency of doctors to call modern medicine an 'inexact science', it is more accurate to say there is practically no science in modern medicine at all."*
> – **Robert S. Mendelsohn, M.D.**

Falls

Here is a prime example of a fall and a bit of stupidity. One afternoon I went to my mother's house to repair her leaning fence that keeps her greyhounds in the yard. It was a warm summer day and I had my Detroit Tigers hat on to limit the sun exposure to my face and melon. I decided the best and easiest method to secure the fence and solve the problem was to nail a 2 x 4 into the fence. Next, I pushed the fence back to vertical and nailed the other end of the board into a nearby tree.

So we did this and it worked great. I turned around and picked up another board a couple of feet away. As I started approaching the next area to be fixed I smacked my head into the 2 x 4 I just nailed up not eight seconds ago. It knocked me off my feet onto my backside. All I could do was laugh and say, *"That's going to leave a mark."*

I couldn't see the board because of my hat. I did continue my job but sought appropriate care afterwards.

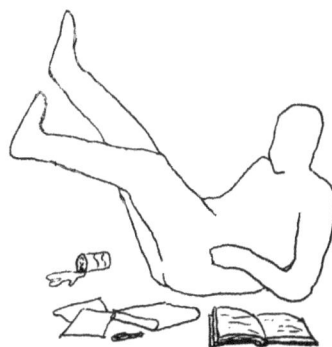

When we slip and catch ourselves or try that new jump on the slopes and take a tumble, this places our bodies under some serious stress and misaligning forces. These imbalances can cause tightening of the supporting muscles, decreased motion and stress to the body; ultimately leading to poor posture, degenerative changes and pain.

Some say it is better to just fall as opposed to contracting certain muscles to maintain your balance and trying to prevent the fall. I equate this with the drunk driver who crashes the car. They are relaxed because they are *"out of it,"* while the people who get seriously injured are the ones who tried to prepare for the impact.

Of course if you do fall you have to be ready to withstand the impact. In that case it is similar to a whiplash scenario. This happens when we fall out of a tree, as a kid, not many sane adults are climbing trees. We're too busy slipping on ice, falling down stairs, overlooking a step, catching our foot and tripping over a child's toy. Anyway, when we fall, there is jarring of our bodies and our heads whip backward.

This will affect your posture. Although there may not be any visible damage or sensation of discomfort at the time, the body has been through trauma. Reread the Whiplash section if this doesn't ring a bell.

The muscles and bones will be in spasm or misaligned, respectively. Left untreated, this is a problem that will catch up to us, as we get older. The abnormal wear and tear will cause tightness or pain that is of short duration at first and will gradually increase its frequency and severity. Doing something about your posture now can make your later years more fun, independent and healthy.

> *"I will have nought to do with a man who can blow hot and cold with the same breath."*
> **– Aesop**

HEAT OF THE MOMENT

A common question I hear is when to use ice or heat. Many patients don't know so they do nothing. As a general rule, ice is for inflammation and heat is for muscle spasms. Inflammation is good to prevent infection but bad for tissue healing. Ice is typically used during the first 24 – 48 hours of an injury. It helps to reduce swelling and numb the area of pain. When applying ice you will feel the coldness followed by a burning sensation, then an achy feeling followed by numbness.

If you don't have an ice pack that doesn't freeze completely, you can use frozen vegetables like corn or peas, or put a 1:2 ratio of rubbing alcohol and water in a Ziploc bag. The alcohol doesn't allow the water to completely freeze and you can add food coloring if you want a funky color. Don't ever use the solid block or solid blue ice pack that goes into your cooler. It is too cold if applied directly and can cause freezer burn.

After the initial 48 hours is when heat usually will be used to help bring in fluids and nutrients to facilitate the healing process. Heat helps to ease muscle tension and reduce joint stiffness as well. Moist heat is regarded as a better therapeutic modality than dry heat because it penetrates the area deeper. Only if your heating pad has a sponge should you use something wet with it. If you are still at a loss for heat try a hot water bottle, take a bath or shower.

Otherwise you could wet a towel and put it in the microwave for a while. When it is finished, place it in another towel so it doesn't burn you. You could also place it in a Ziploc type bag to keep the heat in and place a moist towel around it. Be careful. It may be hotter than you think.

Everyone's tolerance to temperature change is different. Make sure that your spouse's version of heat isn't too hot. Just because they like a thin towel around the heat doesn't mean you will. If it feels like you should be roasting some potatoes while *"the meat"* is cooking, then it is probably too hot. The

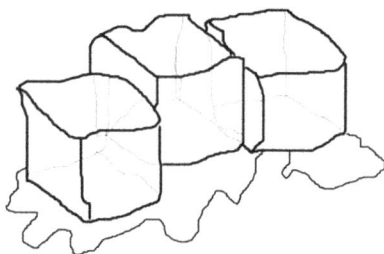

distinct smell of burning skin, especially when it's yours, isn't pleasant.

When using either ice or heat it should only be applied for 20 minutes every couple of hours. Sleeping on the hot pad is not recommended either. When you lie on a hot pad your bodyweight exaggerates the intensity of the heat to a level that can be dangerous or at least cause a skin burn. Likewise for ice. Any longer than 20 minutes will cause your body to have a negative reaction to what should be a helpful modality.

For example, with too much heat your body will try to flush out fluids because too many are accumulating. In other words it will act like ice has been placed on the area. Ever fall asleep with your old standby heat that usually helps you feel relief, only to feel like you were run over by a truck the next morning? That's why.

In some cases you will switch back and forth with ice and heat to flush an area and bring nutrients in and out. Sometimes when you are rehabbing a knee you may use heat before exercising and breaking up adhesions followed by ice to reduce the swelling caused by the exercise.

In any situation, try one and see if it helps. If it doesn't, then try the other. Doing something is better than doing nothing at all. It also helps me when I ask a patient if ice or heat helps and they can say heat makes it worse. That gives me vital clues as to what is going on. Also, follow your provider's instructions. If they say use ice don't decide to jump in to the hot tub with your friends later that night over cocktails. You may look like Shamu trying to get on to dry land due to the pain.

> *"There is great treasure there behind our skull and this is true about all of us. This little treasure has great, great powers, and I would say we only have learnt a very, very small part of what it can do"* – **Isaac Bashevis Singer**

Concussions

Motor vehicle accidents can result in a concussion and so can sports or a slip and fall. More and more we hear about professional athletes getting knocked out of games. The problem is that studies have shown concussions are more dangerous than we first thought and more prominent in younger athletes.

The American Association of Neurological Surgeons describes a concussion as, *"an injury to the brain that results in temporary loss of normal brain function … usually caused by a blow to the head."*

Football players will suffer the most head injuries this year followed by hockey, soccer and lacrosse, which were #2, #3 and #4 on the list of sports resulting in the most head injuries. Football-related injuries have more than doubled over the last five years and helmet to helmet hits were responsible for 65 percent of concussions reported.

During the 2010 NFL season alone, concussion injuries were up by 21 percent. Some of that is because they are more aware of this type of injury than they were before. That is why the NFL is penalizing hits to the head to deter these occurrences and protect the athletes. Too many veteran players are suffering from brain injuries later in life-like some boxers do. But, the big hit still makes ESPN's Top Plays.

The real problem is if you have had one concussion, your chances of experiencing another one are about 35 percent. Many of these player injuries go unreported for various reasons. Examples would be when a young athlete wants to continue playing or a coach or trainer misses the signs of a concussion and is over-anxious to have a star athlete return to the field. Some schools don't even have trainers on staff.

The American College of Sports Medicine reported 300,000 concussions are reported nationally from either sports or recreational activities involving athletes 18 and under, which is about one in every four athletes. They also believe 85 percent of concussions aren't identified at all. A study in the *Clinical Journal of Sports Medicine* also found 66 percent of athletes didn't think their injuries were worthy of reporting.

Playing with a concussion and being hit again can result in death from second impact syndrome (SIS), a condition in which the brain swells, shutting down the brain stem and resulting in respiratory failure. That's why you should always report an injury.

Several studies have found that it wasn't a specific hit to the head that caused symptoms, but an accumulation of repetitive trauma to the head. The repeated collisions cause an accumulative effect on the brain known as Chronic Traumatic Encephalopathy (CTE).

Any trauma to the brain can lead to long-term problems like blurred vision, depression, slurring of words, memory loss and dementia. They found the Hall of Famer Junior Seau suffered from this.

Typical signs or symptoms to look for when evaluating a concussion include: the athlete does not have to lose consciousness, headaches, fogginess, difficulty concentrating, easily confused, slowed thought process, difficulty with memory, nausea, lack of energy, tiredness, dizziness, poor balance, blurred vision, sensitivity to light and sounds, mood changes like irritability or anxiousness.

I'm not advocating against sports, because they are a great learning experience for our youth on many levels. I'm alerting you to the dangers and maybe advocating for better head protection. Don't take chances. Be evaluated thoroughly if you experience a concussion injury.

"Most diseases are the result of medication, which has been prescribed to relieve and take away a beneficiate and warning symptom on the part of Nature." – **Elbert Hubbard**

Symptoms

If you want to know what is going on with your health, just listen to your body. A little ache or pain is trying to tell you that something isn't right. That's how the brain communicates with you. Unfortunately too many people ignore the pain, think it will go away or take a drug to hide the symptoms, like placing tape over your dash board warning light. What do you typically do when your kid calls out for you? Do you ignore them? What about when they stop crying out your name? Do you assume everything must be okay again? Of course not.

I have heard patients say *"I don't like doctors."* Doctors are there to help you. Not knowing if something is wrong is just a silly reason not find out what ails you. Some people with family histories of cancer refuse to see a doctor for appropriate tests because they fear something may be wrong.

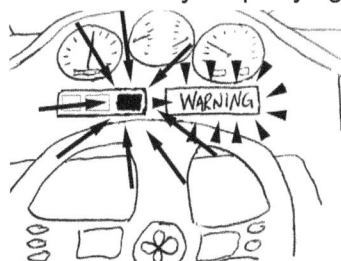

It would be better to know you only have three months so you could tell everyone how much you care about them and maybe even visit the places you've always wanted to see. It might also be smart to find out early so there is a possibility something could be done to save your life.

"Symptoms, then, are in reality nothing but a cry from suffering organs." – **Jean-Martin**

HAVEN'T GOT TIME FOR THE PAIN

So when it comes to your body, what will you do? Is pain normal? No. So why hide it with a medication when your body is clearly crying out something is wrong? A medication may help decrease your back pain, allow a better night's rest or get you through the day, but that pill isn't going to correct any postural problems, misalignments, muscular imbalances or trigger points causing the pain in the first place.

I want to know why I have pain and where it is coming from. Medications don't solve a problem they only pacify the symptom. I also don't want to perceive I am feeling better so I can return to my normal abusive activity level only to collapse on the 4th hole after my chip shot.

I have patients who have ignored enlarging growths on their arms. Some aren't concerned when a mole expands or changes color. Others believe blood in the urine or sciatica will go away. Sounds crazy, but it happens every day with simple backaches and headaches that become worse over several months.

> *"The most important thing in communication is to hear what isn't being said."*
> **– Peter Drucker**

DO YOU HEAR WHAT I HEAR?

Even if you don't have symptoms with your teeth you still go to a dentist every six months to prevent any problems from showing up. Why wait if your body hurts elsewhere? Otherwise the repairs can really be costly. Do you wait to bring your car in when it starts sputtering and blowing black smoke? Probably not.

So if not having any symptoms doesn't warrant skipping your dentist appointment because they may still find a problem, then why do people automatically associate a disappearance of symptoms as a sign they are healed? Just because your pain stops doesn't mean the problem is resolved. Often muscular problems have started long ago from repetitious and stressful movements or from falls and accidents. These will all cause accumulated stress to the body's frame resulting in spasm and tightness.

An example I like to use is Cancer, which is occurring in the body for a while before symptoms show up. Another is a heart attack. Usually its symptoms are the classic shortness of breath, gripping pain in the chest and pain radiating into the arm, but these typically occur after years of poor diet and lack of exercise. Both problems started long before their symptoms forced a doctor's visit.

Eventually if you do something as easy as picking up a pencil your back will go into spasm. You may have not had symptoms but the problem was there all along. You may have experienced symptoms of varying duration that have come and gone a few times over the years and thought you were better. That is until you feel another similar twinge and this time it doesn't go away and has a little more intensity.

If you have a headache from your kid playing his stereo too loudly you can take some aspirin to relieve it. But if you never stop your kid from crankin' his alternative, grunge and machine music too loudly, then you haven't stopped the source of the headache. A quick sledgehammer to the stereo or a discussion with your child will stop the headache, prevent future ones and save your kids ears. Now you've solved several problems.

The next time your body is talking to you or sounding the alarm, listen to it and help yourself. *"If you have time to hurt, you have time to heal."*

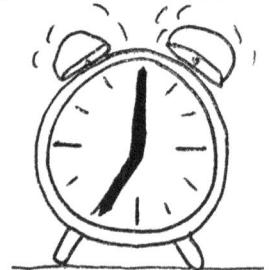

> *"[Medicine is] a collection of uncertain prescriptions the results of which, taken collectively, are more fatal than useful to mankind."* – **Napoleon Bonaparte**

Medications

The pharmaceutical industry was one of the most profitable businesses in the world until a couple of years ago when I believe the oil companies, who have taken over the fleecing of America, dethroned it. Many of the drug companies have been found to spend much more in advertising than in research and development.

Morning and evening news programs are quick to cover a new breakthrough in the treatment of one disease or another. They promote the story that researchers have found that drug X has been shown to promote positive changes and it hits the news wires like it is a confirmed cure.

Later on they discuss how these were accidental findings or finally admit that this miracle is 10 years from having enough research to fully back these findings and be approved by the FDA. Too late. You have already promoted drug X so much that consumers wrongly believe that it may help their condition. If the drug is on the market already people will start using it now for the alleged benefits covered. Investors must be buying stock right before the second announcement is made.

A recent funny news story to be misconstrued was that the divorce rate is down to its lowest rate in 30 years. Wow. Men and women have finally learned how to tolerate each other and love one another at the same time. Nope. Less people are getting married so the numbers are down. What did you take away from the initial announcement? Divorce rates are down.

For years drug companies have had an open forum to promote their drugs to people of all ages for this problem or that one. A recent report found 50 percent of Americans are on some form of medication.

Pharmaceutical representatives, who are usually attractive people, have supposedly been restricted from buying lunches for offices or offering trips as ways to promote the use of their brand of drug and possibly influence their sales. It's about time.

Each night you can see hundreds of commercials pushing one drug after another. How do you expect our kids to say no to drugs when we don't? I was thrilled when these companies had to finally announce some of the more common side effects from their drugs. It is also interesting how the commercial uses movement, changing screens, music, colors, objects or characters to distract the viewer while the precautions are being read. It's big business.

My favorite of all time is a new drug for *"restless leg syndrome"* that calmly mentions the side effects of uncontrollable sexual urges or gambling. You may feel better, but you will end up divorced and broke. Great! When can I get into see my doctor. That's pure genius! Sex and gambling? Hmmm. I wonder if Vegas has known about this all along?

Society is now programmed to *"Nupe It"* or they are *"all Advil,"* if they have an ache. Maybe Bayer aspirin should be a part of your day because it is the miracle drug they keep finding has new benefits for the body. Except the miracle of you being created, somehow missed the page in the instruction manual when it was supposed to include Aspirin in our DNA.

Then drug companies have come up with the powerful, consumer driven method of sales. At the end of each commercial you hear, *"Ask your doctor if, place over-priced drug name here, is right for you."* Patients seek out doctors for a medication because they are convinced it is the cure. Even Veterinarian drugs are being advertised to owners and they have to list the side effects just before they say, *"ask your vet ..."*

Just read a book like The Pill Book. Under the drug Ibuprofen, aka Motrin, Advil, Midol and Nuprin, to name a few, the general information states, *"We do not know exactly how they work ..."* and other medications have comments like *"it may work."* So let's get this straight. The public is taking bunches of these medications that we aren't even sure how they work, let alone know the long-term side effects? Nice.

There was a news story that popular cold medicines that are recommended for kids are actually modified adult doses. No real studies have been done on children so the companies decided to just extrapolate a weight-based dose and it has been okay for years. Well unfortunately some 54 children aged two and under have died during the last 40 years because of these medications.

In 2005 alone around 88,000 calls were taken at the U.S. Toxic Exposure Surveillance System, a national database of poisoning cases, because children had either overdosed or had an adverse reaction to the drugs. The FDA's recommendation now is to avoid giving these antihistamines and cold medicines to children under two because there isn't sufficient evidence that they work or that they are safe.

Remember the law suits because of Vioxx, Bextra and Celebrex? How quickly the mighty fall. How about Oxycontin? They were fined 600 million dollars because they knowing lied to the public about the addictive properties of the drug. So after making billions in profits and causing numerous deaths

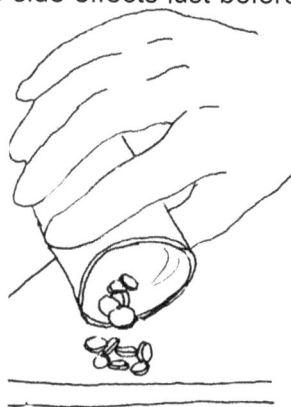

and problems in families across the world, they are now being held somewhat accountable for the damage they have caused to the public. The fines aren't enough. That should be considered pharmaceutical terrorism.

Do some of your own research on the web. Next, talk to your doctor. Have them do some research as they may have access to better sources. Don't take anyone's word as it is written in stone. There are plenty of good medications out there. Just be sure the one you use is what you need. If you have several doctors, make sure that they all have a current list of all of your medications so there is never a harmful interaction.

> *"..The maintenance of health should take precedence over the treatment of disease, ..."*
> **– Robert A. Aldrich, M.D.**

LISTEN TO YOURSELF

If your body hurts or you have symptoms, don't just take a drug to mask the pain, find out why you have the discomfort. It could be very serious. Too many people think that headaches are normal but they're not. Too many people self medicate or have friends and family who play doctor and recommend their meds for them.

If you have chronic headaches are you going to keep trying to decrease the pain with drugs or do you want to eventually try to figure out why you are having them? It could be anything from a vascular problem, a tumor, a musculoskeletal problem, or a food allergy.

The concern I have with all of these drugs is that we over utilize them. A kid will get an ear infection, typically due to a virus, and they are prescribed an antibiotic, which only works on bacteria.

Again part of the fault falls on the public. We are programmed to find a miracle cure for everything, like weight loss, in a pill. We can't always find a quick fix when it comes to our health.

Parents want to give their child something because they would rather do something than nothing at all. People are getting used to the typical antibiotics and need stronger ones. The bacteria are adapting and becoming resistant to the medications we have developed because they are prescribed and used too frequently.

Don't get me wrong, there are some great medications to help people get through their day, to tolerate cancer, help them sleep due to pain or relax muscles in spasm. On CNN, Dr. Drew just said, *"Medications make us healthier when they're worth the risk."* My point is that it would be best to use them as a supportive treatment when possible, instead of only relying on them as the answer.

Analyzing the patient's health with regards to posture, the muscle and skeletal system, diet, nutrition, stress, work and rest are just a few of the factors that could be reviewed to help patients naturally.

> *"The really good physician prevents disease; he cannot cure anything. Because of a lack of knowledge, sickness has become more natural, or more to be expected, than health."*
> **– J.H. Tilden, M.D.**

IT'S A NATURAL THING

If you want to go natural for your treatment or illness, you have many options. Sometimes too many. The key is to educate yourself and become an informed consumer. The Internet provides many avenues to research supplements, as does visiting your health food store. Again companies are advertising their products to you and can make some outrageous claims.

If you do decide to do some research on the Internet, be careful. Many companies will preach unbelievable claims and miracles, mention their bogus research and wrap it neatly around the ultimate goal of selling you their worthless product. Look for sites that aren't selling a product to get a more honest opinion of a product.

I think clean living keeps your mind sharper than Ginkgo Biloba, but it might help anyway. If you've been living hard and not exercising your mind, it ain't gonna dust off any cobwebs and turn you into an information-filled Alex Trabek.

I am a big fan of natural supplements and herbs. I use glucosamine and chondroitin sulfate to help support my cartilage or what's left of it. Echinacea and Vitamin C offer a great boost to my immune system. More importantly I try to eat right, exercise regularly, get adequate rest and wash my hands. It is all part of a healthier lifestyle.

Ask questions before you make any decisions about what you are going to put into your body. Have there been any studies showing clinical data to prove effectiveness? Without research, their statements are just claims.

My motto: *No science, no sale.*

Supplements aren't currently under FDA guidelines because they are not a drug substance. There is a battle being waged in courtrooms against regulating natural supplements. Some of it may be to protect the consumer from deceptive claims, but some of it may be to protect profit margins of pharmaceutical companies and their strong hold on the market. Be informed and become invested in your health.

Healthcare has changed. You have a say in your treatment. Why not try alternative treatments in conjunction with standard care for many of your health problems. If your doctor disapproves of your suggestion, ask them why, see if they are even knowledgeable in alternative care or find a new doctor. You aren't under a contractual agreement with any one doctor. As a patient I want a doctor who is open to trying anything; be it acupuncture, chiropractic, etc. The more opportunities, the more chances for success.

> *"I have never met a man so ignorant that I couldn't learn something from him."*
> **– Galileo Galilei**

IT'S A LEARNING PROCESS

Many progressive doctors are being forced to learn more about natural health because of its popularity and effectiveness in other major countries. For instance, Europe and Australia don't allow drug businesses or insurance companies to dictate healthcare protocol like we do here in the United States. Think about that for a second. They also express more interest in trying healthier alternative approaches to their problems. Partially because there is no way anyone can ignore the growing list of side effects drugs can cause in the body.

I have always told patients I don't care what they try to get better. You want to try muscle relaxers, medical doctors, chiropractic physicians, acupuncture, yoga, physical therapy and chamomile at the same time, I'm all for it. I don't need the credit for helping you regain your health. I take satisfaction from knowing I played a part in it.

> *"If you are distressed by anything external, the pain is not due to the thing itself, but to your estimate of it; and thus you have the power to revoke at any moment."*
> **– Marcus Aurelius Antoninus**

Stress

Well if I could tell you how to avoid it, then this book would be worth millions. Unfortunately all I can do is tell you what to do about it. Stress is always around us in the form of work, family, money, family and of course family. You can always choose your friends. And I would drop those who drain you emotionally. There is no need to surround yourself with dull and unhappy people when there are so many fun and happy ones out there.

I watched a story on a morning television show about a revealing study. It was found that stressful homes may lead to early puberty in women. I thought it was the hormones in our foods, but reducing your stress can also play an important role in your life and the ones around you.

I bet a lot of stress comes from us tax payers having to work until June to pay the government to waste our money. See I feel better just letting my feelings out. Don't keep it all inside. Sometimes you just gotta let it out. Scream, yell or break something. Take your frustration out on a punching bag, chopping wood or a killer kickboxing class. Don't hurt yourself, anyone or anything. Make it a productive release so you can still benefit.

How do I know stress can debilitate you? About eight years ago there was some stress in my life and not only did my blood pressure elevate to 152/90 from 106/66, but my back started to really hurt in the same area it had when I was younger. Perhaps a disc relapse? Maybe. But the stress had found my weakest spot.

I decided to drive five hours to Boston to see my father for the weekend so we could talk. I felt great all weekend up until the point I returned home and woke up the next day. Even sitting 10 hours didn't bother my condition. Now finishing off a bottle of Grey Goose together might have helped but I'm not advocating trying that for your pain. It was being away from the source of my stress.

The bad thing about stress is that it builds up in the most vulnerable part of your body. For example, some people say they carry stress in their shoulders. I believe stress hits our body equally but causes tightness and pain at our weakest link.

If you tried to lift a heavy box off the ground and you had previously sprained an ankle, that ankle is the place I would expect to limit your lift. It needs to be treated and rehabilitated to bring it up to the same level as the rest of the body.

Tight muscles can lead to changing the normal motion of our spines by distorting our posture. With altered movement comes additional stress to other regions of the body. The tight muscles caused by stress can lead to restricted motion, headaches, soreness, exhaustion and much more.

Another bad side effect of stress is that when the body is under pressure it releases a hormone called cortisol. Cortisol is released by the body to give you a burst of energy for the fight or flight response, increased memory function and increased immunity; but, it does raise the pain threshold.

Sometimes when your body has a metabolic disease or you are constantly under high levels of stress, can you produce too much cortisol at levels that may cause your body to gain weight and fat. Cortisol helps break down muscle tissue to be converted into glucose for energy. It also helps store foods as fat. So if you are under really intense stress, then it may have the possibility to ruin a great workout by destroying your muscles for energy. Provided your doctor does not believe you have a metabolic problem, the best thing you can do for yourself is find ways to relieve your stress.

According to the Mayo Clinic, when a healthy individual produces cortisol it is not in a quantity that would substantiate the need for cortisol blocking pills. No research shows that reducing these "normal" cortisol levels will produce weight loss. You've heard the diet commercials claiming to block cortisol but there is no research to show these products

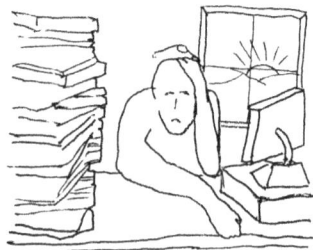

do what they even claim they do. There are new regulations against them for exaggerated claims.

> *"True enjoyment comes from activity of the mind and exercise of the body; the two are united."*
> **– Alexander von Humboldt**

IT'S TIME TO PUMP YOU UP

If you like working out, make time to get to the gym so you can burn off some of that extra energy. Take out your frustration on the iron or a spin class, not your co-workers or loved ones. The extra focus could really help you push through a sticking point and increase the benefits of your hard work and sweat. Exhausting yourself in the gym or enjoying the outdoors are two great ways to gain some peace of mind and get an awesome workout.

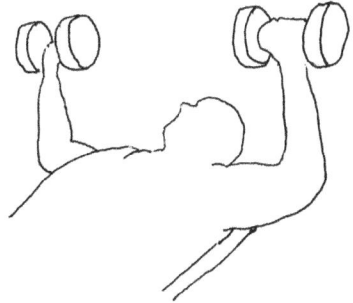

Speaking of outdoors, try a nice walk through a wooded trail to enjoy the nature around you. Perhaps you are more adventurous. Grab your mountain bike, your rock climbing gear, skateboard or snowboard and hit' em hard. Doing something you love is an easy way to forget time and any problems you are dealing with.

> *"The creation of something new is not accomplished by the intellect but by the play instinct acting from inner necessity. The creative mind plays with the objects it loves."* **– Carl Jung**

HONEY YOU SHOULD DO LIST

You can find quiet time for yourself by becoming absorbed in a good book or perhaps do your own writing. There are a lot of categories of books to choose from and one has to be appealing. If not a book, pick up a magazine that might cover a topic that interests you.

Crosswords, Jumbles and Sudoku are simple, and mentally stimulating games you can play to pass some time. Regardless of the weather or setting, this can be a fun activity. If you are a gadget person, then how about Tetris on your iphone, Blackberry (*"crack berry"* as my wife says) or game boy? Better yet, bust out the X-Box or Wii games.

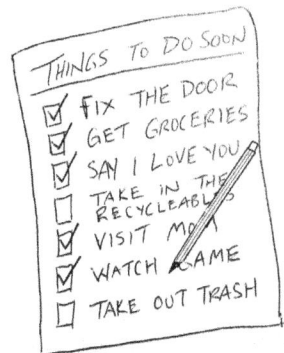

Maybe you have a project like a birdhouse you wanted to work on but haven't made the time. Well, make the time and enjoy working with your hands.

Pretend to design your dream house but make it functional for birds.

A tree house or fort for the kids would be a fun project. My fort as a teenager was awesome. It had three different rooms, saloon doors, carpeting and couches, electricity and the homemade, barrel wood stove for year round use.

Possibly sewing or knitting is your thing. Patch some old jeans or create something new for you or a loved one. Time flies when you do something you really enjoy. Maybe you are a seamstress and can make quilts or bears. Get wrapped up in that and have some fun. You can even make your holiday gifts and feel good about doing something from the heart. That's a win-win.

In the same crafty vain as sewing, a lot of people really get into scrapbooking. Join a club and learn some nifty techniques for putting your photos in order and decorating the book as well. I've seen some cool ones that have sayings next to your pictures. Some appropriate, some not so, but it can be funny.

So you never won the Academy Award in high school. Have you given up your dream or the thrill of being in front of a live audience? Many local churches and theaters have open casting calls for musicals and plays. You could participate in one of those and have a blast meeting fellow actors. So go break a leg.

Nothing spells calm and stress relief like a good round of golf. Okay, well at least there's the outdoor part. I like to play the scenic route. By zigzagging my way around I have a greater chance to enjoy all of the course, and not just the grassy fairways where everyone else is.

Whatever sport is your weakness, just do it. Visit the batting cage or the driving range to take out some aggression from work or practice by whacking the balls a mile. Better yet play catch or kick a soccer ball with your kids or take them to a game and introduce them to your passion. Sports can be a lot of fun either alone or in a group, like a softball game or going to watch a pro game. Play ball!

Maybe you're the consummate gardener. There's nothing like your own vegetable garden. No pesticides and no chemicals. Growing up I loved eating fresh tomatoes and cucumbers right off the vine. That's some good eating. You can get out in the clean air and gardening is exercise too.

If not vegetables, how about flowers? A beautiful planting is a wonderful thing to see anytime of the day or year. It can lift your spirits and the colors are amazing. The earth is like your own canvas in which you can decide what colors to cover it in.

"I don't know anything about music. In my line you don't have to." – **Elvis Presley**

ROCK ON

For me it's music. I love to play guitar and sing. There have been days that I have disappeared into the basement for three hours just wailing away and ruining my vocal cords. Wow do I feel good. Grab a new CD and crank it up.

What about that drum set or piano that has been in the corner for years? You remember how great it was to play. I bet a couple of lessons or a DVD lesson might help you play better and peak your interest again. Maybe even try to put the old band together like in the Blues Brothers.

Maybe you need to take all of your CDs and load them on to your new MP3 player. That can take some time and is something you will enjoy when you finish. The easy way out would be to check the Internet for places you could download music. It might cost a little but you can have your player filled with great music in no time. Then sit back and enjoy.

Sometimes just kickin' back and listening to some great tunes from our youth can transport us to a different time. It can bring back some terrific memories and remind us of old friends. In fact, why not get back in touch with a couple of old buddies? Talk about the glory days and maybe plan a get together.

How about checking out the live scene? Where is your 80s hair band playing? Take a drive or plan a fun trip to see one of your favorites with some friends. I once drove four hours to meet my college roommate Andy in NYC for a Toto show. I drove back that night. It was fantastic, silly, and costly. We would do it again in a second. That's easy to say as we have made such a run five times!

You could even check the local papers for a place to hear blues or jazz over a glass of wine or cold beer. Nice and relaxing for a music lover. If you enjoy entertainment or would rather be a part of it, find a karaoke place. It's fun to sing seriously or to *"ham it up,"* go up with a group of people and belt out a Grease hit or just have fun listening to others.

Lose your inhibitions and let loose. Sometimes we have to forget what our age is and just have a good time. When is making a fool of yourself and getting people to laugh a bad thing? If more people would realize it is okay to laugh and have fun we might have less hatred in the world. There really are better ways to spend your time.

Some studies have found rock'n roll energizes you naturally, like for a great workout. Other reports have even suggested that laughing and singing could add five to 15 years to your life. Either way it will definitely add life to your years. Singing seniors from the Levine School of Music in Washington were found to have less need for medications, fewer doctor visits, better posture, improved lung capacity, stronger voices, less depression and higher energy. Maybe it's time you started singing a different tune.

> *"Two roads diverged in a wood, and I took the one less traveled by, And that has made all the difference."* – **Robert Frost**

HIT THE ROAD JACK

Maybe you enjoy driving. Plan a fun trip for an exciting meal, a great show or just to sing in the car where no one can hear you. We're all American Idol rejects. Find a great back road with lots of fun curves or beautiful scenery. Or take out the Harley and put the hammer down. Feel the wind against your body and let the engine roar.

Nothing can beat a little bit of sunshine. It is proven that too much time in darkness can drive a soul crazy. I know because the saying in Syracuse is *"never a sky in the clouds."* I remember months when we would have about 18 hours of sunlight. That's in a month. You just want to hit yourself with a mallet. If we backfill the Great Lakes I think that will prevent the clouds, the rain and snow. Fisherman, sailors and wildlife may object!

Sometimes a change of scenery, like a trip to Arizona, the Caribbean or Alaska might be needed. We all get stuck in our everyday grind and it can become monotonous. It would be like eating the same sandwich for lunch every day. We need a little variety in surroundings now and then.

> *"A life is not important except in the impact it has on other lives."* – **Jackie Robinson**

DANCE, DANCE, DANCE

One of the hottest shows on television is Dancing with the Stars. People are crazy for it. Maybe you should take that someone special for a Rumba or practice your John Travolta moves with an audience.

Dance is used by many tribes as a form of celebration and communication. Some dance is a sexual mind game. I have to admit, my wife wanted to take dance lessons for our first dance at our wedding reception. She didn't want to just stand there with me. She definitely didn't want me to break out my running man or cabbage patch dances. Not yet anyway.

Sure I stepped on her dress at the reception but we kept going and looked pretty darn sophisticated. The classes were intimate and we practiced at home. We had quality time to spend with each other, got some exercise and had fun. I hate to say she was right, in print, but she was. Our instructor said that couples that dance together, stay together. He may be on to something. Although I teased her the entire time I know we will do it again.

Get your partner or some friends and go boogie. Disco is making a return so check to see which club has their disco ball turning and have fun. Bust out your funk, hideous shoes and silk shirts and go dance the night away to the timeless sounds of the Bee Gees.

> *"Be courteous to all, but intimate with few, and let those few be well tried before you give them your confidence. True friendship is a plant of slow growth, and must undergo and withstand the shocks of adversity before it is entitled to the appellation."* – **George Washington**

STAND BY ME

Plan a fun outing with some close friends. Life is difficult and we are fortunate to meet people who complement us and have similar interests. These people are your support group in times of need.

Your friends have probably been there for you when you needed advice and you have been a shoulder of strength for them when they needed one. Friends are the people you can count on when things get crazy. My wife spends special time with just her girlfriends and I have little weekend getaways with my college buddies.

Well, if all heck has broken out and you're not in Kansas anymore, call a high school friend, some of the gang from college or the couples who you can invite over for dinner. Pick an activity from a show, a game or even a simple happy hour. Enjoying their company is medicinal. Probably just as much as letting them know in person or with a card how much you value their friendship. A hug is pretty cool too.

> *"The real man smiles in trouble, gathers strength from distress, and grows brave by reflection."* – **Thomas Paine**

OUTSIDE THE BOX

Do something for someone else. Is Christmas about giving or receiving? How great is it to make something or find that perfect gift for someone special. You feel wonderful inside. It doesn't even have to wait for a holiday. Think of someone else who may have it a little worse because a loved one is sick, a bad relationship ended or they're having a run of bad luck. Cheering someone up will absolutely turn your spirits around.

Some examples of good deeds include: brushing off the snow for someone who doesn't have gloves or a scraper; picking up your neighbor's trash can from the middle of the road and moving it to the sidewalk; helping a neighbor bring in some furniture or groceries; sharing some freshly picked fruit or vegetables from your garden. Simple ideas like these could change how a lot of people function in this world.

Give someone a compliment. Maybe a friend got a new haircut, lost some weight, or has a nice outfit on. Let that person know. Too many times we think things and don't say them. Granted sometimes it is wise, but if you have something nice to say about someone, let them know.

Tell them they are doing a good job. Tell your significant other how much you need them and how much they mean to you. Maybe give a few hugs to people you care about. Human touch is healing. Nothing feels like home like a good compassionate embrace from someone who really cares about you. If you're really daring, offer a hug to a stranger. You will lift their spirits and yours.

My wife and I just spent some time in Florida and for some reason the starfish were washing up on shore. Now knowing they have a greater survival rate in the water, unlike the people that walked by, we picked as many up as we could each day and put them back in the ocean. They're starfish, not alligators. They don't bite. They may not make it, but it felt good to do something for something that otherwise had no hope.

When enough people asked why we were doing it, we explained why not? If I get lost I hope someone is kind enough to help put me back on the right path. The starfish couldn't move back into the water fast enough in the heat. Some people joined in. Imagine if doing some good in the world could always catch on like that.

In that same line of thought, contribute to a charity that means a lot to you. Maybe someone has an illness and could use some extra cash, or you hope to help wildlife that has been affected by the destruction of their habitats or pollution. It is truly better to give, than receive.

Last but not least, how about flowers? They get you out of trouble but how do they make you feel when given for any reason? Flowers can put a smile on someone's face. They have a nice aroma and are bright and colorful. They are sure to lift anyone's spirits. You could even just buy some for yourself. Nobody will love you, like you, so be good to yourself.

> *"The church was not merely a thermometer that recorded the ideas and principles of popular opinion; it was a thermostat that transformed the mores of society."* – **Martin Luther King Jr.**

CHURCH AND STATE OF MIND

Some individuals have found that becoming more involved in their faith may help them forget their problems. Church can be a deeply personal and resolving place for you alone or to share thoughts with others. Being able to talk to others of a similar faith and who have similar beliefs can be comforting and supportive. It can have a calming effect on the mind, body and spirit.

Churches also have lots of projects and fun events to bring people together. You can become more involved and divert your focus from you or your stress. Now make a choice to regroup and direct your energy to be constructive for someone else who is having a tough go of it.

There are some studies that suggest prayer has helped people regain their health or decreased the chances of complications after surgery. The studies go back and forth on whether or not it helps. I say the more people think positive thoughts about you or me, the better.

In 2002 I encouraged all of my doctorate students to say *"Go Red Wings!"* during the time the game was being played. All that positive thinking may have paid off when the Wings won their 10th Stanley Cup Championship.

Regardless of who you seek out or where you go for guidance, peace of mind or faith, or who you believe is in charge up above, all forms of religion have their place. Respect each other's beliefs and the world can be a happier place.

> *"There are days when any electrical appliance in the house, including the vacuum cleaner, offers more entertainment than the TV set."* – **Harriet Van Horne**

IT'S SHOW TIME

Laughing is not only a great way to tighten up your abs, but it is also a great way to forget about your problems. Maybe you need to watch your favorite show; like a rerun of Seinfeld and Scrubs, or turn on the Comedy Channel for The Daily Show or Tosh.O. Make time to see a show that makes you laugh.

Ten – 15 minutes of laughing can even burn up to 50 calories according to a recent Vanderbilt University study. Some say it reduces pain and lowers blood sugar levels too.

There are some morning shows with interesting ideas or stories that could be beneficial to you regarding health, children or relationships. There are even shows that try to help people with their problems like Oprah and Dr. Phil. Sometimes it is comforting to see other people struggle with similar problems. It can help you talk about them and maybe even lead you to seek help.

If you need a show to capture your attention, then any one of the law or police dramas should be the ticket. By diverting your attention you can temporarily escape from the real world.

> *"To be free of destructive stress, don't sweat the small stuff and by realizing that all stuff is small."* – **Author Unknown**

CALGON TAKE ME AWAY

Ladies already know about this next idea because they have been hiding this way from their families for years. A warm bath can relax and ease muscle tension and have a calming effect. Light a few candles, grab a magazine or a good book and open a bottle of wine.

Enjoy the solitude. Maybe add some smooth jazz in the background and just unwind. Many people have Jacuzzi tubs or hot tubs. Although not as quiet, they can provide a chance to have the body massaged, relaxed and toasty warm. Not a bad combination. How did guys decide their escape would be in the *"other room"* of the bathroom? That was poor planning.

Why not self indulge? I hate to say shop, because this will come back and bite me, but some people enjoy a little retail therapy. Now shopping isn't always about buying, but maybe there is something you need, or have wanted. Look into it and make the purchase. As long as you aren't buying a Lamborghini and putting the family in debt, it may cheer you up.

Better yet … spa day. Schedule some time to hit your favorite spa where they pamper and spoil you rotten, *"Yeah Baby."* Does a hot stone massage, haircut, manicure or pedicure sound like your cure? You'll be looking and feeling good! Call your Ya-Yas and make it girls' day. Some people say it is better to look good then to feel good. How about both? *"Marvelous."*

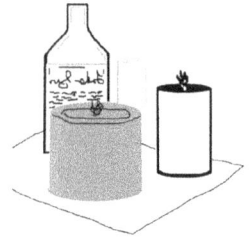

> *"[Sleep is] the golden chain that ties health and our bodies together."*
> **– Thomas Dekker**

RELAXATION

How about listening to the sound of morning dew dropping off the leaves as the birds awaken to the warming rays of the sun. That sounded so peaceful and tranquil I almost went to sleep.

Pure meditation can ease your mind and body. Light some incense for the aromatherapy enjoyment and soothe your soul. Take the morning off and sit on your deck with some warm coffee and listen to the world waking up. Or spend peaceful moments cuddling with a loved one.

Maybe a power nap will work. I love to go home on my breaks from work and curl up with a couple of my cats to take a real *"cat nap."* That works wonders for me. Even at work, if I have a break, I may shut the door for 15 minutes and drift away into a subconscious state. I go into Darth Vader, deep breath mode, startle myself awake; ready to join the Jedi fully recharged.

A recent study by the Harvard School of Public Health and University of Athens Medical School found that a midday nap reduced the rate of death due to coronary heart disease in men and women by one

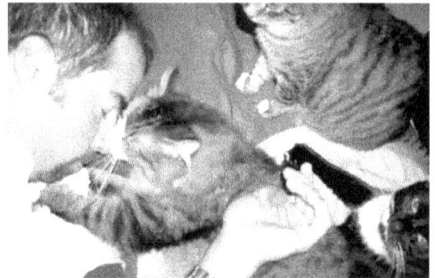

third. It may also be a way to help cope with stress, but it definitely sounds like a 30-minute siesta, a few times a week is just what the doctor ordered.

When we are sleep deprived we can get cranky. I know, and simple things can bother us more. Either try to plan for a better night's sleep or close the door and shut your eyes for 10 or 20 minutes. It might be the snooze you need to make you feel recharged.

Meditation is also a possibility. It is a way to bring peace and inner calm to your soul. Deep breaths and relaxation are part of this ritual, which is said to open up the mind and liberate it.

> *"Animals are such agreeable friends-they ask no questions, they pass no criticisms."*
> **– George Eliot**

ALWAYS HAPPY TO SEE US

I am a big fan of having pets. They are so thrilled to see us when we come home from work or even when we come back from getting the mail. They truly love us.

I have cats now and they have great individual personalities and quirks. I come home and they come to greet me and make noises. One of them rolls around and squirms he's so happy. Sometimes I think they might be happier to see me than my wife. Just kidding, Honey.

Just add a little catnip and watch 'em wrestle and run. When I had dogs, it was always fun to play catch, wrestle or take them out for a walk. Animals have been proven to extend the life of the elderly and provide unconditional love. Some have even saved their owners' lives. They make great companions.

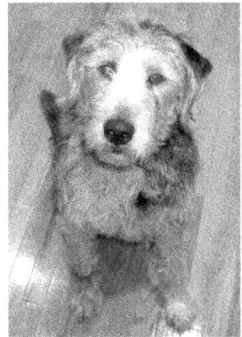

Enjoying your pets is a fantastic way to cheer you up as you give them some well-deserved attention. If you need a pet, there are many advertised in the paper; or check with your area animal rescue center or veterinarian.

Whatever you find to help you through your day or life, the key is to know when you need a break and do what is best for you. This helps prevent an overload of daily stress and allows your body to remain healthy and ready for anything.

There is a great book about a cat that changed two women in their ways of thinking about cats and now brings them joy every day. He even brings warmth to millions of people due to his story of survival. It is called *"What's the Matter with Henry? The True Tale of a Three-legged Cat."* By Cathy Conheim and B.J. Gallagher. What can I say, I cried reading it.

"A smile is the shortest distance between two people." – **Victor Borge**

KEEP SMILING

It takes a greater number of muscles to frown than it does to smile. So to conserve energy, relax and smile more. If you need help, think of something funny. Read something that is amusing or watch a comedy like an old Marx Brothers movie. A smile is a better look too. No one likes a sourpuss. Besides, smiling could really tick off the boss or annoy the person who is making your life miserable. Like yawns, a smile can be contagious and could help people change their attitudes.

True story. One of my old high school teachers who was a patient of mine had a discussion with my homeroom teacher from 8th grade who said his back was bothering him. She told him to come see me, and he asked her, *"Is he still smiling all the time?"* What a great way to be remembered. Granted, I have huge chompers. I can't keep them in my mouth. I've seen smaller teeth on farm animals. But smiling is a great way to be remembered versus the kid who always fought or never did his homework.

"Art is the desire of a man to express himself, to record the reactions of his personality to the world he lives in." – **Amy Lowell**

CREATE SOME MAGIC

Do you like to doodle while you're on the phone? Did you paint or draw when you were a kid. Why not take a few classes in art and re-whet your appetite for canvas, watercolor and charcoal.

If you've been to any museums you know there are lots of different styles and one might bring out the inner artist in you. There's Cubism, Realism, Impressionism and don't forget Not-A-Clue-ism. That's the one with a line on an 8 foot canvas or the paint looks like your child did it in three minutes. The pressure is off. Beauty is obviously in the eyes of the beholder.

I have disappeared in my basement for what seems like months. My pool table has become my art table where I create art pieces of different sizes, mediums and colors. What a great way to release your inhibitions and let your imagination run wild. I often tell my wife regarding my creative side, *"I can't control it, I can only hope to contain it."*

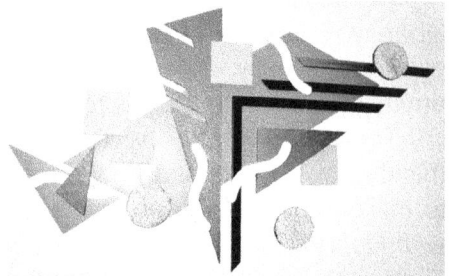

> *"The fact that the mind rules the body, is, in spite of its neglect by biology and medicine, the most fundamental fact which we know about the process of life."* – **Franz Alexander, M.D.**

The Mind

William Arthur Ward once said, *"If you can imagine it, you can achieve it. If you can dream it, you can become it."* That's positive thinking. Many people are limited by their own mind. Paralyzed by the fear of failure, or maybe the possibility of success. What makes some people take chances and shoot for the stars? How do they get the nerve to take that first step and break out of their comfort zone?

The mind encompasses our ability to process things using our capacity to reason, our convictions, emotions, determination, thoughts, faith, intelligence, courage and learned experiences. We have the ability to rationalize and predict what may happen if we do something. We can use this to accomplish anything we want to if we put our minds to it.

Top athletes visualize their sport in their minds. Baseball players can see the pitch coming in before crushing the ball. Golfers mentally practice their swing. Seeing, is also believing. Playing out a scenario in your mind lets you prepare to conquer it when the time comes.

If you were a Magnum P.I. fan you will remember he always mentioned his little voice. This was the voice in his head that would warn him of danger or help guide his intuitions when he tried to solve a case. All of that is true. Each of us has an inner voice that can help us recognize potentially dangerous situations or even act as a premonition. We just have to listen to it. It's the thought that you may have left a burner on or didn't lock the door. I'm waiting for mine to come up with the winning lottery numbers.

Some patients have undergone hypnosis before surgery and have never experienced any pain during the procedures. Sometimes if we believe in something intensely, it can have a positive effect on our health. That is why some research tests drugs against placebo pills, which are nothing more than sugar pills. The patient believes they are taking the new miracle drug and convinces his body to respond favorably to it. The power of the mind should never be underestimated.

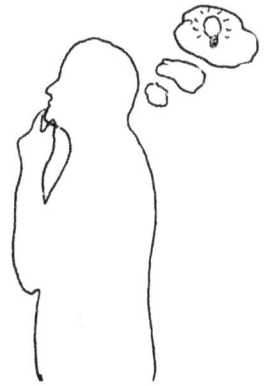

> *"A painting in a museum hears more ridiculous opinions than anything else in the world."*
> **– Edmond de Goncourt**

I CAN'T HEAR YOU

Did someone forget to tell Buster Douglas he couldn't beat the invincible Mike Tyson? He didn't get the memo. How many times does one football player say something negative about an opposing team only to have that team's coach make copies and post it in the locker room? It motivates the players to succeed.

Try thinking big. Step out of your comfort zone. Make opportunities out of situations and learn from your past. *"Everyone is responsible for his or her own actions."* Think positive. Be positive. Surround yourself with positive people, books and music. This is the land of big dreams and opportunity. That's why people love to come to the United States.

Set your mind on a goal and map out your path. How will you get there? What steps do you need to take? How long will it take you? Are you being realistic?

Randy Pausch was the professor who lectured on living life to its fullest even though pancreatic cancer was ending his. He mentioned how brick walls aren't there to prevent you from getting there; they are there to be broken down by your will and sheer determination to get through them. He also discussed how you can either live life like Tigger or Eeyore. Eeyore always saw the worst possible scenario while Tigger was upbeat, adventurous and fun. Who do you want to be?

How about Susan Boyle? She tried out for the British version of American Idol as a 50-year old who didn't possess the superficial physical qualities Simon or society embraces. That was until she unleashed her angelic voice upon the world. Now who's laughing?

Last example. There was a boy who never got to play on his high school basketball team partly because of his size, but mainly for another reason. He was named manager of the team due to his enthusiasm and heart. He was just one of the guys and was there for every practice and game. He had played for years at home and worked hard at this sport because he loved it.

One day his coach decided to put him in for the remaining four minutes of the game. After missing his first shot badly, and then a blown layup, he persevered by scoring 20 points like Michael Jordan. He knew he could play and he knew he could shoot. He has autism and his name is Jason McElwain. Now he is referred to as J-Mac by ESPN and many sports authorities. I get choked up every time I read his story or see the video. He is fantastic. A true winner.

The whole idea is that the coach gave him the opportunity and J-Mac took full advantage. He made these shots at his house and was ready to do it in a game. As he stated, *"I was hotter than a pistol."* Disney and others are begging for the rights to this magnificent story.

Whether your goal is to regain your health, be a better person, express your feelings more, lose weight, start exercising again, get promoted or spend more time with the family, you can do it. You have to believe in yourself. If you don't, why would anybody else? Make it happen. Shoot for the stars. You might just land on the Moon.

> *"It is better to sleep on things beforehand than lie awake about them afterward."*
> **– Baltasar Gracian**

Sleep

We all need rest. Some people need more than others. Remember trying to get up for school? Some of us still go through it with work. Just a few more minutes. Where's my snooze button?

My college roommate Andy used to hit the snooze button six to eight times each morning. All I could think was, why not just sleep soundly for another 45 minutes and get up once, instead of having to wake several times in a morning? As if once isn't bad enough. Some people are morning people and others aren't.

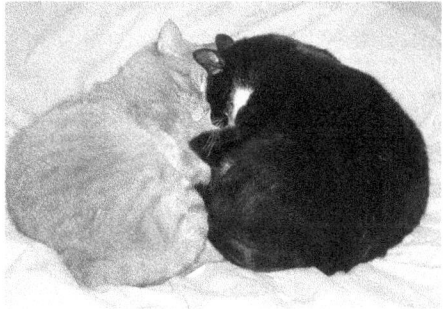

Your pets sleep. Animals in Africa sleep. Even fish sleep. Not that many of us get enough good quality R & R, but we should be getting six to eight hours a night on average. So up to one-third of your life is going to be spent zonked out. Make sure it is on a good quality mattress and maybe even with someone you like. If you are sleep deprived you are more likely to have trouble balancing your blood sugar and will have a greater tendency to gain weight. So make time for some sleep.

Activity levels, work habits, children, age, stress, snoring and the type of mattress can all affect the amount and quality of sleep. Sleep is extremely important because this is a time when we reduce the outside stimulation, diminish our movements and shut down for repair. Your body uses this time to rebuild and form new tissue. This is why bodybuilders have to make sure they rest if they want to get bigger. It gives their body time to recuperate and grow.

It also gives your mind a chance to play out a scenario or work out a situation. You can actually learn from your mistakes. Dreaming allows us to battle internal conflicts and find resolutions. People who are sleep deprived may actually make riskier decisions or have a lack of good judgment, according to a study by Duke University and the National University of Singapore. I find that when I am trying to get back to sleep I have a multitude of thoughts, hence the reason I am typing at 4:38 am. That and the cat was lying on my head.

My whole point is, what is the value of a good night's sleep? How much would you spend to know that you are going to be able to relax and feel completely rejuvenated when morning comes? Many hotels try to charge us $200 – $400 in some places. For mathematical reasons, would you consider paying $100 a night to get a great night of sleep?

What are you sleeping on now? Have you flipped your mattress religiously? As my Mom suggested to me several times, like only mothers can do, she said to use a marker and number the four sides. That way when you flip it you always know which number should be at the top of the bed next. Not a bad idea. I don't think you can even flip the new pillow top mattresses.

Does your mattress sag in the middle? Have you ever tried placing boards underneath it to firm it up? Does it look like you are in it, when you stand there looking at it? Is it 12 years old? Twenty? The time to let it go could be now.

I know money is tight and we all have our priorities for where the funds need to be allocated. I want you to think about making your health your main concern. If you can't function then the whole family's ecosystem can't function. It's like when Mom gets sick, the house and family fall apart and become less organized. She is the grease that keeps the wheels turning.

A new quality mattress will probably cost around $1,000 or more. If that setup lasts you 10 years, it only costs you $100 a year for 365 days of pure heaven. Now we previously decided a hotel would be worth $100 per night if you slept well. Now you could be getting the same great sleep at home for $0.27 a night. If there are two of you, that's 14 cents each.

I would love to tell you to shop around when you are searching for a mattress but it seems that companies produce the same mattress with different model numbers so you can never check for the best price. Search online too. There is plenty of room to move when it comes to the prices of mattresses. Businesses probably do the same thing with appliance and TV model numbers so you can't effectively comparison shop for them either.

"Some national parks have long waiting lists for camping reservations. When you have to wait a year to sleep next to a tree, something is wrong." – **George Carlin**

TIME FOR BED DEAR

So now that we know how important sleep is, what about when you can't fall asleep or stay asleep. Insomnia and sleep disruption are common problems for many of us and medications are often prescribed to help. I would recommend discussing your options with your doctor because of the side effects and potential drug interactions with medications you may already be taking. Let's discuss the possible solutions that nature provides.

Some of the reasons we don't get to sleep range from our schedules, eating habits, lack of exercise, stress and more. Insomnia will most likely strike each of us at one time or another, but for some it is a way of night. These unfulfilled nights of rest can lead to more stress, poor work, bad relationships and health problems. Let's discuss causes so we can eliminate them from our days.

Alcohol is one common source of sleeplessness. It may seem that the liquid depressant would calm you and sooth you to sleep. However, while it initially makes you tired, it is then converted into sugars and can keep you wired a few hours later. Not to mention the frequent bathroom trips from all of the fluids won't help you sleep either.

Likewise, having too much water or any fluids later in the day could lead to a lot of trips to the toilet. As we get older, or after women have kids, we all have an increase in our number of trips we need to make each night. Reducing fluids later in the day could help keep you in bed.

Many people unfortunately still smoke and that is a stimulant, which will interfere with falling asleep and staying in dreamland. It may seem calming but it isn't to your body or mind, and is an addictive behavior. Your body may disturb you at anytime during the night because of its need for more nicotine. With chronic smoking comes the *"smoker's cough,"* which sounds like the lung, then the liver and the intestines, are all coming up.

Along that same line of coughing would be getting sick with a seasonal bug. There may be no escaping a cold so if it happens, be prepared. You may need cold medicine, liquids to stay hydrated, and Vick's to help clear your nasal passages. Propping the pillows up could help keep your sinuses draining and prevent acid reflux. There are sprays and lozenges for your throat; however I have always found gargling apple cider vinegar with warm water worked longer.

Most people know that caffeine can give you a little jolt so maybe ease up on the soda, coffee or tea, unless it is decaf or a tea that claims to be formulated to help you sleep. If you like the evening coffee, have it at least an hour or more before trying to settle in for the night.

Setting a routine can be helpful. If you come home from work late and need to get some work done that is okay once in awhile. But if you make it a habit your body will reset its clock to be awake. That internal clock functions around the 24-hour cycle of our sun. So constant bright lights can mess it up.

When that happens, these circadian rhythms, meaning *"around the day,"* that control your sleep/wake cycle or regulate body temperature, can malfunction. That's part of the reason why traveling out of your time zone can give you *"jet lag."* Most of us wake up before the alarm because our bodies learn our routine. I told you your body was neat.

So try to complete what you can and wind down at a reasonable time. When I would try to get my son to sleep I would lower the lights, quiet things down and maybe even make a warm bath or heat his blanket up. Try curling up with a book under your blanket or by the fireplace. Put on some relaxing music.

Reading puts me to sleep, but you can't read a Stephen King novel and expect to sleep like a baby. Try something that is middle of the road like a magazine or a book about an interesting topic, as long as no one is chasing people with axes or guns.

Changing your bedroom or sleep environment may also help. Maybe your room isn't conducive to sleep. Do you need the room darker? Could you try an eye mask? How about the sound of a fan or an ambient noise machine that can sound like a stream or an ocean shore? That white noise can be as mindless as counting sheep. It just distracts the brain so you can relax. I sometimes wear earplugs so I can shut out external noise from neighbors, cars or my cats. As long as you don't mind inner white noise like listening to a seashell, you'll sleep soundly.

Speaking of the bedroom. I have a whole section devoted to picking a good mattress as well as the best sleeping positions that can help put an end to neck, back and body pains. What I haven't mentioned is that as an animal lover sometimes you've got to cut the cord. Cats and dogs are great. They love us unconditionally, snuggle and provide heat.

However, they also take up room and we are forced to contort our bodies because we don't want to disturb them. Heck my mom sleeps with at least two greyhounds. They're like small Clydesdales. I have to remind myself my cat sleeps 18 hours a day so it's okay to have him sleep elsewhere for a night. Animals can scratch, lick, bark or meow and fuss. This can keep you awake so try breaking away for a night.

Considering many people are unhappy with their partner or marriage, this can lead to unrest. If it is a silly fight, try to iron things out before going to bed. Having solved the argument could result in peaceful thoughts. If the problem is greater than that, you might try staying at a hotel or friends house, until things become more conducive for sleeping without your mind racing. Speaking with a specialist might help ease the situation and help lead to resolution.

Another source of interruption is the phone. Unless you are a doctor on call, expecting an emergency update from family or work for the fire department, turn off the phone. It never fails that when you finally just start to drift off to la-la land, the phone rings. My college roommate and I would laugh at how automatic it was. If I laid down for a nap, the phone would ring within five minutes. That's when I learned that my sleep is more important than unwanted sales calls.

Sometimes the battle of the thermostat in the household can keep you from sleeping. If the room temperature isn't right, you may find it difficult to relax if you are uncomfortable. Try adding an extra blanket or piece of clothing to stay warmer. How many times have you fallen asleep next to the heat of a roaring fire? If you respond differently to heat lose a blanket at night to cool down some, open the window slightly or turn on a fan.

Coming home and eating late may contribute to trouble falling or staying asleep. Of course we can also look forward to weight gain as well as some restlessness. Consuming food too close to bedtime can cause an upset stomach or acid buildup. Like the old saying, wait 20 minutes before jumping in the pool; I advise eating your last meal about one to two hours before bedtime. Likewise, sometimes you may need a light snack to quiet some hunger pain. Keep a snack next to the bed so you don't have to get up and get exposed to light. Try to pick something healthy like some nuts or berries. Not cookies or sugary goodies.

Watching TV may seem like a good idea but who can relax when the news is filled with people killing each other for $20, your 401K has called 911 or someone abducts an innocent child. So you turn the station to your relaxing over the top crime show or scary movie, but realize they will make your mind active if you sleep. Next is the game and Syracuse is headed into only the 6th overtime against UConn. How exciting! Oops. Right. Find a show that is calming or shut the darn thing off.

My favorite, and I'm so guilty of this, is the falling asleep TV watcher. The spouse or roommate shuts off the TV, changes the station or even worse says, *"Why don't you go to bed?"* The typical responses are, *"I was just resting my eyes"* or *"I was watching that."* Take a hint from your body. Again, it knows what you need. If it is trying to shut down, don't fight it and get your second wind.

Another problem is many of us do computer work or may just be shopping and playing games online. Like TV, the computer is a stimulant, especially if you are online playing games for hours. I've done it. Next thing you know, it's 3 a.m. and when you close your eyes you can still see the game being played out.

As previously mentioned, sometimes during the day you may get a bit tired and decide to nap. Naps are great. They can rejuvenate you. That's why they call them power naps. If you can't sleep at night, don't give in during the day. Try to get that tiredness to carry over for when it is actually time to shut it down for the day.

Exercise is great for your body. It can rev up your metabolism and get you going when you do it first thing in the morning. That's a potential problem for people who prefer to workout in the evening. Try not to workout too late. Your body will be all pumped up and it will not be able to relax. I commend you on the effort but try waking up a little earlier to workout. Then when the evening comes you will have deprived yourself from sleeping in and may start to recover it at night, like you should.

Well one of the things you could try to relax into better sleep is meditation. Try closing your eyes and using imagery to create the most peaceful places in your mind. Maybe it is relaxing on a beautiful, sunny beach in the Caribbean or snuggled up with someone special by a fire, reading books together. Whatever it is, make it calming so you can distract your mind from thinking, *"Darn, I'll never get to sleep and I have so much to do tomorrow."*

That type of stress can wreak havoc on your nighttime snooze. In this book I cover ways to try to relieve some of the stress we all face. Find what works for you if you have a bunch of things keeping you awake. Remember, supplementation of a full range of B vitamins can help combat stress in the body.

When I am awake at night and thinking, rolling over to look at the clock to determine how many hours of sleep I'm not going to be getting, it just gets me fired up. If you know what I'm talking about you could try turning the clock around so the bright numbers aren't staring back at you. Seeing the time can be aggravating and make things worse. The alarm will go off anyway so there really is no need to know what time it is every time you roll over.

You could also write down all of the things you need to do. It will remove any fear that you may forget what needs to be done. Sometimes jotting things down can relieve your anxieties. Having a list is never a bad thing.

Herbal supplements like chamomile, lavender, kava kava, lemon balm, passionflower, valerian root and St. John's Wort have been shown to help some people get to sleep. Make sure there are no interactions with anything you could be taking already by simply asking your doctor or healthcare professional and doing some of your own research. Some of these aromas can also be found in candles, oils, incense and lotions.

Melatonin supplementation has been researched as a sleep aid because melatonin levels naturally increase in your body as darkness falls, and reduce when it gets lighter. Supplementation should help raise your levels and trick your body into sleep, but studies have not had overwhelmingly positive results.

How about some massage, acupuncture or acupressure? Working on the body can release stress, stimulate points of the body that are associated with your brain and even increase serotonin levels, which helps promote sleep.

A natural substance that can raise serotonin levels is Tryptophan. One by-product of its breakdown is L-Tryptophan, which will then change into serotonin. Although it doesn't work for everybody, think about this. Warm milk and turkey can raise your Tryptophan levels. That is why Mom always said to drink a warm glass of milk before bedtime. Also, how many times does Thanksgiving Day look like a disaster zone after dinner when everyone is zonked out?

If you see a specialist, keep a diary of you sleep habits, food, exercise and daily routines. I hope some of this can lead you in the right direction because no one likes to be cranky, tired or unproductive.

"Smoking is one of the leading causes of statistics." – **Fletcher Knebel**

Smoking

What are you thinking? Don't! Enough said. Unfortunately many people still smoke and kids still think it is cool. Hey if your parents can do it and they have always told you they know what is best, why can't you?

I don't care if the cigarette companies advertise that they have light cigarettes, low tar (that sounds healthy, eaten any asphalt lately?), all natural ingredients or fiber. Smoking is terrible for your body period! End of discussion. You're either pregnant or you're not. It doesn't go both ways.

As far as I can remember, each house has a chimney to remove the smoke and deadly fumes. If smoke wasn't bad then seal up the chimney and close the flue. Keep your windows closed when you smoke in your vehicle and don't throw the darn butt in the streets. I'm going to start throwing my apple cores on your yard. Hey and they are biodegradable.

As a kid it never made sense that smoking was bad, but second hand smoke wasn't. It doesn't make sense. I thought this as a kid and the government continues to waste millions of our tax dollars, like they do so well, on research studies to prove the blatantly obvious. Smoke is deadly period. Doesn't matter if you're smoking alfalfa sprouts. Remember stop, drop and roll?

"Question. Firemen wear oxygen masks so they don't breathe in ... (BZZZ) ... What is smoke? I'll take common sense for $400, Alex."

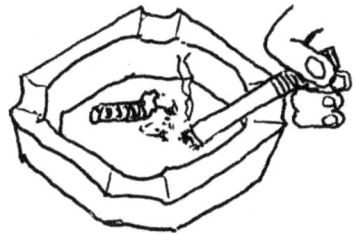

When you smoke you may not realize it but everything you are near, like your clothes and hair, smells like an ashtray. The odor is strong. Some states have adopted a position to make smoking in indoor facilities illegal because other people, who have chosen not to smoke, are forced to breathe in the second hand smoke. Now non-smokers can actually go out to a bar or restaurant and come home without stinking. I used to leave my clothes in the garage because I couldn't stand the smell of them or myself when I returned home. I had to take a shower to clean the smell off me.

If you wish to smoke, that is your choice. However, over 125 million non-smoking Americans continue to be in places like vehicles, work environments, public places and homes where they are exposed to second hand smoke.[52] People should not have to breathe in your smoke if they are in a common or public place.

When possible, the non-smokers should also make a conscious effort to avoid those places that do allow smoking like bars and restaurants. It's a dual responsibility, not just for the people who continue to smoke. To minimize your exposure, go elsewhere.

When exiting a building that has all of the smokers huddled up by the doorway or inside the vestibule like a gang, hold your breath when you wade through the cloud of toxins. You could also stay upwind of people at open air events if they are smoking, like parents at a kid's soccer game. That may be more beneficial than you know. Want some revenge? Eat lots of beans and that will give you a chance for retaliatory fire. Haha.

Smoking decreases your lung capacity and destroys your health. I have always mentioned, once, to any patients who smoke, the best thing I could do for them beyond relieving their pain, would be to get them to stop smoking. I can't emphasize that enough.

Around 30 percent of all heart disease deaths in this country are directly related to smoking.[53] The Centers for Disease Control found not only does smoking effect almost every organ in the body, but it is responsible for almost 440,000 deaths a year, or nearly one of every five deaths.[53] There are over 4,000 chemicals released into the air and close to 50 of them are known carcinogens.[54,55] No one should breathe that.

Besides lost labor due to illness and death, healthcare for conditions related to smoking combine to a staggering cost of more than $175 billion a year.[56] It is the leading cause of *"preventable"* death[57] in the United States. It also effects circulation, skin, your voice, arthritis of the spine, osteoporosis and your children's health.

In the *Archives of Pediatrics and Adolescent Medicine* a study found that second-hand smoke would kill approximately 6,200 children as a direct cause of their parent's smoking.[58] Will it include one of yours?

When expectant mothers smoke during pregnancy, babies have died due to low birth weights, sudden infant death syndrome, respiratory infections, asthma and burns. Smoking has also been linked to behavioral problems in kids.

There is even a threat to kids known as third-hand smoke. Remember coming from Uncle Charlie's house or the bar and wreaking of that cigarette smell? University of California researchers have found the smoke residue on clothes, skin, hair, car seats, carpet and more can be potentially dangerous for months, even though there has been no recent exposure of smoke. Walking on the carpet for instance, can send toxins back into the air and potentially enter the lungs and cause breathing problems like Asthma or worse, Cancer.

So if you can smell the odor of smoke in a house or car, it can harm your child, and you. Kids who slept in rooms of smokers had three times the level of nicotine in their body then those that slept in another room. Airing out the house is the only hope to reducing that smoky smell and some of the dangers.

When I hear a new patient say hello to the office manager I can usually determine if they are a smoker. The signs are visible and audible. You may not notice it but your voice can start to sound raspier than Demi Moore's.

I never understand why people who have had bypass surgery, have diabetes or have to travel everywhere with an oxygen tank, are determined to still go outside for a smoke. They're wasting their doctors' time and shortening the time they have with their families. I just talked with two people who have had one or two heart attacks and still have no rationale for why they still smoke. They weren't scared enough the first time, but the next time could be complete with their fatal warning.

My parents smoked since they were kids in Brooklyn. They were tough kids, hanging in the gangs, with greasy hair and rolled up packs of Lucky Strikes in their white t-shirts like Henry Winkler and Sly Stallone in The Lords of Flatbush. Now my father has had his share of heart problems and he has finally quit smoking. I hope it's not too late. I would like him to see my kids graduate from college. My mom just quit cold turkey after forty plus years.

I know quitting isn't easy. Quitting causes weight gain because the drugs in the cigarettes increase your metabolism and keep you thinner. You also need to satisfy the oral fixation and tend to put food in your mouth. When you notice your cravings creeping up like an unrelenting monster, try to chose nicotine laced lozenges or gum to curb your cravings. Crunchy foods without a lot of calories would be good like celery, cereal, carrots or almonds.

> *"It is better to learn late than never."* – **Publilius Syrus**

IT'S NOW OR NEVER

After your last cigarette, your lungs and heart will start to repair damaged tissue and your nose may smell food a little more distinctly. That's in the first few days. Even before this your blood pressure will drop, poisonous gas levels will drop, body temperature will rise, nerve endings grow and your chance of a heart attack decreases.[59,60]

After one year smoke-free, you will notice greater lung capacity, sinus changes and less coughing. Plus, your risk of developing heart disease is cut by one half. Beyond that, the risk of lung disease or cancer can be dropped in half after 10 years of quitting and heart disease is almost that of a non-smoker after being clean for 15 years.[59,60] The sooner you quit, the sooner your body will start to repair itself. What are you waiting for?

The government has raised taxes and the prices of cigarettes so high that by quitting you could save enough money to pay for that new gym membership, a new game for the family, or boost your rainy-day slush fund.

The effects on your lungs and your health are much more severe than 10 or 15 pounds you might gain. So to counter weight gain, go exercise and start eating more sensibly. You can quit. You can do this. For you and your family. You will even save a bunch of money. How much is a pack now, $8? You may choose to quit due to finances.

"Every great advance in natural knowledge has involved the absolute rejection of authority."
– Thomas H. Huxley

Vitamins

These are over-the-counter (OTC) substances you can take to *"supplement"* your diet. This doesn't mean you take a handful of vitamins and live on Hostess Cupcakes and Devil Dogs. If you're eating habits are deficient in one vitamin or another, this is a way to ensure that you are getting enough into your system. It is an insurance policy in case you aren't as well rounded an eater as you ought to be.

Taken incorrectly, or in dangerously high doses, vitamins can be detrimental to your health. Linus Pauling took mega doses of Vitamin C and lived to be 93. His opponents to this theory of the importance and benefits of high dosages of Vitamin C often lived to 60. However, there is no need to go to extremes. Use common sense.

I prefer to take a vitamin that has lots of good herbal ingredients, vitamins and minerals, no binders and fillers. I take one in the morning and one later. This way my body can dispose of the rest I don't need, and pick up another dose 12 hours later when my levels may have changed. I'm not taking two or three at once, dumping excessively high doses into my body. Instead I'm trying to maintain my levels of vitamins within my body.

If you have difficulty swallowing pills you have a few options. Look for small pills and not the horse-sized ones. Try taking the pills with a swig of a thick liquid like a shake or yogurt. Some stores have vitamins in a liquid format so you can add them to cereal, coffee or soup.

Some vitamins have minerals that help in their absorption and make them more effective. Vitamin E and Selenium or Calcium and Magnesium are examples of this union. Let's look at some vitamins and see why they are good for us and where to get them naturally from foods.

Kids also can benefit from taking vitamins and minerals unless your kids munch on raw broccoli and walnuts. Choose wisely because companies sneak lots of sugar and fillers in there and kids don't need that either.

But first I want to briefly discuss another supplement that has been out there for years and has been helpful in treating arthritis. You may have heard of shark cartilage and that supposedly sharks don't get cancer. So people thought it would be great to kill sharks for their cartilage. Plants don't get cancer either. Perhaps sharks don't get cancer because they don't consume steroid filled meats, soda, bioengineered sugars and preservatives. Maybe we should change our diet first instead of looking for a magic bullet.

Another version would be purchasing glucosamine and chondroitin sulfate in a 3:2 ratio. The dose is usually 1500 mg of glucosamine sulfate to 1200 mg of chondroitin sulfate. The molecules are different sizes but both have been found to be helpful when rebuilding cartilage and easing some types of joint pain.

Think of it as trying to build a block wall. When you supplement with these two sulfates you are bringing more blocks into a usable area to make rebuilding easier. When your body needs to start to rebuild and repair new joint cartilage, you will have easy access to the items your body needs.

Some patients notice a difference instantly. Others notice a difference three to four months later. Then there are those who realize they did benefit from the supplements but only after they stopped taking them. Sometimes you have no response, but it can't hurt to try.

If you have any arthritic complaints you should try it. I have seen it help knees, ankles, necks and hands. It has no side-effects and no negative interactions with any medications. Give it a chance.

VITAMIN	BENEFIT	SOURCES
Vitamin A	• Growth and repair body tissues • Fights bacteria & infection • Healthy eyes & skin • Helps with bone & teeth formation	• Red, yellow, orange and dark green vegetables • Nuts • Dairy • Eggs
Vitamin B1 (Thiamine)	• Carbohydrate metabolism • Healthy nervous system • Appetite regulation • Growth & muscle tone • Healthy heart	• Watermelon • Peas • Avocado • Whole grains • Pork & organ meats
Vitamin B2 (Riboflavin)	• Required for carb, fat & protein metabolism • Form antibodies & red blood cells (RBC)	• Milk & dairy • Avocado & kiwi • Organ meats • Enriched grains

VITAMIN	BENEFIT	SOURCES
Vitamin B3 (Niacin)	• Helps the digestive system • Important for healthy skin and nerve function • Aids in conversion of food to energy	• Poultry, fish & beef • Nuts like almonds & peanuts • Peaches, kiwi, bananas cantaloupe & watermelon • Avocado, tomatoes, peas, mushrooms, potatoes, corn
Vitamin B5 (Pantothenic Acid)	• Helps aid metabolism of food • Helps formation of hormones and good cholesterol	• Oranges & bananas • Avocado, sweet potato, corn, lima beans, broccoli, carrots, cauliflower
Vitamin B6 (Pyridoxine)	• Helps form antibodies • Formation of RBC • Maintains nervous system	• Chicken, beef liver, fish • Bananas, watermelon, • Avocado, peas, carrots • Sweet potatoes, spinach
Vitamin B9 (Folic Acid)	• Needed to produce RBC • Helps formation of DNA	• Fortified cereals, enriched grains, nuts & seeds • Lima beans, spinach, asparagus, broccoli • Kiwi, blackberries, orange, strawberry, bananas, cantaloupe
Vitamin B12	• Formation of RBC • Maintains nervous system • Energy production	• Fish, red meat & chicken • Dairy products • Eggs
Vitamin C	• Important antioxidant • Healthy bones & teeth • Wound healing	• Red berries, grapefruit, kiwi, oranges & guava • Red & green peppers, tomatoes, broccoli, spinach

VITAMIN	BENEFIT	SOURCES
Vitamin D	• Formation of bones and teeth • Proper formation of bone	• Dairy products, eggs • Sunlight • Saltwater fish
Vitamin E	• Powerful antioxidant • Formation of RBC • Wound healing • Helps prevent and treat wrinkles	• Vegetable oils, • Dark green leafy vegetables • Nuts, seeds & legumes • Whole grains & oatmeal
Vitamin K	• Blood clotting • Regulates blood calcium	• Dark green leafy vegetables • Oatmeal, other grains, eggs • Spinach, broccoli, soybeans
Coenzyme Q10	• Super antioxidants like Vitamin E • Aids circulation, increases oxygenation by blood • Stimulates immune system • Great for heart disease	• Mackerel, salmon, sardines • Beef • Peanuts • Spinach
Bioflavonoids	• Increase strength of capillaries • Enhance Vitamin C absorption	• Peppers, buckwheat • Black currants, citrus fruits • White material under peels • Grapefruit, cherries, oranges

> *"When you are right you cannot be too radical; when you are wrong, you cannot be too conservative."* – **Martin Luther King, Jr.**

I'm Not Anti-Oxidants

Antioxidants deserve more attention because they help to remove free radicals or unstable molecules, which can lead to cancer and even premature aging. They are unstable in the sense that they have an incomplete number of electrons around them, which makes them more reactive then their balanced counterparts. Humans typically produce oxygen-containing molecules, which will then try to steal electrons from other molecules. This is how the damage occurs. It looks similar to rust on a car or an apple that turns brown.

Antioxidants can stabilize these radicals and help prevent any future damage they could cause. A new study by the Department of Food Science at Louisiana State University Agricultural Center in Baton Rouge just discovered that black rice has the same antioxidant power as blueberries. Better yet, it has more fiber, less sugar, can lower cholesterol and costs less. Rice is nice!

Most people know about Vitamins A, C, E, Beta-Carotene and lycopene. Let's take a closer look at some of the more important ones you may not have been aware are so beneficial. These can be bought for tremendously high prices or you simply eat a balanced diet and get your antioxidant power from having solid nutrition.

Beta-Carotene can be found in orange foods like apricots, cantaloupe, dark greens, kale, mangoes, papaya, peppers, pumpkin, spinach, squash and sweet potatoes. It is a powerful antioxidant.

Lycopene is found in apricots, pink grapefruit, papaya, guava, tomatoes and watermelon. It can guard against aging of the skin, may prevent Cancers of the prostate and mouth, diabetes, cardiovascular disease, osteoporosis and male fertility problems.

Lutein has been touted for helping the eyes and can be ingested by consuming a diet with lots of dark, green leafy vegetables like collard greens, kale and spinach.

Phytochemicals are nutrients from plants and there are lots of different ones. For example, Flavonoids, like Resveratrol and Quercetin, are believed to be really powerful antioxidants. These lifesavers are found in apples, black-berries, blueberries, cherries, cranberries, grapefruit, grapes, pomegranate, red wine, soy and strawberries.

Glutathione is produced in the liver and aids your metabolism and your immune system. It can be found in fresh fruits, meats cooked rare and raw to uncooked vegetables. Heat can remove the glutathione content. That is why cooking your food less or eating it raw is healthier. Great sources are apples, asparagus, avocado, carrots, grapefruit, spinach and tomatoes.

Studies have shown oral supplementation is not well absorbed so the recommendation is to increase its precursors or eat foods to help its production occur naturally in the body. Things like N-Acetyl-Cysteine, which has been shown to help glutathione production in cases of acetaminophen overdose. Also vitamin C, Undenatured Whey Protein, selenium, milk thistle and Alpha-Lipoic Acid (from Omega 3 fatty acids) have been shown to boost levels of glutathione. Foods like asparagus, broccoli, avocado, spinach, garlic and fresh unprocessed meats can get you there as well.

Some research has found glutathione to be helpful in treating Parkinson's disease, Liver Cancer and lowering Blood Pressure in Diabetics. The bottom line to all of this is to eat a well-balanced diet that includes lots of variety and color in your foods. The less over-cooked your food is, the better it is for you. Eat smart.

"Chance is always powerful. Let your hook be always cast; in the pool where you least expect it, there will be a fish." – **Ovid**

Does This Smell Fishy To You?

People talk about Omega 6 and Omega 3 essential fatty acids, but do you know why? We can't make them on our own so we either have to eat a diet rich in these nutrients or supplement with fish oil caplets. There are plenty of sources of foods with Omega 6 in them but few with Omega 3.

Omega 6s are found in raw nuts, seeds, legumes and oils such as borage oil, flax seed oil, grape seed oil, sesame oil and soybean oil. Because people crave carbohydrates and snack of foods high in refined oils, many people are consuming too many of these types of fatty acids. That can be a problem. We need to cut back on these, and balance our levels by increasing our Omega 3 intake. Keep reading and I will explain.

The main components of Omega 6 fatty acids are Linolenic Acid (LA), Gamma - Linolenic Acid (GLA), Dihomogamma Linolenic Acid (DLA) and Arachidonic Acid (AA). These function to increase inflammation, blood clotting, water retention and can raise blood pressure.

However research suggests supplementation of GLA alone can be beneficial in opening blood vessels, regulating water loss, promoting healing, healthier skin, reducing menstrual cramps, lowering cholesterol and boosting the immune system. Some studies have found it also decreases arthritis pain, fights cancer and may help diabetics.

Omega 3s are found in flax seeds, walnuts, pumpkin seeds, sesame seeds, avocado, Brazil nuts, dark, leafy vegetables, olive oil and fatty, cold-water fish like Alaskan salmon, mackerel, sardines and anchovies. If you are going to add cold-water fish to your diet, get wild caught fish from the coldest waters available and broil or bake them. They are rich in Omega 3 fatty acids, where some farm-raised fish do not have healthy levels.

Farm-raised fish just hang out, may not be fed chemically free grains and don't develop healthy meat from their lack of swimming against currents. They end up with less protein, their meat is gray until colored, they have a higher fat content and contain unhealthy Omega 6 levels. A 2004 study in *Environmental Science and Technology* reported higher levels of polybrominated diphenyl ether (PBDE) in farmed salmon than in wild salmon. PBDE cause reproductive toxicity and may also cause cancer.

The main components of Omega 3 fatty acids are Alpha-Linolenic Acid (ALA), Eicosapentaenoic Acid (EPA) and Docosahexaenoic Acid (DHA). These function to: increase heart health, lower cancer and Alzheimer's risk; reduce allergies, Rheumatoid symptoms and PMS symptoms; as well as, improve memory, mood, your eyes, skin, hair and brain function. Where do I sign up for this?

Studies recommend we have a ratio of Omega 3:Omega 6 around 2:1 to 10:1, instead of 1:10 – 20 like we do. Consuming Omega 3 and Omega 6 in a healthy ratio can really help us fight disease and stay healthy. The wrong ratio can lead to an inability to utilize the Omega 3 fatty acids ingested and cause symptoms such as depression, obesity, hyperactivity and violence. In fact, a 2002 study in *The British Journal of Psychiatry* found prison violence dropped 37 percent just by supplementing inmates' diets with Omega 3.

A cool finding from a 2006 *Surgical Neurology* article found including appropriate levels of Omega 3 essential fatty acids in your diet can eliminate any need for pain drugs that patient's routinely take to help reduce discomfort from an arthritic spine.

Did you know there is an Omega 9? The main component is Oleic Acid (OA). A good source of Omega 9 is olive oil. It helps to reduce the risk of heart disease and arteriosclerosis. Pure EPA contains a healthy blend of all three Omega 3 EPA, Omega 6 GLA and Omega 9 OA. If you try this as a supplement, make sure your source of Omegas is from cold-water fish and it is clearly labeled with what kind it includes.

The difficult part of choosing fish from any area in the world now is due to pollution. For years we have been warned to not consume too much predatory fish because they keep accumulating dangerous levels of mercury. Over months and years fish continue to accumulate the poisonous metal in their bodies from the fish they eat and it never leaves, until it is passed on to you.

Since the huge BP oil spill in the Gulf and the Nuclear contamination of the waters off the coast of Japan, where are we supposed to get healthy fish? These are times I think more about eating grains and nuts for my Omegas.

> *"I would feel more optimistic about a bright future for man if he spent less time proving that he can outwit Nature and more time tasting her sweetness and respecting her seniority."*
> **– E. B. White**

Minerals

This table will look at some of the more common minerals, the benefits they provide and some sources of food that can add that particular mineral to your diet.

MINERAL	BENEFIT	SOURCES
Calcium	• Strong bones & teeth • Regulates heartbeat • Helps muscle & nerves function	• Dairy • Seafood like salmon & sardines • Dark green leafy vegetables • Almonds, broccoli
Chromium	• Metabolism of glucose • Metabolism of fats, carbs, & protein	• Beer & brewer's yeast, • Brown rice & whole grains • Cheese & meat
Copper	• Nerve function, hair growth • Formation of bone and RBC • Healthy nerves & immune system	• Beans & lentils • Nuts • Seafood & beef • Chocolate
Fluorine (fluoride)	• Strong teeth & bones • Helps prevent Osteoporosis	• Salt water fish, gelatin, tea • Fluoridated water
Iodine	• Metabolism of excess fat • Normal thyroid function	• Iodized salt, saltwater fish • Seaweed, kelp
Iron	• Production of hemoglobin • Oxygen carrying factor of RBC • Keeps immune system healthy	• Fish, liver, meat, chicken • Dark green leafy vegetables • Whole grains, nuts, eggs

MINERAL	BENEFIT	SOURCES
Magnesium	• Healthy heart & arterial linings • Aids metabolism and bone growth	• Dairy products • Meat, fish & seafood • Fruit, nuts, dark green leafy vegetables
Manganese	• Normal bone growth • Normal cell function • Fat and protein metabolism • Healthy immune system & nerves	• Nuts, seeds, legumes • Avocado, blueberries, fruits • Whole grains, eggs • Coffee, tea, cocoa • Dark green leafy vegetables
Molybdenum	• Normal cell & nerve function	• Dark green leafy vegetables • Beans, legumes, grains
Potassium	• Healthy nervous system • Maintains fluid & BP/HR • Regulates water balance • Regular heart rhythm • Muscle contraction	• Fish, meat & chicken • Oranges, bananas & avocado • Whole grains, nuts, legumes • Vegetables & dried fruit
Selenium	• Works well with Vitamin E • Antioxidant	• Fish, meat, shellfish, chicken • Grains, eggs & tomatoes
Sodium	• Proper blood pH • Regulates water balance	• Table salt, dairy products • Any food, especially canned
Zinc	• Wound healing, normal growth • Prostate gland functioning • Aids taste & smell	• Brewer's yeast, whole grains • Fish, eggs, meat, chicken, soy • Legumes & seeds

Section II

In Search of the Healthy Grail

> *"Exercise ferments the humors, casts them into their proper channels, throws off redundancies, and helps nature in those secret distributions, without which the body cannot subsist in its vigor, nor the soul act with cheerfulness."* – **Joseph Addison**

Weight Problems

It's in the papers and it's on the news. There are pictures showing men and women from various races, with their bellies hanging over their belts and thighs so big they waddle when they walk. Now it is becoming a learned behavior by our youth. They too are exercising less, eating more and becoming increasingly heavier as a result. None of this is healthy.

So the population is getting heavier and unhealthier by the year. We are being categorized into two groups. One is obesity, which is being heavier than the government standard only because of increased fat. Men are typically in the 20 – 40 percent body fat range, while women tend to be in the 30 – 50 percent range. Part of this is because of genetics and males having more muscle than women.

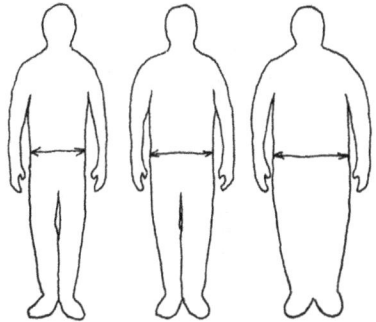

The second is when someone is overweight. The composition of the body is then taken into consideration and the excess weight can be due to muscle, water, bone or fat. Being considered overweight is based on a set standard for weight according to a certain height, known as the Body Mass Index (BMI).

Consider now a bodybuilder who is muscle bound and in good shape. Because muscle weighs more than fat their weight is much more than what is recommended for their height according to this index. Should they be classified as *"overweight?"* Most of us can look in the mirror and figure out if we need to lose a few pounds. This *"look at yourself"* scale is good for the vast majority of people.

According to the National Institute of Health (NIH) the number of overweight people has risen 20 percent, while the number of obese people (based on fat) has more than doubled, during the same time frame. Some reports show the number of kids overweight or obese, doubling in the last twenty years and the number of overweight teenagers tripling.[61] These numbers aren't good.

The rising numbers, put a strain on our healthcare system. It has been found that this increase in our overweight and obese population is driving health-care costs higher. They estimated 92 billion dollars a year was the cost to the healthcare system.[62]

There are more costs that could be added if you consider the amount of lost work production that accompanies the treatment of these health problems. The CDC also estimates that the working class from 17 – 64 years of age cost approximately $4 billion in lost production due to missed days, doctor's visits, and restrictions related to obesity.

Due to lifestyles, laziness or employment, many of us don't eat well or get the exercise we should. Some people may not care, but poor diet and lack of exercise are almost ready to overtake smoking as the number one cause of preventable deaths.[63] Time to change your tune.

The more weight our bodies carry the more stress there is on our joints, muscles and spines. Remember each additional 10 pounds equates to 50 pounds of pressure on the knees and 100 pounds of pressure on our backs. There is also a direct correlation between proper weight and abnormal stress to the spine and posture. Obesity and inactivity affects internal health manifesting in heart problems, diabetes, reduced flexibility and ranges of motion.

There are other situations that can cause weight gain like tumors and water retention. In some cases your thyroid, an organ in your neck, could be unhealthy and sending the wrong information to your body. It is part of the Endocrine System, which is responsible for releasing the right amount of hormones to specific organs in your body to regulate mood, growth and metabolism.

Conditions like Hypothyroidism, in which your thyroid is functioning less than optimally, will slow your metabolism regardless of any exercise you do to try and raise it. Another example of an endocrine disorder would be Cushing's Syndrome. In this disease the body releases far too much cortisol, which encourages the storage of fat within the body.

If you have any health concerns, or can't lose weight on your own, your medical doctor can order some blood work and run tests. Lab work will help identify or further confirm your condition. Tests also help your doctor determine how to treat your condition and establish treatment, supplements, medications or therapy that may help you.

Sometimes we reward our kids with sweets when they do something well. *"Finish your Brussels sprouts and you can have dessert."* If I got As on my report card we went for a hot fudge sundae. The technique works. Sometimes we even reward ourselves as adults if we've worked hard or have been under stress. A nice brownie or ice cream cone always makes the day better. Those calories can add up. This type of reward may have some consequences to your well being so choose wisely and make healthy choices.

My colleague Mark comically postulated the reason people get heavier as they age is because they have higher paying jobs and can afford to buy more food. There could be a slight bit of truth to that but I thought it was pretty funny when he said it.

"You are the bows from which your children as living arrows are sent forth."
– Kahlil Gibran

TEACH YOUR CHILDREN WELL

Parents can lead by example. Maybe it's time you got off the couch too. Don't just come home and spend the evening on the couch in front of the idiot box. Interact with the family, work on a project or shoot some baskets with the kids.

Don't let your children play games on the TV or computer for four hours a day. Make sure they are involved with something active. Limit their time with electronics and enrich their lives with outdoor activities and sports. As kids we used to ride our bikes around a 4.5 mile block that would give the Tour de France riders a run for their money. And we survived without helmets.

Times have changed. Now you need protection and have to worry someone is going to grab your kid. What have we become? Anyway, next time you buy gifts for a child make sure they are geared toward exercise like a Nerf football, Frisbee, rocket set, or kickball.

There are however some new computer games that really are interactive. Decathlons in which you have to do all of the events, baseball and golf games that require you to swing to hit the ball, or dance revolution, which can all burn some calories as you test your footwork on the dance floor. They're also a lot of fun for people of all ages.

I just played boxing with my nephews and after a few rounds I was a sweaty mess. I almost called 911. If everyone started boxing like that they could lose weight and have fun with the family at the same time. You might even claim the Heavyweight Championship. Are you ready to rumble?

Kids often eat what we feed them; well, after their picky years. If we put unhealthy foods on the table or in the pantry, then there's a good chance it will be eaten. And, probably not in the intended serving size. Teach your children about good nutrition and portions. Just like anything else you teach them, they will use these life lessons to make healthier decisions.

> *"Censorship, like charity, should begin at home; but, unlike charity, it should end there."* **– Clare Booth Luce**

YOU MAKE THE CALL

Too much weight can wear out the knees and hips. When that happens we will hobble because of the pain. That motion will have a negative effect on the rest of our body since it is all connected. Please don't make me sing *"the knee bone's connected to the hipbone"* again.

Sometimes people will need one knee replaced. But if the other one is the same age, why doesn't it need to be replaced too? Because there has been extra stress to that joint in particular, which has worn it down over time. It could be your job, a shorter leg, lugging babies or tight muscles that have caused more weight to be carried on one side.

In addition, people who are classified as overweight and obese, and have been influenced by poor diet and inactivity, have an increased risk of diabetes, high blood pressure, high cholesterol, sleep disorders, asthma, depression, heartburn, joint problems, and poor health status.[64,65,66] Even at an early age, obese children have been found to have cardiac profiles regarding heart rates, blood pressure and cardiac output that were higher than non-obese children of the same age.[67,68,69]

Adult onset diabetes is now becoming so common in adolescents and children due to their increasing size[70] that it is being estimated that one of every three children born in the year 2000 will become diabetic in their lifetime.[71] The number of kids taking meds has increased due to Diabetes Type 2, which is known as adult onset Diabetes.

Our country is the leader for many great things, except when it comes to the *"Human Race."* We continue to get bigger and *"badder,"* when referring to our health anyway. One estimate is that more than 34 percent of the American population over 20 years of age is overweight. Sadly almost 33 percent of the population is obese, meaning they have large amounts of fat on their bodies, which can have a deadly effect on their health and their families.[72]

Even more disturbing, is that the CDC and NIH have found that close to 20 percent of our kids 6 – 19 are overweight. Some estimates regarding our kids' weight were even 10 percent higher. Females who were overweight as children have a 10 – 30 times greater tendency to be an overweight young adult.[73,74] Another predictor that is being researched is the skin fold test done on the back of a child's arm. It may be more accurate in determining the percentage of fat in a child, as well as, the likeliness they will be overweight as an adult.

In general, overweight kids who reach six years of age have a greater than 50 percent chance to become overweight as an adult [67], but when they reach their teenage years, the number increases to 70 – 80 percent.[75,76] Having at least one obese parent will also increase the likelihood of future obesity in the child.[68] Don't just set the table, set an example.

> *"Children need models rather than critics."* – **Joseph Joubert**

GIVE ME THE GOOD STUFF

What are our kids eating in school? Grease-laden crap! Pizza with fries. Cheeseburgers with fries. That cafeteria lunch is a great place to make a difference in your child's health. Pack them a healthy lunch a couple of days a week. Maybe meet with your school and see if they can make any changes. A child's early years are when poor dietary habits can start the development of heart disease[77] and osteoporsis.[78]

Many areas around us just got rid of some of the soda machines in schools. AWESOME! That is a great start considering carbonated beverages have been found to deplete the calcium levels in the bones of teenage girls making them more susceptible to fractures[79] and developing osteoporosis later in life. It isn't healthy for boys either.

If you want to monitor what your kids are eating, why not try a web site like www.mylunchmoney.com? For a small fee they will keep tabs on what your little angels are buying. You just log on and view who was sneaking cookies instead of broccoli.

The carbonated soft drink has become Americans' number one source of calories. The soda giants marketing departments spend $200 million or more in advertising to target their audiences[80]. Whereas only $1 million is spent by the U.S. governments to promote the importance of consuming five vegetables a day.

These drinks can either add up the calories by themselves, create a feeling of hunger that tricks you into eating more, or may even take the place of more nutritious foods and drinks. Unless you're planning on wrestling off your dinner and expending serious calories, you can put the sporty, sugar-filled drink back into the refrigerator too.

MythBusters found cola to be an effective rust remover. Imagine what that *"battery acid"* is doing to your teeth and your insides! My father-in-law just switched to minimizing his soda intake and replaced it with drinking water again. He can't believe it. The aches and pains in his joints have disappeared, probably because less sugars means less inflammation in the body, and he isn't eating all the time. He's losing weight and not even trying.

Although sodas can't be totally blamed for diabetes, there has to be some responsibility placed on the individual to know their genetic tendencies. People need to watch the amount of sugar they take in, limit their calories and exercise regularly. However, there have been strong links to diabetes for consumers

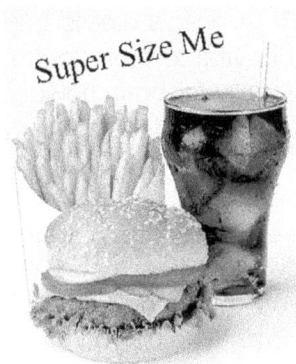

drinking one to two soft drinks a day[81]. The occurrence of diabetes was twice as great in those who drank one per month. Which category are you in? Where would you like to be?

A child's diet is important for many reasons. A brief list would include that it is vital to their health, enhances athletic ability, maintains alertness, supplies energy for brain power, creates good habits early on and because kids in school can be ruthless about weight.

Imagine your child, or remember how kids who were tall, fat, developed early, skinny or basically a little different, were treated. Comments to the *"fat kid"* were cruel and hurtful. How does that influence children as they grow up? How do their classmates respond to the attractive girl or the star athlete? Who do you think goes through school with confidence and is popular with the other kids? Who do you think is suffering from low self-esteem?[82] How does that affect their education and future? Some kids contemplate suicide due to the constant teasing about their weight.

> *"All excess is ill, but drunkenness is of the worst sort. It spoils health, dismounts the mind, and unmans men. It reveals secrets, is quarrelsome, lascivious, impudent, dangerous and bad."*
> **– William Penn**

YOU ARE YOUR OWN WORST ENEMY

Everybody loves the holidays. They are fun and cheerful, and overindulgence runs rampant from Thanksgiving to Easter. That's five months or almost half the year, we celebrate with gorging ourselves and eating unhealthily. It's so easy to put on weight in preparation for winter months … *"even a caveman could do it."*

We kick off our food fest with Halloween. It is a great way to make every dentist busier and richer. All that sugar and sticky, chewy candy is enough to fill the appointment book for months. Not to mention the stuff we buy for the neighborhood, just happens to be our favorite. So if no one shows up, who do you think will eat all those empty calories? Guilty as charged.

Thanksgiving is next, the big meal consisting of turkey, gravy, mashed potatoes and all the sides, followed by too many desserts. We eat appetizers waiting for the real feast and then sit down for the meal. Next are the six pies to be consumed soon after dinner. More sugar filled calories. In between all this are the naps, because we ate too much or the sugar content was too high. Eating too much and then napping are a great 1-2 punch to gain weigh.

Christmas and New Year's parties last the entire month or longer. We bounce from one office party to another family or friend gathering. December is basically alcohol, sweets and over indulgence for thirty days. Next we have the Super Bowl and a full day of gluttony at its best. Next we consume

Valentine's Day candy, St. Patrick's Day and Easter candy accompanied by another huge meal. This coincides with winter when we are typically less active in general. I know some of us can throw in a few birthday cakes along the way too. That is a lot of food.

The economic drive for the public to buy sugary crap, and gifts, for these holidays is well beyond the original meaning of any of these holidays. Combine that with a decrease in activity and excessive calories, and terrible ones at that, and you have the recipe for big weight gain. It is no wonder we get unhealthier every year.

There is no magic pill or quick dieting scheme that can provide you with safe, long-lasting weight loss. The one scientifically proven method I want you to consider and adopt is exercise. Maybe add a workout or increase the time and effort you expend in the gym when you are in there. This can also help to offset any additional special event or holiday calories that may be headed your way in the future.

Incorporate a little self-control with your eating habits during this vulnerable time period. Try a bite of this, nibble on that, skip on seconds and have some water on the rocks a couple of times during the party. This way you aren't denied the satisfaction of trying the various foods or knocking a few cocktails back. You just aren't adding as much to your bottom line, so to speak.

In general, if you decide to have a nice dinner out, use the same principles. You don't have to eat all of the bread at the table. Those are empty calories. It doesn't mean you can't have any. Just don't eat the whole loaf. Besides, why fill up on bread when the good stuff is about to come? When you order, look for leaner meats or things without heavy sauces. There may even be symbols next to healthier meals on the menu, or at least an opportunity to make a substitution, like egg beaters for an omelet; or skip the fries and opt for a fruit cup instead. Order drinks if you want but remember those calories add up too.

If dinner comes with any pasta or rice, try to keep it on the side because you know it may be made with heavy sauce or butter. Get your salad dressing on the side, like any sauce, so you can add it and the lettuce isn't drowning. Flavor your salad; don't flood it. You don't have to eat everything on the plate. If you take some home, you can have a great lunch tomorrow.

I may even order dessert and split it with my wife. We enjoy a nice dinner out, with a dessert, and have reduced the total calories we could have eaten by using some self-control.

"Expose yourself to your deepest fear; after that, fear has no power, and the fear of freedom shrinks and vanishes. You are free." – **Jim Morrison**

I SECOND THAT EMOTION

Speaking of control, a lot of people have trouble resolving or coping with feelings like depression, stress, loneliness, relationship problems, anger, health issues and low self-esteem. Eating can be used as a relief to a situation or as a reward. The problem is it may cause *"dis-ease"* in your waistband and overall health. The longer this behavior goes on the more likely this behavior will become a habit that will be difficult to break.

It is believed that almost 75 percent of all overeating is caused by your emotions. It is normal to eat due to your emotions once in awhile. When it happens constantly then there is a problem. This type of eating can lead to consuming junk foods, or large quantities of food, as a way to bring comfort to the individual. Examples include having to deal with financial difficulties or unhappiness with work that may lead you to snack when you get home late, or keep you awake and wandering to the fridge during the early hours. Food can satisfy a craving and cause the body to feel better just from the action of eating, or from the chemical changes foods can produce within the body.

There may be certain triggers that compound this problem. In particular social environments you may be inclined to eat more, like at office parties or weddings where your stress levels are higher. If you are stuck at home due to an injury, illness, etc., you may start eating out of boredom. At a movie you may have to pass the popcorn and candy aisle and figure, heck, why not? Also when we dine with others we often see what other people are ordering, which can sway us from our normal style of eating.

If you try to control these urges and find a solution to relieving any of these stressors that induce overeating, you may beat this. Check the section on stress. Maybe there is an idea that you can use to help distract your false hungers and create true balance in your diet.

> *"Some scientists claim that hydrogen, because it is so plentiful, is the basic building block of the universe. I dispute that. I say that there is more stupidity than hydrogen, and that is the basic building block of the universe."* – **Frank Zappa**

IF YOU SMELL WHAT THE DOC IS COOKING

The food pyramid was originally created by the USDA and was developed to help people understand the importance of different food groups and what quantity they should be consuming them in.

The first version was divided into blocks that made up the pyramid. Each block represented a food group. The lower the block, the more significant it is as it made up the base of your diet. At the peak were sugars, fats and oils as they should be included in your diet in moderation.

The next food pyramid was a design that included a stairway. On the side, a person was running up it to acknowledge the importance of including at least 30 minutes of moderate exercise in your daily life. In an average adult diet of 2,000 calories a day the government recommended 6 ounces of grains, 2.5 cups of vegetables, 2 cups of fruit, 3 cups of dairy products and 5.5 ounces of meats and beans.

Now a simpler pyramid is being tried which people will be able to make sense of more easily. It is the shape of a plate with the amount of space each food group should take up on your plate. Vegetables and grains were drawn to occupy the largest portion of the plate. Next, one quarter of the plate should contain proteins and fruits. Dairy would be in the form of milk, yogurt, cheese, etc. They do not even mention fats, oils or sugars.

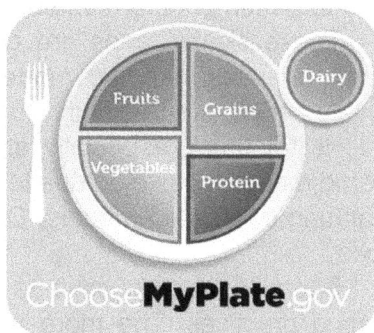

Do you remember the old adage, *"You are what you eat?"* I have always been amazed at how we put ourselves last. Consider how much care is given to our vehicles and not to our bodies. I see people flooding to the garden stores for Miracle Grow soil or another type of enriched topsoil. This way their plants get the nutrients they need to grow big and strong.

With that fancy car, how many hours are spent washing, cleaning, waxing, and polishing to make it look great, turn some heads and protect it from the elements. There is a feeling of pride when you step inside, turn the key and let her roar down the road. You stop at the gas station and fill up. Not with just any gas. Even though prices are up, you still put in the highest grade available.

"Imagine if you used the same thought process and pride when it came to your body."

> *"I've been on a diet for two weeks and all I've lost is two weeks."* – **Totie Fields**

Dieting

Eat this. Don't eat that. Eggs are good, then bad, and now good again. How many times have you heard not to eat fat? And then someone says it is okay to eat fats and proteins, but skip the carbohydrates. Too much protein is bad for your kidneys. Eat more protein to burn more calories. Don't eat at all. Suppress your diet with this pill. Eat seven times a day to fuel your body. Tell me what I can pop to allow me to eat the same junk food I always have and get lean. How about a pill that replaces exercising? The acai berry is a miracle berry. Nope. It's just another over-hyped fruit you haven't heard of before for moneymaking purposes. If it sound too good to be true, then it probably is.

Of course the public is confused. Every three months there is a new fad diet or exercise promising to shed fat so you can get that *"lean, sexy body you've always wanted."* The media loves how thin the Hollywood women and other famous people are and too often put them on our TV screens to admire.

These skinny icons are glorified and hailed as such beauties, like the models in Europe. Except finally people are beginning to realize how unhealthy this is for them, especially after several actresses had health problems and some models even died due to complications from Anorexia. In fact, Europe was banning emaciated models. One restaurant offered free meals to models as a joke.

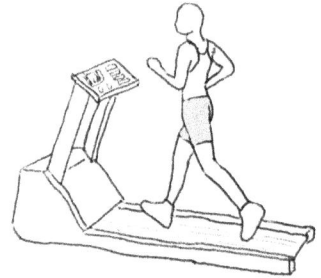

Because models have to remain so thin they have mastered unhealthy eating practices. The more magazines and news stories that promote these *"skeletons,"* the more our young accept the misconception that skin and bones is healthy and an acceptable option. This affects young girls and women everywhere. Even boys feel the pressure to remain skinny. It is not about eating too little or over-eating; it is about learning how to eat right. Anything else is unhealthy.

Someone once said to me that dieting is the only sure way to gain five – 10 pounds. Most weight is lost during the first six months of a diet, except 30 plus studies reviewed by the University of California show that after five years almost 70 percent of the people are likely to be heavier than when they started their diet.

The public isn't learning healthy habits. They are looking for the quick fix, resorting to their old habits and putting the weight back on, and then some. Repeatedly attempting to diet stresses the body and can lead to permanent damage to your organs.

> *"It's so much easier to suggest solutions when you don't know too much about the problem."*
> **– Malcolm Forbes**

IT'S GONE TOO FAR

Anorexia has stricken many Hollywood girls. Too many young actresses have made the headlines for extreme and sudden weight loss. In the blink of an eye they literally and figuratively become half the women they used to be. They proclaim they have been working out and eating right, only to collapse and later plunge back into the headlines for health problems from starving themselves thin.

One woman who spoke out about her battle with Anorexia in the news was Chloe Lattanzi, the daughter of Olivia Newton John. She came forward and spoke out to help young girls. She will struggle with Anorexia for the rest of her life. The damage to her body is permanent.

Anorexia is a disease. You don't recover from it like a cold. It will always be with you. It sometimes develops due to stress, fear of being fat or being perceived as fat, depression, unhappiness, low self-esteem or loss of control. Othertimes it is due to family conflicts.

One of my patients who suffered from this disease, now has control over her life. Every day is a battle and her doctors continue to monitor her health. When she was young her parents put her down, making her so self-conscious about her weight. Her misperception of her body led her down this path.

She has spoken out and was on Oprah and in print discussing her battle so others could learn from her disease and understand the consequences. She struggles every day and is winning. She now looks great and is healthy!

A person suffering with anorexia may become obsessive with counting every calorie, working out excessively, using diet pills or even inducing vomiting. Besides weight loss, signs may include fine, down-like hair growth on the face, back, arms and legs, denying being hungry, loss of hair on head and irregular or absent menstrual periods. Other symptoms include dry, flaky skin that may be yellowish and possibly tooth enamel discoloration or erosion.

Similarly, Bulimia is another outlet for weight loss that people turn to for similar reasons or conditions as Anorexia. It may also occur after failed previous dieting attempts. It too affects women more, but men may also turn to this as a solution.

Secretive eating, excessive exercising, self-induced vomiting or purging, and the use of laxatives and diuretics characterize Bulimia. With repetitive vomiting, the stomach acids that usually dissolve foods become exposed to the enamel of the teeth. This can lead to discoloration, erosion of the enamel and the acids

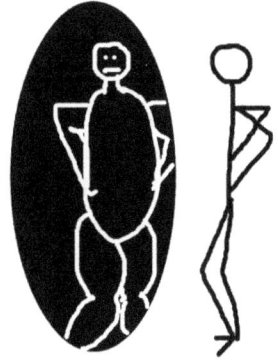

may damage the esophagus of your throat.

Other signs may be excessive eating and never gaining weight and using the bathroom frequently during or directly after a meal. Visually a person may develop chipmunk cheeks from throwing up due to expanding the salivary glands.

The intake of food is initially comforting to people but then their self-disappointment and loss of control forces them to rid themselves of the food anyway possible. This re-establishes their control over their bodies.

What is the toll on the body from enduring this abuse you ask? A best friend of mine lost his beautiful sister-in-law due to Anorexia. So death is the ultimate side effect. Depending on how long the individual remains in this self destructive eating mode they can expect liver, heart and kidney damage, as well as, gastrointestinal problems and electrolyte imbalances from not eating or taking laxatives, and developing ulcers from throwing up.

Tyra Banks spoke out against the unrealistic pressure of women to be super thin, especially after a terrible shot of her made headlines. On her show she blasted the media and the public for saying she was fat or ugly. This photo and negative press was just more damage to women all over the world and hurts their self esteem. Tyra is a beautiful woman who is proud of who she is as a person, what she looks like and has done something positive to help women everywhere. You go girl!

On an awards show Britney Spears was ridiculed after she made a TV appearance in her classic skimpy outfit. They called her overweight and made fun of her. If you think about it or look at the videotape, her lip-syncing may have been off but her body looked fantastic. I challenge anyone who has had two kids to disrobe in the public eye and show your body. There's no option for photoshop. She looked amazing. She looked like most women hope to look. She was judged unfairly and it was covered horribly by the press.

Guys you can witness it too. On some shows like *"Babewatch,"* they would spray tan abdominal regions on guys. You've seen what they can do with painted on clothes; well they can hit the abs, arms and legs too. Nothing really for the hair on the head though except the Ronco spray paint. Oh well.

So if seeing thin models and actors everywhere isn't enough to stress you out, how about clothing manufacturers that change ladies clothing sizes to include a size zero. Doesn't that mean you don't exist? Now when you shop and you are an *"average sized woman"* you're supposed to find comfort buying a size large? Not likely. That will resonate poorly with almost every woman in the world. That crushes their self-esteem and confidence. Nicely done fashion world.

There are simple principles to eating and dieting. We will cover them and you will understand them and be able to implement them into your life. You can take that to the bank!

> *"They can fix anything they can convince you, you need fixed."* – **Dr. Jay M. Lipoff**

SNAKE OIL SALES

People! There is no short cut. Stop wasting your money! These are billion dollar industries that are preying on your insecurities and desperation. Could be breast size, your cellulite, graying hair, a lack of hair, age defying creams or your big, ugly teeth. Heck your dang pan doesn't boil water right either. Watch enough of these commercials and you might feel so insecure, you will decide to never leave your room.

The only reason companies keep conjuring new ideas, and flooding late night TV with commercials is because people want a magic bullet. Like the spark-o-matic pain reliever, it was just a gas barbeque grill lighter. They swore up and down how great it was, backed it with *"research,"* sold millions and eventually were busted for false advertising and inaccurate claims. But they made their millions because it sounded so good and TV lends products validity.

How many times can we continue to see a new and improved version of existing products? I'm starting to think the stuff I've been buying all these years is junk. Think about this for a second. There is no Easter Bunny. And there's no trick to getting in shape and staying healthy.

Where is the intervention to protect the public? Where is the FCC, FDA, SWAT, ATF, or the A-Team to prevent these companies from ripping off the American people with gimmicks and lies? Actually some of these bogus companies are being hit with huge fines for their false advertising. Fines are in the millions but it happens years later after they ran a successful money making scheme. The people who were taken, do they ever see any of that money recovered?

There still needs to be a regulating system before any product hits TV. A new drink product just hit the market promising to help you lose weight. It has been covered on the news as junk, yet it is still allowed to hit the stores and will likely make millions. Next was the yogurt to help maintain your digestive system. With some clever advertising and brilliant marketing, it's a hit. Now they get accused of making false or misleading claims. These practices need to stop.

"The wise man should consider that health is the greatest of human blessings. Let food be your medicine." – **Hippocrates**

YO-YO DIETS / STARVATION DIETS

This is when someone who diets for a while by not eating, or by eating a very small amount each day. That doesn't sound too smart, does it, considering your body is relying on food for energy?

So they stop eating any calories and start to lose weight. Of course that's what happens. However when there is no energy source for your body to survive, your pancreas secretes glucagon, a hormone that will break down muscle tissue (protein) into glycogen and then convert it into glucose so it can be used as energy. This is known as Gluconeogenesis. The more you do this, the more efficient the body becomes at breaking down muscle tissue as a source of energy.

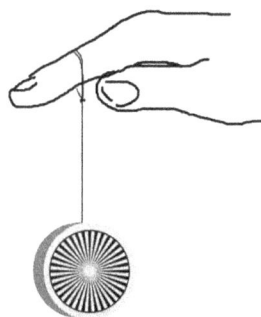

As this process happens water will be released as a by-product and excreted from the body. Much of a diet's first success is due to water weight being lost. That's why you can lose so much weight during the first couple of weeks but remember you are also losing important muscle protein.

So when you first started dieting you were 70 percent muscle and 30 percent fat. As your body struggled to survive, it broke down a lot of muscle and some fat. When you are done with your diet; your weight loss has slowed, you are happy with the results or you can't stay on this diet any longer. You are now at your desired weight and composed of 55 percent muscle and 20 percent fat.

In the process of starving yourself, the body adjusted to your limitation of nutrition. It reset and slowed down your metabolism, the rate your body processes food and turns it into energy. So the first thing that happens when you start to eat again is that the body won't know what to do with all of this food. As more calories are being consumed than the body was used to, it will store the perceived surplus as fat for another day.

The more you return to your normal habits of eating, the more the weight comes on. But this time it returns as fat. Now your body composition becomes 60 percent muscle and 40 percent fat. The more people keep trying this form of dieting, the more their composition changes.

You will end up with a higher percentage of fat and lower percentage of muscle tissue, even though your clothes fit as they did before your diet started. So you might get on the scale and think because you are lighter, that means you must have successfully lost weight, but muscle weighs more than fat. If you have a greater concentration of fat than when you started your diet than of course you weigh less. You have less muscle tissue.

Sumo wrestlers skip breakfast. Then they workout and go to lunch. Because they are so hungry they overeat. Then they take a nap. Memo to self; two things not to do: skip breakfast or nap after eating. Check. Got it!

"To eat is a necessity, but to eat intelligently is an art." **– Francois De La Rochefoucauld**

LIQUID OR JUICE DIETS

I'm a big fan of getting more fruits and vegetables into the American diet. Jack LaLanne, who was one of the all-time greatest fitness gurus, has always touted the benefits of juicing to the public. Juicing would be healthy as part of a balanced diet, but alone it depletes the body of needed fiber. Fiber is needed to help in the transportation of fat through the digestive system and slows the affect of sugars in your body.

There are two types of fiber. Insoluble fiber doesn't dissolve in water and keeps you regular. It is found in foods like whole grains, vegetables, seeds, tomatoes, nuts, bran and zucchini. It speeds transition of food through the digestive tract and maintains a healthy pH in your intestines, which can reduce the likelihood of developing colon cancer.

Soluble fiber dissolves in water, can lower your cholesterol and slow the spike that occurs with the intake of too much sugar into the body. Eating foods like beans, yams, berries, broccoli, carrots, bananas and apples will provide you with this type of fiber. It helps to decrease cholesterol levels in your blood and regulate blood sugar levels in your blood. This is especially important for people with Diabetes.

Many research studies have found that raising your dietary fiber intake is beneficial for both sexes with regards to Type 2 Diabetes, Heart Disease, Diverticulitis, and Irritable Bowel Syndrome, and to a lesser degree Colon Cancer.[83]

If you need to be bonked on the head like in the V-8 commercials than by all means drink your fruits and vegetables juiced. Maybe add some fiber powders to the mixture. An apple a day, and many other foods can keep the doctor away. Try some.

"He who takes medicine and neglects diet wastes the skill of the physician."
– Chinese Proverb

CARBOHYDRATE & FAT BLOCKERS

These are the magic pills that limit the damage you do to your waist when you eat too much of a bad thing. Do these pills work? To some degree they do. They recommend eating in moderation. Well that works to keep weight off anyway. They are supposed to attach to the unwanted fat molecules and make some of them too big to be broken down so they are passed through the body.

Research has shown much higher doses are needed for them to be really effective and there is no guarantee that they will work. Some of the makers of these products have been hit with false advertising lawsuits because they can't substantiate their claims. The side effects from these can be, bloating, cramping, nausea or gas.

Good fats may also be blocked in the process and that is detrimental to your health. Some important vitamins that are fat soluble include A, D, E, and K. If there is not enough fat in the body to break these down, you can develop a deficiency in these vitamins leading to a whole other group of problems.

A study published in *The Journal of Nutrition* found pectin can reduce liver cholesterol and blood cholesterol levels. The highest concentration of natural pectin is found in the peels of citrus fruits like grapefruit, lemons and oranges. Other good sources are apples, plums, carrots, lettuce and spinach.

"The only way to keep your health is to eat what you don't want, drink what you don't like, and do what you'd rather not." – **Mark Twain**

ATKINS DIET / SOUTH BEACH DIET / ZONE DIET

These first two diets limit your carbohydrate intake in one way or another. Without carbs, you break down fats for energy, known as ketosis, and also break down muscle to make glucose, known as gluconeogenesis. You lose water weight because it is a by-product of the production of glucose from muscle.

Having the right carbohydrates is okay. Complex carbohydrates found in whole grains, vegetables, fruit, beans, yams, oatmeal, and dark green vegetables for example are healthy.

Complex carbs are consumed hours before sporting events to provide an energy source during the event. That is why runners are lean and eat plenty of complex carbohydrates the night before marathons.

Too much protein can mean too much saturated fat from meat. Saturated fats can increase your chance of Heart Disease and Cancer, while high protein diets can also stress your kidneys.

The Zone Diet focuses on the Glycemic Index, which ranks how quickly common foods will be broken down into sugar and what affect that will have on the body's insulin levels. This is a clever way to determine which foods will do a body good. If you stick with foods that cause less of a roller coaster ride with your metabolism, you will help your body avoid hunger pains and not overeat.

When sugar enters the body, the pancreas secretes insulin to counter the sugar, like a checks and balances system. Too much sugar in the blood can lead to Heart Disease and Type 2 Diabetes, which is when your body still produces insulin but it is an inadequate amount or the body has minimal to no response to it. Type 2 Diabetes is often associated with a lack of exercise, being overweight and a poor diet.

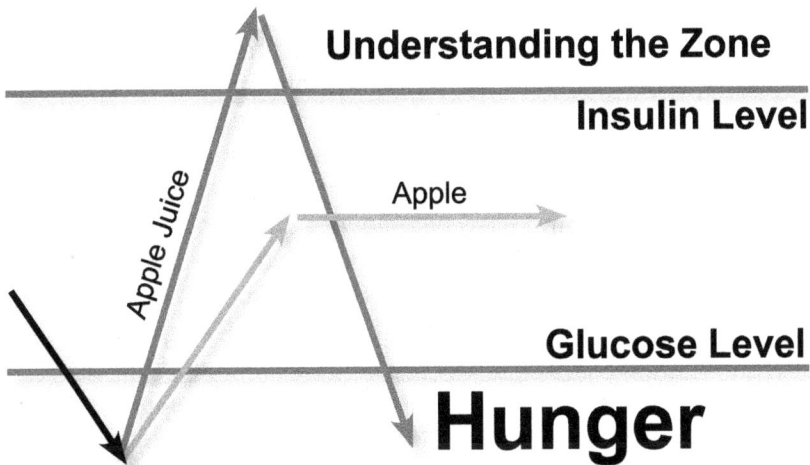

Understanding the Zone

Insulin Level

Apple

Apple Juice

Glucose Level

Hunger

Look at the palm of your hand. Your pinky finger is the floor of the zone, or glucose level, and the pointer finger is the ceiling of the zone, or your insulin level. At all times we should try to keep our glucose levels in the middle of these four fingers. When we get hungry, our blood glucose levels drop below the bottom floor (pinky) of what we consider the zone. The dark arrow on the left demonstrates this.

If we eat an apple, our glucose levels rise to below the pointer finger and stay beneath the ceiling of this zone. This is because the fiber in the apple helps to slow the absorption of sugar and regulates it. The lighter arrow shows the initial rise in blood sugar levels but then evens out to keep your hunger balance within the zone.

If we have a glass of apple juice we send our glucose levels through the ceiling (pointer finger), because there is no fiber to regulate how fast the sugar hits our blood stream. The juice is pure simple carbohydrates and causes the pancreas to over react. This is shown by the medium-colored arrow.

Too much insulin is secreted to counteract the immediate effect of the sugars in our blood. The insulin amount is so great it drops our glucose level back below the floor of the zone. We feel hungry again in a little while. This can cause over eating. We may also feel tired. Ever get slapped with a wave of exhaustion after eating a meal? That's a sign you just ate too much sugar or foods that are high in simple carbohydrates.

Sugars also cause our bodies to slow their metabolism and the insulin converts the excess sugar to be stored as fat. This is how a snack that doesn't have a low Glycemic Index could cause your diet to stumble. You could be doing everything right and then eat a large chunk of birthday cake. The havoc the excess sugars can cause your metabolism can throw it off the track you had been working hard to maintain.

Simple carbohydrates like corn flakes, white bread and juice, have a high Glycemic Index and can lead to other symptoms. For you bread eaters, pumpernickel bread has been shown to have the least effect on the body in relation to the Glycemic Index. Otherwise go with a hearty whole wheat bread. Don't believe the ingredients. Check the weight of the bread. Lots of good grains will make the bread heavy and filled with flavor and benefits.

You may have experienced the *"sugar high"* wave or had it happen to your kids. There's a big birthday party and your kids have snacks, cake and sweetened drinks. They become full of energy and out of control. Being tired usually follows this up, along with possible mood swings. Does this sound familiar?

This is why a bowl of Frosted Sugar Cubes for breakfast makes children in school hyperactive, non-attentive, tired and even diagnosed with ADD. Don't give them the toaster ready, sugar-filled and topped, dessert pastries either. If they say they don't have time to eat properly, then make them get up earlier so they do.

In summary, although some of these diets might work temporarily, they can have damaging side effects. They become very difficult to stick with, which is why diets only last so long. The goal for success is to make a permanent lifestyle change in how you eat, what you eat, when you eat and what you do to help keep your body running on all cylinders.

There is a healthier way to lose weight besides reducing the calories you eat during the day. There is no magic pill you can take to watch those pounds slip away. Starving is definitely not an option. What can you do? I want to give you simple ideas you can implement in your everyday habits to make a difference in your health, posture and life. But first, back to the shenanigans.

"To be always intending to make a new and better life but never to find time to set about it is as to put off eating and drinking and sleeping from one day to the next until you're dead."
– Og Mandino

EATING FOR YOUR TYPE

Some diets have made their money touting that you need to eat a specific way depending either on your blood type, your pH or body shape. Let's look into these and see what the real story is.

A diet specifically designed for your blood type tries to uncover what foods are best absorbed depending on your blood. The belief is that blood types evolved over time. Certain blood types have developed to tolerate meat, some should stick to vegetables, while others can eat any combination.

There is research cited to support this theory in the book if you bought it. However I had trouble finding anyone who supported this diet in any way. Every comment I reviewed claimed the research cited was bunk and no real clinical trials have ever been performed. Personally if you add some cautious eating and exercise to anyone's lifestyle the result will be weight loss. If you have had personal success with this diet, stick with it.

The pH of your body is a way to identify the Hydrogen activity in a certain region of your body. Your body is neither acidic (increased hydrogen activity), nor alkaline (decreased hydrogen activity), it varies depending on what each organ or body part is needed to do. For example, to fight off bacteria and disease, your skin has an acidic pH.

There is some benefit from having the proper pH within your body because it regulates the effectiveness of how the body performs its daily functions. To attempt to eat to make your entire body one way or another would be disadvantageous to your health. If you forced your body into more of an alkaline state, what would that do to your skin's immune function, your digestion, the absorption of nutrients, etc?

Instead of trying to eat for one pH or another, how about you try to eat a balanced diet that contains foods from all categories and let your body function the way it was designed to. If you had a digestive problem and you had too much acid production, or too little, then you could try to eat foods that would be less aggravating to your system. Then maybe you could control stomach acidity without the OTC chemical solutions so readily advertised and offered to the public.

The diet for your body type is next. I could find little information regarding the benefits of eating or exercising specifically for your body type or proof of the effectiveness of this strategy.

People are grouped into different shapes, which are classified as types of fruit ironically. The pear shaped person has normal shoulders but widens at the waist. The apple is a person who holds most of their weight in their torso.

The kiwi is the guy with hair all over his back and the banana is a skinny person hunched over and not *"a-peeling"*. I'm kidding about the last two.

If you have ever seen any of the shows like *"The Biggest Loser"* you will see all kinds of body types. When they exercise and eat properly they all transform their bodies. Instead of being confined to one specific strategy utilize the one constant in all of these plans. You need to eat wiser. Now eat a balanced diet and incorporate some exercise. It's as easy as that.

"What is food to one, is to others bitter poison." - **Lucretius**

GLUTEN FREE DIET

Gluten is a small protein found in grains like barley, wheat and rye. People with celiac disease found avoiding gluten helped keep their bowels happy, stopped stomach pain, diarrhea and facilitated weight loss. It is estimated 1 in 133 people have celiac so it is pretty common. Research also found 5 – 10 percent of the U.S. population may have some form of sensitivity to gluten.

Processed foods like cookies, crackers and muffins are your obvious culprits. Gluten can be found as a thickening or texture agent in ketchup, ice cream, breads, salad dressing, barbeque sauce, cereals, soup, spice blends and a whole lot more. That is why it is difficult to maintain a gluten free diet. Hollywood has made it popular but many have personal chefs.

By demand, more stores are offering a greater selection of gluten free products but there is a price. Some have substituted higher amounts of sugar. Also being gluten-free and avoiding grain sources can cause an absence of much needed vitamins because grains are enriched. Obviously, take a good vitamin and fiber supplement to fill in your nutritional gaps.

I spoke with a friend who decided to include a gluten-free crust at his pizza shop. Unfortunately, he explained he would have to get a completely different oven and area with separate utensils to truly be gluten-free. He's right.

If you order a salad and it comes with bread crumbs and you remove them, the smallest crumb can trigger an intestinal nightmare. They call that cross-contamination. Even oatmeal has to be processed in a separate building that hasn't been used to make any type of wheat products.

Some foods naturally have no gluten, like rice or corn. So there are cereal options for you breakfast eaters. Other foods include: fresh vegetables (no gluten-based wax); fresh meat, fish and poultry; nuts; eggs; soy; fresh fruit; potatoes; water; milk; buckwheat; flax and quinoa to name a few to pick from.

Research goes back and forth with this type of diet but if you have allergies, food sensitivities, or autism it might be worth a try. Have your doctor test you for a gluten allergy. Otherwise I would avoid processed foods and eat a variety of healthy, fresh, organic, undercooked foods from different cultures.

> *"One should eat to live, not live to eat."* – **Moliere**

Rules To Successful Dieting

In order to succeed with a diet, you must understand that it is a change of lifestyle in which you are making certain sacrifices to achieve personal goals; in addition, to becoming a healthier person. Be consistent with your dedication to your health.

Dieting is not about restricting your food. It is about eating healthier, making smarter and more educated decisions about what you put into your body and what you feed your family. Exercise needs to be an important component of your health strategy. Move it to lose it!

*"The **ME PRINCIPLE**. You can eat whatever you want, in **M**ODERATION, with a steady diet of **E**XERCISE!"*

> *"In general, mankind, since the improvement of cookery, eats about twice as much as nature requires."* – **Benjamin Franklin**

SLOW AND STEADY

A safe diet is one on which you lose around one to two pounds a week even though you may lose more initially. That is a reasonable, healthy goal to set for yourself. Most likely your weight has been increasing over months or years and now you have decided it is the time to lose it. The additional pounds didn't come on over night and they aren't going to disappear easily either.

Maybe it is the 20-year reunion; an upcoming wedding or you want to improve your health, posture and life in general. It doesn't matter. The fact is you need encouragement; a realistic plan, determination and you must be patient.

A simple rule is to burn more calories than you put in. If you eat 2,500 calories and only use up 2,000 for energy while you walk, work, play, etc., than you will have a surplus of 500 calories. Over a week, that is 3,500 extra calories that haven't been used and will wind up on your body as one pound of fat. Over the course of one year that could add up to 52 pounds of excess weight.

If you reverse this and use up 2,500 calories and only eat 2,000, then your body will use fat and convert it into energy and you will lose weight. You still have to eat, just smarter. Don't be overly restrictive and add some exercise to your day. A couple of great sites are on the web to help you count calories like www.fitday.com and www.calorieking.com. There are probably other sites similar to these. For a small fee, you type in what you eat and it will count calories. It keeps track so you don't have to and displays it all on screen for you to follow.

A spouse still bringing home Krappy Kreme doughnuts is not going to help your waistline or anyone else's in the family. If it is there, then you have a greater chance to eat it. Get them to change their eating habits with you. Clean out the foods you no longer want and donate them to the local food pantry. Then those foods don't sit there and become a temptation calling to you in a moment of weakness.

Try to get your family or a neighbor involved, or to become cheerleaders for your mission. Participating is really beneficial for everyone and can increase your commitment and success. The more people involved the better your chance of success. When you are a little resistant or tired, your workout partner may just offer the coercing you need to get you back out there.

Other ideas would be to pick the time of day you have the most drive to workout and stick to it. The AM workout is best for your body and you won't have the *"I'm too tired at the end of the day"* excuse to fall back on.

The morning workout can rev up your metabolism and get you running hotter throughout the day. You may actually feel a little euphoric after completing your routine. It is amazing how doing something you know is good for you can lift your spirits.

Figure out a schedule for the week. Planning is part of the key to success. In your plan, vary your exercises to keep things fresh. Varying your routine is more effective way to burn calories and build muscles.

Make it easy to stick to your plan. If you work out at home, set up the equipment for the next day's workout, each time you finish. You don't have to search through the house to find your shorts or a sweaty t-shirt. I leave my shoes right on or by the treadmill. If you go to the gym after or before work; keep a bag ready or in your vehicle so everything you need is right there and waiting for you.

Remind yourself your new schedule is making you healthier, will transform your body, and give you more energy. You can do this.

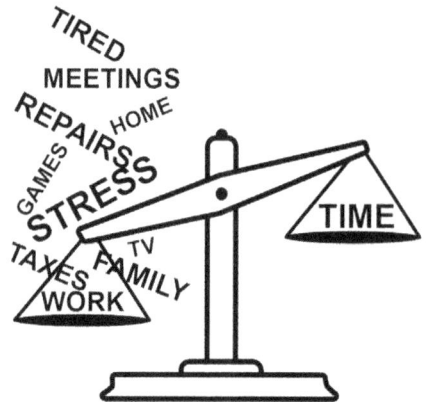

"There is no safety in numbers, or in anything else." – **James Thurber**

SCALE BACK

There is no reason to hear the resonating sound of the numbers that ring up on the scale like a Sunday morning church bell. Hello! Look at me!

Don't watch the scale. Staring at a red stoplight doesn't make it go green any faster either. Everyone knows you have to blow on it. Anyway, micro managing your weight is a surefire way to become discouraged. Each of us can take a long look in the mirror and know if there are any extra pounds that could be lost. Seeing numbers on a scale isn't necessary.

It takes time. Your weight could fluctuate rapidly in the beginning but slow down after a few weeks. You could lose five pounds and gain two the next day. It doesn't mean you are doing anything wrong. Also if you are building muscle and replacing fat, your body will be heavier due to the change in your body's composition.

You may notice a slight difference in the way your clothes fit first. Someone at the office might ask if you've changed anything about your appearance or if you have lost any weight. A belt may need to be switched to a different hole.

As your weight drops you will have increased energy and better self esteem. Now you've got it. Take it slow but be persistent and it will pay off.

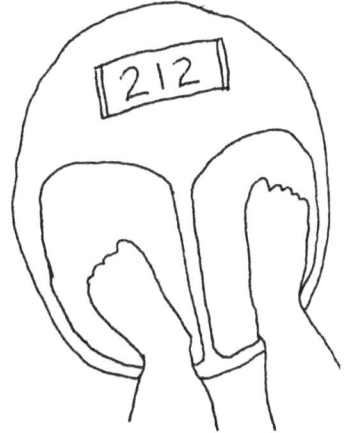

"Nobody realizes that some people expend tremendous energy merely to be normal." – **Albert Camus**

KICK START MY HEART

Each of us has a metabolism that burns food at a specific rate. The faster our metabolism, the more our food is converted into energy and the less fat gets stored. Also if you are burning "hot," then you will burn more calories at rest and may even be able to eat a little more due to your caloric demands.

Your metabolism can be affected by several factors: your activity level, body type regarding the percentage of muscle you have, genetics, your age, how often you eat, your self-discipline, what you eat and what you drink. These are just a few things that can all play a part in regulating your metabolism.

With all these options and more, there are loads of things you can do to burn off extra calories. Let's take a look at some of them so I can help you reach your goal.

"Life goes on within you and without you." – **George Harrison**

TURN UP THE HEAT

There are some foods that can actually help you kick your metabolism into overdrive. Hot sauce, cayenne pepper and anything that adds some spice to your meal can raise your metabolism by up to 20 percent. BAM! Ever notice how fast hot food runs through you? That's the velocity of spicy ferocity. Turn it up! *The Journal of Agricultural and Food Chemistry* recently reported that red chili peppers might actually stunt the growth of fat cells.

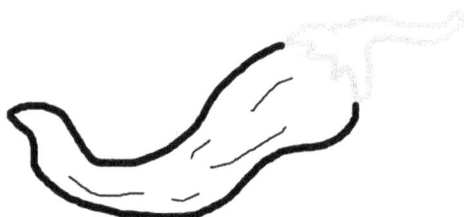

Drinking ice water is an easy way to make your body burn calories because it has to heat up the water to your body's temperature to use it. You already know how important it is to drink 8 glasses of water each day. Well if you knock back eight cold ones it can burn around 200 calories in addition to all of the other health benefits. It's a win-win.

Okay cinnamon may not boost your metabolism but it has been shown to be pretty healthy. Studies have shown that this great spice can help to control the rate glucose enters the blood stream and how it effects the body. This spice has been shown to help diabetic patients with balancing their glucose levels. In addition, it can help lower your bad cholesterol levels. Don't just sprinkle it on your oatmeal or applesauce, put a healthy dose on your foods and enjoy the benefits.

Some other great foods are celery, foods high in protein, green tea, cabbage and grapefruit. They can elevate the rate at which you burn some calories. For the really desperate, or dedicated, depending on how you look at it, you can split your foods up before consumption.

Your body processes food more efficiently when they are ingested separately. You could eat your protein at one sitting and your complex carbs at another, but that takes some real dedication. It also takes the fun out of eating. My suggestion here is to not go overboard. Just eat sensibly.

> *"Everybody gets so much information all day long that they lose their common sense."* **– Gertrude Stein**

SHOP SMART

Half the battle can be won at the store. It is really simple. If you don't buy it, you can't eat it. Replace your old standbys with healthier alternatives. Look for leaner cuts of meat, healthier breads, low fat and low calorie foods and better drinks. Read the labels for the nutrition and junk manufacturers hide in your foods.

Look in your cabinets right now and see what options you are making available to yourself and your family. Look at the labels and read the nutritional values. If it doesn't look like it's healthy than remove it from your house and let's start fresh. If you can't pronounce the ingredients remove that too. Once you conquer control and become portion savvy then, if you want to, you can consider reintroducing these items into your house.

When you go shopping, make sure you have eaten first. If you go while you are hungry, a lot of foods are going to look great in your cart. Having eaten beforehand will allow you to control your urges and keep you from buying foods and snacks you don't really need. Prepare a list and stick to it.

Also when you shop, ask yourself how a pudding with real milk or Cheez Whiz can sit on a shelf that isn't refrigerated. Or when looking at weirdly colored ketchup, snacks, etc, think, *"Are those wild colors really good for my kids?"* Too many preservatives and dyes.

> *"We are indeed much more than what we eat, but what we eat can nevertheless help us to be much more than what we are."* **– Adelle Davis**

CHOW TIME

My Mom drives me crazy with this. *"I'm not hungry. I don't have time to eat in the morning. I just need my coffee."* She has shut down her metabolism to that of a snail. If you have slept for six to eight hours, your body should be hungry. So Mom, if you're listening, if you skip breakfast you are 3.5 times more likely to be overweight. I can't wait to eat. I'd eat my right arm if it wasn't attached and I didn't need it to hold the fork.

You should eat your biggest meal in the morning. It is the foundation for your day and you have all day to work it off. Eat less as the day goes on and you become less active. People, who don't eat in the morning or afternoon, either stuff their face at night because they are starving or dinner becomes the body's one meal.

Your body will slow its metabolism in response to that one big meal because it learns that nutrition shows up once a day. Your body slows down and takes in its one meal and stores much of the food as fat so there will be an energy source for another day. Imagine getting to fill up your car only once a month. You would limit the amount of travel you did (slow your metabolism) and conserve what gas you had (store food as fat) to ensure an energy source for another day.

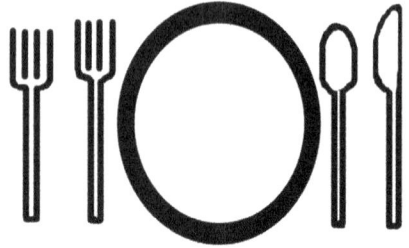

Likewise; eat dinner around 6:00 pm so it too can be digested or worked off. If you need a late night snack, try fruit, vegetables, protein snacks or no fat snacks to start. If you want dessert, don't eat a 400-calorie meal and instantly follow it up with something yummy to the tune of another 400 calories. You will add to the total amount of calories eaten at that one time. That's too many calories at once.

The problem for most of us is we work too hard, come home too late, have errands to run and by the time we sit down to eat its 8 or 9 o'clock. We eat, then wind down and get ready to sleep on a full stomach while our metabolism slows as night approaches. There is no need for the buffet of calories at this time because we have no caloric needs.

> *"It is not these well-fed long-haired men that I fear,*
> *but the pale and the hungry-looking."* – **Julius Caesar**

FEED ME SEYMOUR! FEEEEED ME!

If you wanted to count or watch your calories each day, you could average it out. In order to lose one pound of fat a week you have to eat 3,500 calories less. Or you need to expend 3,500 more calories than you normally would, considering your normal intake for the week.

Let's say you wanted to only eat 2,000 calories a day. If you consistently only eat that amount, you will reset your metabolism for that many calories. Initially you will lose weight but then the body will re-establish itself and maintain your weight. The idea is to oscillate the amount of food so the body has to work every day to process what you give it and burns hotter.

One day have 2,200 calories, the next 1,800 and the next 2,000 and so on. This way you will average out the week the way you wanted to without slowing your metabolism or allowing it to adjust.

If you can add exercise to your week, you could burn 2,000 calories walking the neighborhood for 30 minutes, five days a week, and only reduce your food intake by 1,500 calories. That would equal 3500 calories or one pound.

> *"What difference does it make how much you have? What you do not have amounts to much more."* – **Seneca**

ENOUGH IS ENOUGH

Don't eat too much at one meal. About 300 – 400 calories per meal should keep you satisfied if you eat the right things. Eat 3 – 6 smaller meals throughout the day and you'll never feel hungry. Any more than 400 calories is like putting a large log on a fire instead of small sticks. Sticks, like small meals, burn fast and hot. A large log, or meal, will smolder and take forever to burn.

I tend to eat at 7 am, 10 am, 1 pm, 4 pm, 7 pm and sometimes a light snack around 10 pm. By eating at regular intervals it helps to keep my glucose levels balanced and allows my body to keep functioning like it normally should.

Check the calories associated with the foods you eat. You will be shocked at how many calories are typically consumed with each meal. I'm not trying to get you to eat with a protractor and slide rule. You have a calculator in your head. Just make a mental note as you put foods into your mouth.

Many diet companies that have eating programs try to teach you how to watch calories, equate food with points to regulate carbs, fats and proteins or try to teach portion control. By understanding what goes into your system you can control how much you put in.

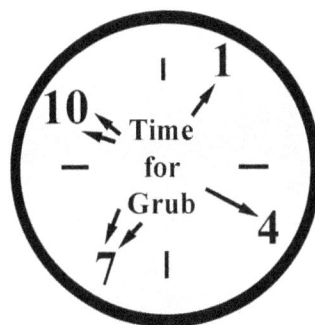

> *"We have no more right to consume happiness without producing it than to consume wealth without producing it."* – **George Bernard Shaw**

YOU GONNA EAT ALL THAT?

Be smart about your eating and portion sizes. When we are hungry we tend to take more than we need. Think about what you put on your plate. Some people like to only go for one serving while others like to eat 80 percent of what they put on their plate. Then there are wives who give the extra to their husbands who can get bigger simply to avoid wasting food.

If you consume too much at one sitting then you have a good chance to store the extra calories as fat that your body keeps available if it needs energy later. In fact, if you eat too much and the content is mainly fat, it is easily converted into body fat that can be stored. If you consume too much protein or carbohydrates, it takes more energy from the body to convert it into fat for storage. So it is better for you if you are going to eat, to have a few extra shrimp. It still doesn't give you a license to overeat. Calories are calories. Think before you chew.

The *"Freshmen 15"* happens when students have free access to all kinds of food. They can eat lots of fried foods and desserts, regularly and in great quantities, with no one telling them not to. It is all about self-discipline, which few of us have at that age.

> *"No amount of experimentation can ever prove me right;*
> *a single experiment can prove me wrong." –* **Albert Einstein**

SEEING IS BELIEVING

Read the label for portion size. Many companies give you a false sense of security about an item by telling you it only has a certain number of calories per serving. For example a bottle of soda may only have 140 calories per serving, but there are 2.5 servings per bottle. Who drinks half of the bottle?

In fact many people drink that with a meal and add to the total amount of calories for their meal without even realizing. Sometimes there are only 120 calories in chips and crackers, if you eat 10 chips.

I remember going to a seminar with my colleagues. The refreshments they provided at this bodybuilding and natural fitness seminar included no fresh fruit, only juices but my favorite was the variety of muffins. Sure they looked good and the wrapper read only 270 calories. The recommended serving was ½ a muffin.

Once again this is about portions and self control. That is why I always say you can eat whatever you want in moderation because the calories are what add up to extra pounds. If you can eat 12 chips, a lean turkey sandwich on pumpernickel bread with mustard and a glass of water for a total of 400 calories, then you've got it. Wait a minute. You had chips??!! I'm kidding.

> *"The cost of a thing is the amount of what I call life which is required to be*
> *exchanged for it, immediately or in the long run." –* **Henry David Thoreau**

COUNT ME IN

Fats, proteins and carbohydrates all have a calorie value for each gram of them you eat. For instance, fat is 9 cal/gram, while proteins & carbs are just 4 cal/gram. Because fats have such a high calorie count, they are denser and give you that full feeling.

A simple rule to try and follow would be to look for foods with labels that have 10:1 total calories to, fat calories. For example: 100 total calories, with 10 calories from fat. You will get plenty of fats from cooking your food or eating more nutritious foods if they contain healthy fats.

Protein increases your metabolism by 30 percent, but eating too much protein can damage your kidneys and still lead to weight gain. Protein sources are: meats like fish, beef, chicken, eggs, turkey and pork, and vegetables like soybeans or tofu, grains like rice, quinoa flax, and nuts. This is a second energy source when you eat a balanced diet. It should be served on your plate like a side order to your carbohydrates instead of occupying the majority of your plate.

Here's a neat math problem. You buy lean hamburger meat that is 95 percent lean. In a portion there are roughly 150 calories. There are approximately 25 grams of protein (x 4 calories per gram = 100 calories from protein), there are 0 carbohydrates and 5 grams of fat (x 9 calories per gram = 45 calories from fat). So if the total number of calories is 150, almost one third of the meat, 45 calories, comes from fat. A lot of meat fat is saturated too, which isn't healthy for your arteries or your heart. Limit the red meat in your diet or eat very lean pieces.

Nutrition Facts/Datos De Nutrición

Serving Size/Tamaño por Ración 1/2 cup/taza (120g)
Servings Per Container/Raciones por Envase about/acerca 26

Amount Per Serving/Cantidad por Ración	
Calories/Calorías 110 Calories from Fat/Calorías de Grasa 20	
	% Daily Value*/% Valor Diario*
Total Fat/Grasa Total 2g	3%
Saturated Fat/Grasa Saturada 0.5g	3%
Trans Fat/Grasa Trans 0g	
Cholesterol/Colesterol 0mg	0%
Sodium/Sodio 410mg	17%
Total Carbohydrate/Carbohidrato Total 18g	6%
Dietary Fiber/Fibra Dietética 8g	32%
Sugars/Azúcares 3g	
Protein/Proteína 6g	

2 grams of fat @ **9** calories per gram = **18 cal. from fat** (roughly 20 total) 18 grams of carbohydrates @ **4** calories per gram = **72 cal. from carbs** 6 grams of protein @ **4** calories per gram = **24 calories from protein** **18 + 72 + 24 = 114 total calories**. (As you can see, it's not perfect math but it gives you an idea on how to determine where your calories come from.)

> *"...when you have eliminated the impossible, whatver remains, however improbable, must be the truth."* – **Sir Arthur Conan Doyle**

DON'T BELIEVE THE HYPE

Many diets tell us to stay away from carbohydrates. The problem is certain carbohydrates are good and some not so good. Simple carbohydrates are the source of all this crazy talk. These foods like candy, table sugar, white flour and pasta are more calories than nutrition. We call them empty calories. It is easier to eat two cookies than two chicken breasts and there are more calories in the cookies.

Remember when too much sugar, or a food easily converted into sugar, enters the blood stream too fast, you start a roller coaster ride with the balance of your insulin and glucose levels. The pancreas overreacts and secretes too much insulin as a counter measure and sends glucose levels down. When your glucose levels drop really low you feel hungry again or tired. This leads many people to overeat or become tired after lunch while at work.

You need complex carbohydrates like whole grains, fruits, vegetables and beans. These break down in the body slowly, providing you with vitamins, minerals, and fiber that help you feel fuller for a longer period of time. Anywhere from 40 – 60 percent of your calories should come from complex carbohydrates.

Carbohydrates are your primary energy source for your body. Absorption starts in the mouth. That is why it is important to chew your food completely. Without complex carbs, your body will break down muscle into glucose for energy.

> *"The cost of living is going up and the chance of living is going down."*
> **– Flip Wilson**

FAT CHANCE

Fats are important for your body to function properly. They are: an insulator for vital organs; transport for Vitamins A, D, E & K; a long-term energy source like with aerobic exercise; and they support the nervous system.

We should get 10 – 25 percent of our calories from healthy fats but unfortunately we are at 40 percent. There are several types of fat, which is where the confusion starts. They all contain the same amount of calories so decreasing fat in your diet can help you lose weight. Saturated fats are solid or semi-solid at room temperature and should be only seven percent of our diet. One way to think of saturated fat is when bacon grease cools and becomes a solid again.

Oils remain liquid because they are unsaturated. Hydrogenation bonds hydrogen to these oils. The molecules are super-heated and contorted into the bad "trans" formation from the normal good "cis" form. Partially hydrogenated oils are used to make donuts, cookies and breads, to increase their shelf life, and also fried chicken and French fries. Both inhibit the body's ability to regulate cholesterol, are difficult to digest and become stuck in our blood as cholesterol. Experts agree we need to avoid trans fats that form this way and the above types of foods are a major source of the trans fatty acids consumed in the US.

In general, trans fats are far worse than saturated fats, but both of these fats can slow your metabolism, increase your weight, have been linked to higher coronary Heart Disease, lower good cholesterol levels (HDL) and higher bad cholesterol (LDL). Other diseases being researched for how fats impact them include: Diabetes, Liver Disease, Obesity and Cancer.

Foods like palm oil, coconut oil, chocolate, non-lean meats, whole dairy products and butter have saturated fats and should be consumed sparingly.

The healthier fats are unsaturated. Polyunsaturated fats are found in fish oils, walnuts and dark sesame oil. Monounsaturated fats have been found to be beneficial to heart health, lower cholesterol levels and less inflammation. These fats can be broken down in the body. Sources are organic canola oil, extra virgin olive oil, soybeans, almonds, most other nuts, avocado, fish such as salmon, shrimp and chunk light tuna, and lean meats including bison and ostrich.

> *"Estimated amount of glucose used by an adult human brain each day, expressed in M&Ms: 250."* – **Harper's Index**

YOU'RE SO SWEET

Eat your calories, don't drink them. Eating an orange is much healthier than drinking its juice. Juice is a simple sugar or carbohydrate and your body needs complex carbs and fiber. The simple juice causes that spike in your insulin levels whereas the fiber from a whole fruit keeps you in *"the zone"* and in check. However, drinking 100 percent juice is far better than the imposters companies put on our shelves as healthy.

All those mislabeled, cute 10 percent juice drinks for kids, sodas, sports drinks, elderly drinks, etc, are just full of calories. Read the labels. They are water with sugar, high-fructose corn syrup and junk. People who drank their carbohydrates were compared to those who ate the same amount of calories in solid food versions in the form of jellybeans. The people who drank their calories showed a significant weight gain.[84]

Some drinks aimed at kids like Ovaltine boast how great they taste and that they are good for you because they have a vitamin dissolved in their chocolate drink mix. Whoopty-doo! Stop the presses. Then why does it contain sugar as its first ingredient? If sugar is ever in the first three ingredients then try something else. It's crap! Read the ingredients, not just the label. Marketing is trying to convince you and the kids that this is a healthy alternative to something else. It's not.

Here's the only catch. If you are exercising vigorously then a sports drink may help replenish your energy sources because your body needs the carbs and electrolytes for fuel. Those simple carbs can satisfy this need for an immediate energy source and help replenish your system during physically, demanding activity.

This is the only time it is recommended because your body has a need for the simplest form of sugars it can utilize immediately and following rigorous activity. Without carbohydrates, you deplete muscle tissue for energy. That's why some guys work out for years and never get bigger. They forgo replenishing the body and end up losing muscle as the body converts it into an energy source.

In fact, after each swig, top your drink with water. This will increase the amount of water you consume each day and offset what you lose as you sweat. But drinking these sugary drinks all day does nothing but add calories to your day.

Now soda has been shown to cause an increase in calcium and bone demineralization or loss. What is more concerning is that it's happening to teenage girls. As if Osteoporosis down the road isn't enough, dumping sugar water like this into your body only adds to the problems. Each person in America consumed around 575 cans of soda in 1997 and the soda companies responded to the demand by producing more than 56 gallons of their health depleting nectar for every person the following year.[80]

> *"The ingredients of health and long life, are great temperance, open air, easy labor, and little care."* – **Sir Philip Sidney**

CHEAP AND NASTY

There are many different sweeteners today thanks to companies looking for cheaper alternatives to boost profits. They can help to cut calories too. The USDA reported that in 2001, each person consumed 147 pounds of various types of sweeteners.

High fructose corn syrup (HFCS), which was introduced in the '70s, is a highly concentrated sweetener and makes up over 62 pounds of the total consumed. Fructose in small amounts in fruit is fine. We are consuming a concentrated version of it in large amounts because it is used in jams, cereals, bread, wheat crackers, chips, protein bars, dairy products and ketchup. Two-thirds of its use is in sodas.

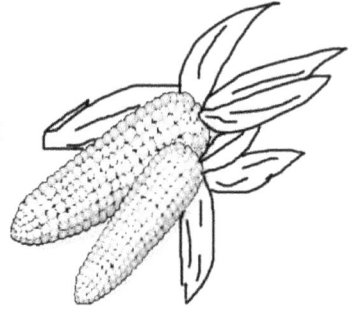

Interestingly, HFCS correlates to an increase in average weight among Americans ever since its introduction.[85] In fact it has increased its usage over 1,000 percent from 1970 to 1990, greater than any other substance, and comprises more than 40 percent of all sweeteners added to foods and drinks.[86]

In addition to that, one recent study in *The Environmental Health Journal* found 9 out of 20 samples of HFCS to contain mercury. Next the Institute for Agriculture and Trade Policy detected mercury in nearly one third of the 55 common household products manufactured by Quaker, Hunt's, Hershey's, Smucker's, Kraft, Kellogg's, and Yoplait. Sadly the FDA sat on this for a couple of years.

The problem is that there is no insulin response to high fructose corn syrup. With glucose there is an insulin response and that increased insulin level can suppress appetite.[87] Insulin also increases the release of leptin,[88] which controls appetite,[89,90] into the body Without an insulin response there is no increase in leptin, which allows you to continue ingesting unlimited calories without feeling satisfied and ultimately will cause weight gain. Large amounts of fructose will also increase the storage of calories as fat, a process known as lipogenesis.

Check your foods and say no to high fructose corn syrup. Products guilty of hurting your health include: bodybuilding products like EAS, cereals like Special

K and All-Bran, Ensure for the elderly, Go-Gurt for kids, Sunny D, Gatorade G2 and the list of fake nutritious foods goes on and on. Some baby formula's first ingredient is corn syrup solids. Don't forget your sauces and dressings too, like pickle relish, Cool-Whip, barbeque sauces, Ketchup, salad dressing and more.

Then the corn industry ran commercials with one person refusing to consume food or drinks because it contains high fructose corn syrup. They comment, *"You know what they say."* The other person replies, *"What, that it's made from corn?"* Television magic at its best. They should have lie detectors on people when they say this stuff. However public pressure is making companies change.

More and more are placing a *"No High Fructose Corn Syrup"* on their labels because consumers are smarter and they demand better. Otherwise sales drop.

Further evidence was a study published in Behavioral Neuroscience by Purdue University found the artificial sweeteners in just one can of soda a day can reset your metabolism and cause you to overeat. In addition, it can increase your risk of diabetes and stroke. *"Drop the pop."*

If you were going to use a form of sugar, I would stick with natural forms that nature has provided like honey, maple syrup, organic and real sugar, fruit, molasses and brown sugar. I like to be sweetened naturally, and in moderation. In general, consuming less processed foods of any kind is smarter. I realize they were designed to reduce tooth decay, calories and cause less blood-sugar spikes. I'm not sure we get all the facts from big companies until there's a problem with sweeteners like Aspartame, Acesulfame K, Maltodextrin, Sucralose, etc.

A problem with sugar for us old folks is that it can increase the inflammation within our bodies. Along with high-fat meats, processed meats, like cold cuts or hotdogs, junk food and sodas, this can increase joint pain. So if you have arthritis or inflammation, eliminating these foods and following a healthier, balanced diet can make you feel young again.

"No amount of artificial reinforcement can offset the natural inequalities of human individuals." – **Henry P. Fairchild**

WHAT A CROCK

Some companies are advertising protein drinks, like Boost and Ensure, to our youth and elderly, that are nothing more than water and sugars as the first three ingredients. I think they recently stopped using high fructose corn syrup. Some healthcare professionals recommend it because it's easy. Does this sound like a drink you want any person drinking? How about someone who is sick and needs quality nutrition? Better read some labels.

You can get 13 grams of protein and 8 grams of carbohydrates by just drinking an eight ounce cup of milk. In their defense, Ensure High Protein does have a better nutritional profile. Another quick source of protein would be to check a health store out, or go online and research protein powders, which actually give you protein minus the sugar and corn syrup. You still need to read the labels and ingredients.

When the food or drink contains words like all natural, granola, fruit, whole grain, diet, fat-free, no unhealthy fats, low carb, etc., slowly back away from your cart, bring your hands up and turn the label around. These containers have been found guilty of misleading the public. Don't believe them. Everything from cereal to drinks to snacks, are part of the scam. It's more about marketing than substance. They are more concerned with making a dollar than making you healthier. I'm pretty sure whole grain Lucky Charms is not really a part of a balanced diet, or a recommended one.

Read the labels for: sugar as one of the top ingredients; as well as, partially hydrogenated fats and oils; white or bleached flour; things you can't pronounce; or the serving size small enough that it wouldn't feed a hamster.

Fruit snacks are all sugar. Cut up the fruit into fun, small pieces and eat the real stuff. Don't be taken by big company's false claims on their products. Their goal is to sell. Like dangling a worthless toy in front of a kid that you can only get in an *"un-happy meal."* It's about marketing a product.

For instance, a Hostess fruit pie sounds healthy because it has fruit. Wrong. How about 400 calories and 200 from fats? Gulp!

Speaking of blatantly lying to the public, milk can no longer say it helps you lose weight. Apparently there is no research to back it up and doctors across America complained enough to have this fraudulent statement stopped. Heck if they were going to say something deceiving for sales, I would have said it helps you grow hair back. That would get some sales. Of course it is only helpful if you have hair that is black and white. Mooo.

> *"I believe in getting into hot water; it keeps you clean."* – **G. K. Chesterton**

GIVE ME SOME WATER

Drink plenty of water each day. If you are thirsty, then you are already dehydrated. Over 70 percent of the body is made of water. The body can use anywhere from ½ gallon to 1 ½ gallons of water each day, depending on your size, temperature, environment and physical requirements. This helps prevent dehydration.

If you have trouble drinking water, you can try bottled, steamed, tap, wet, mineral, natural spring, distilled, hose or bath water. Chances are bottled water came out of some dude's hose on a farm in the Adirondacks, if you're lucky. So fill your own bottles and reduce the plastic waste. Drink your tap water, as it is generally cleaner than *"fancy"* waters in many studies.

If you need to, squeeze some lemon or orange into it to give it a little flavor. It's water. It isn't going to taste like lemonade. Otherwise they would have called it, well, lemonade. Coffee and tea are not water. They are diuretics, which mean they help your body rid itself of excess water.

If the bottled water you're drinking says anything or uses catchy phrases like healthy, magic, muscle or energy before the word water, it's not water. I don't care what it reads; it is filled with sweeteners and crud. Go natural. *"If it ain't clear, it ain't water."* The only time water should be colored is when it is in your toilet bowl to help disinfect and clean the bowl. You don't want to drink that either.

When someone is lost, the most important thing to stay alive is to have a source of clean, drinkable water. We can survive by breaking down our bodies for energy. Without water our normal body functions and organs stop working. Water plays important roles: in breathing, circulation, temperature regulation, digestion, waste removal, lubricating joints, protecting and insulating the body, and maintaining flexibility in muscles, ligaments and joints.

Water also helps mobilize fat for energy, can suppress hunger, helps to flush your body of harmful toxins, and is vital to your health. An easy way to monitor how much water you need is to check the color of your urine. If it is colorless or light, then you are drinking enough. If the color is dark yellow, then you would be wise to add some good old H2O to your day.

In fact, those plastic bottles you buy water in are not only polluting the planet, but seeping harmful bisphenol-A (BPA), a toxin into your body. Many health problems are being linked to BPA, like Autism and Cancer, so chill your own water and get safer stainless steel containers. Eating, buying and drinking foods that come in plastics, like Tupperware containers, aren't safe either.

Supposedly if the number on the bottom of your plastic reads 5, 4, 1 or 2, then it is okay for you. I would stop eating and drinking out of plastic altogether, especially hard plastic. I would hand wash them and never microwave or put them in the dish washer because of the intense heat will release harmful toxins.

BPA also lines canned foods. It has been found to seep estrogen containing compounds into those foods inside the can and can cause genetic changes, sterility and worse, to you and your kids. Most recently, researchers from Goethe University in Germany and the University of Rochester, NY found these hormones can have a negative effect on our reproductive hormones. It's scary stuff. Hey, I'm just a messenger. I'm as frustrated with the situation as the next person.

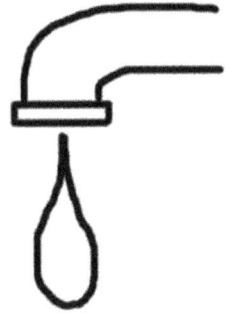

"I have taken more out of alcohol than alcohol has taken out of me." – **Sir Winston Churchill**

EASY ON THE SAUCE

Most people like to consume some alcohol when they go out for a drink or enjoy a party. It helps us to relax and kick back. The problem comes when food is close at hand. Eating while drinking alcohol should be avoided because it decreases our self-control. You may eat a lot of calories you normally wouldn't.

In addition, alcohol slows the metabolism. So if you have been working out and eating right to reset your metabolism to burn more calories, you may just set yourself back. Some alcohol comes with a mixer. Tonic water, soda, daiquiris and other mixers can make one drink contain 300 calories or more. That's why all those fruity drinks you have on a cruise or sunny beach can add up to extra *"luggage"* on the way home.

Alcohol also dehydrates the body. So mixing in a glass of water into the rotation will help decrease the amount you drink, and take the edge off of a hangover by rehydrating the brain.

As a side bit of information, a recent study found that women who drank two to three drinks a day had a higher incidence of breast cancer.

"Anyone can do any amount of work provided it isn't the work he is supposed to be doing at the moment." – **Robert Benchley**

DON'T HIT THE SNOOZE

Never eat a meal and take a nap. You are loading your engines and then allowing the food to sit there and not be used. What do you think will happen to it? Remember, eating and sleeping are what sumo wrestlers do to help them get big. Ever look around and see the waistlines of people who have sedentary jobs? The chances of gaining weight if your job requires more sitting than moving around is very high.

Try to be active. Walk to lunch and walk back. Get up a few times and run some errands or go to the water cooler for some exercise, liquid refreshment and the latest gossip. Otherwise try to limit your intake of food if you know you are going to have to go back to work and sit. Ever have that sleepy-time feeling after lunch. Eat quality foods with minimal simple carbs to prevent it.

> *"If more of us valued food and cheer and song above hoarded gold,*
> *it would be a merrier world." – **J. R. R. Tolkien***

I NEVER INHALED

Eat meals slowly. This allows sufficient time for the brain and stomach to decide when you should be full. Eating too fast never allows that communication to happen when it should.

Chewing each bite 30 times can improve nutrient absorption by up to 50 to 80 percent and give your body a chance to feel full so you'll eat less. This happens because you have broken down large pieces into smaller pieces so the body utilizes them more efficiently. You will tire out the muscles of mastication, or chewing. If they get tired you are also less likely to keep eating.

Try not drinking until after you swallow your food. This will ensure you chew and breakdown your food more completely, and can help you eat less. Some people take a bite of food, swig some of their drink and swallow. They never had the satisfaction of eating or chewing and will probably eat more than they should because of it.

I love to eat. It is a wonderful time and I look forward to preparing a healthy meal, when I can. I am doing something good for my body and that makes me feel great. Try it and savor the moment instead of rushing through it like a nasty chore or interruption to your day. In other countries they set aside time during their work day to enjoy a wonderful meal with friends and colleagues.

> *"Never eat more than you can lift." – **Miss Piggy***

LOVE SNACK, BABY LOVE SNACK

Snacks are the filler between when we have time to really relax and eat a meal. I need a snack at around 10 am and 4 pm. That's because I eat smaller meals throughout the day. When I am working on patients I have to come up with an easy snack so it is quick, otherwise I get cranky when I get hungry. You wouldn't like me when I'm cranky.

Nuts and seeds are perfect for snacks. Raw has less salt and all of the healthy goodness we want. Roasted nuts lose 15 percent of the healthy fats they started with. Choose foods like raw almonds, pumpkin seeds, sunflower seeds, walnuts, cashews and flax seeds. If you need them roasted and lightly salted, they are still better than some of the alternatives like candy or chips. You can even roast them yourself and control what goes on them like wasabi, cayenne, garlic salt or a barbeque mix.

Fresh fruits or vegetables may do the trick. I also keep an ample supply of protein drink mix and protein bars on hand for on demand needs when real food isn't an option.

> *"I like children. If they're properly cooked."* – **W.C. Fields**

IS SOMETHING BURNING?

Don't overcook your vegetables. Over cooking can deplete the healthy nutrients you are trying to get from these foods. Some research also suggests that foods too hot or browned are difficult for the body to digest and process. Raw is much better. Yummy.

Hey, grow a garden so you know exactly what is on your food and in it. Now we have to wash our fruits and vegetables with hydrochloric acid. It seems to remove coloring, waxes and pesticide residuals.

It is difficult to say what is in our meats too. The faster meat sources are brought to market the quicker money can be made. I have seen chicken breasts that must have come from a Pterodactyl. I sure wouldn't want to be the one trying to catch it. Some meats are sprayed to look redder than they are and you don't want that in your system either.

Try steaming, stewing or slow, crock pot cooking your foods to preserve important vitamins, minerals and their natural nutritional value. Blackening foods on a grill or in a pan has been found to contain carcinogens. Whether you are steaming, micro waving, grilling or sautéing your veggies, just don't overdo it.

> *"It is the quality of our work which will please God and not the quantity."*
> – **Mahatma Gandhi**

SUPER ISN'T ALWAYS SUPERIOR

Our society has bombarded us with bigger drinks and meals at the fast foods restaurants. I consider these *"fat"* food restaurants. It is tough to walk away from a deal that means you get more for your money. Except when the price we pay becomes evident in our waistline.

We have more buffets than streetlights. My favorite in Syracuse is the Old Country Buffet located right next to a diet center. Now if you're a client of that center, and still lose weight while they dangle food right next to you, you are strong willed. I give you credit.

Over the years we have increased the size of the plates we use to eat. Now when you put food on it, you tend to put more than you need because the plate looks empty. Get rid of these enormous platters and buy some smaller dishes. It might help you eat less. Also decreasing the utensil size may help. If you eat cereal with a big spoon it may take 20 spoonfuls, but with a smaller spoon it could take 30 and trick you into eating less.

"Supersize Me" was an enlightening film if you haven't seen it. I just watched a commercial similar to the movie's outcome in which the customer asks for a

¼ sized heart attack, a side of thunder thighs and some cavities to go. Nice! That kind of convenience and speed comes at a price. Your health.

Large **$.75**

$.50 S~~uper~~ Stupid -sized

Similarly, a recent study from Sweden researched what would happen to people if they ate fast food twice a day for four weeks and decreased their activity level. They found the average person gained 16 pounds and had significant damage to their liver because of the high content of fat in the commonly consumed fast food items. The fat levels were so high the body could not process the amount of fat and ended up storing it in the liver's cells. Moral to the story is to limit the amount of fat and calories with every meal.

But seriously, I have a whole problem with just their marketing schemes. When has your burger had whole leaves of lettuce and rings of onions on it and not the chopped up versions? Why do they gently lay the insides of the sandwich and pile it on high in the commercials? Anytime I've had no other options and had to resort to ordering a sandwich, it looks like it was sat on. Why do they cut the sandwiches at an angle when they show it? To make it look bigger and more appetizing. It's never as good as the commercial anyway, so why bother.

How many times can the pizza be recreated? Twice as much cheese. Three times the meat. Extra dipping sauce. Eight times the calories and fat, is what they should say. Not so appetizing anymore is it?

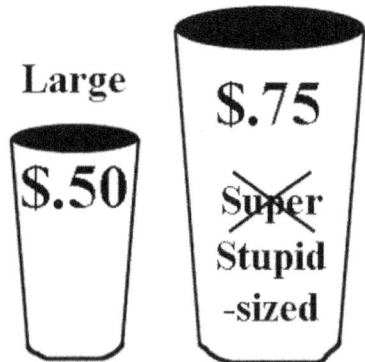

"You don't have to cook fancy or complicated masterpieces - just good food from fresh ingredients." **– Julia Child**

THE REPLACEMENTS

We didn't like them in football and we don't like them in our foods. You are better off eating real foods in controlled amounts. Use the sugar instead of an engineered substitute. I trust what makes sense. Nature. Real maple syrup, old-fashioned brown sugar and honey are examples of sweeteners us older folks used to use in moderation. We survived and are thinner.

I have heard too many reports how an item is safe to eat; or it's okay but causes gas, only to hear of people getting sick from that very food months or years later. They have engineered fats now with a side effect of gas production or diarrhea. For the love of your family, and everything in this world that you cherish, don't eat the item that produces extra gas. We already produce about ½ a gallon a day as is. No need to kick that into overdrive.

A Purdue University study was released in *The Journal of Behavioral Neuroscience* and found artificial sweeteners cause overeating in rats. They reported that because there is no calorie intake with these sweeteners like the body normally expects when digesting sweet foods, they kept eating. The body becomes confused and over-consumes more calories to meet its expectations. The study reported the weight gained was mostly in the form of fat too.

Some skeptics replied that the test was on rats so it isn't transferable to humans. Funny, because why do they test all of those poor animals with drugs and shampoos if there is no relation to the effects of these chemicals on humans? A 2005 University of Texas Health Science Center survey found people who consume one diet soft drink a day had a 41 percent greater risk of being overweight.

I have always taught moderation. If you want to drink a reasonable amount of soda per day, just be aware of the other foods you are eating at that time, so you don't fall into the same trap as the rats.

> *"Health nuts are going to feel stupid someday, lying in hospitals dying of nothing."* – **Redd Foxx**

YOU'LL GET NOTHING AND LIKE IT?

Fat free snacks are sometimes a good alternative to satisfying an urge, but beware. Just because it says fat free doesn't mean it is calorie free.

Calories are as much a major source of obesity as eating fatty foods. You don't have all the fat in some of your favorite snacks but you will be shocked at the number of calories. Also watch out for those partially hydrogenated fats. They are no good either.

Remember if you need to eat something bad, watch the calories and eat it earlier in the day as opposed to at bedtime. This way you have some extra time to work it off.

I had a Girl Scout try to sell me cookies and proclaimed they are healthier, after I told her they aren't too healthy. She said they have no trans fats now. I showed her the box and taught her how to read the nutrition guide and that in fact, the partially hydrogenated fats in the ingredients are a trans fat. Remember, trans fats stop Leptin from being released in your body, which in turn prevents your stomach's auto shutoff from being initiated when it's full. Now you'll likely eat too much. Because Girl Scouts of America only gets about 50 cents per box, I would rather give the Scouts 20 bucks, than have to purchase 40 boxes of cookies so they could raise the same money.

> *"Nothing will benefit human health and increase the chances for survival of life on Earth as much as the evolution to a vegetarian diet."* – **Albert Einstein**

NOW THAT'S SOME GOOD EATIN'

These fruits and vegetables are some of the tastiest, healthiest and most awesome foods you can never get enough of. This is my gotta have it category of foods. Great fruits and vegetables like apples, blueberries, broccoli, spinach and other dark leafy vegetables, cantaloupe, cranberries, dark grapes, grapefruit, strawberries, tomatoes, and yams. How about a nice dark green salad with blueberries or cranberries, chickpeas, broccoli, fresh tomatoes and spinach?

I also eat a wide variety of foods like oatmeal, hummus, black rice, pumpernickel bread, some soy products, almonds, hot and spicy foods, dark chocolate, chicken, seafood and an occasional red meat. If I am drinking socially I stick with dark beer, red wine or Vodka on the rocks with a splash of flavor. I'm not a big drinker so I prefer full-bodied taste and quality over quantity.

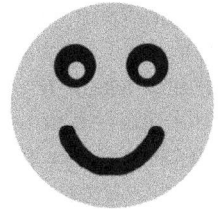

> *"Man does not live by words alone, despite the fact that sometimes he has to eat them."* – **Adlai E. Stevenson Jr.**

THAT'S THE FLAX, JACK

One food that deserves a little extra attention is flax seed and flax oil. Flax was used by the Roman Empire and Hippocrates as a medicine, due to its healing properties. Companies don't like flax oil because it costs more to produce, has a short shelf life and isn't as profitable as the ones filled with hydrogenated oils which can last forever.

Buy flax oil in small, dark containers and keep it cool, away from light and air. It can spoil quickly. Heating this oil can deplete the healthy essential fats that make flax so healthy. You can mix it into yogurt, cereal, into shakes, on salads, or just give me a straight shot, Bartender. It can actually help the absorption of foods.

Flax oil and seeds have been shown to promote heart health, improve colon function, increase your immunity, promote healthy skin, stabilize blood sugar levels, they are precursors for brain growth and can increase your body's metabolism. Now you can even buy it as a powder, which makes it easier to add to anything. It tastes like wheat germ.

Chia seeds, yes, like the ones used for a Chia Pet, have the same health benefits as flax but contain higher amounts. They add a fun crunch to your food without any flavor. You can add both types of seeds to anything you want. Once again, nature's miracle to your health's rescue.

"Do not go where the path may lead, go instead where there is no path and leave a trail."
– Ralph Waldo Emerson

ON THE ROAD AGAIN

When traveling, try to bring some healthy foods along so if you or the munchkins get hungry, you have something nutritious. Unfortunately what you can bring on airplanes has been severely restricted. I used to bring things like water, unroasted & unsalted almonds, cherry tomatoes, sunflower seeds, protein bars, dark chocolate, apples and bananas. Not all at once. They wouldn't let me on with my shopping cart.

Bringing snacks when travelling by car, bus or train is a lot easier, but choose wisely. Kind of like when I said: *"If you don't buy it, you can't eat it."* Well, shop just as smart when it comes to snacks on a trip. Pretzels (they even have pumpernickel now), baked chips, carrots or celery, nuts or whole grain crackers might fulfill that urge for crunching.

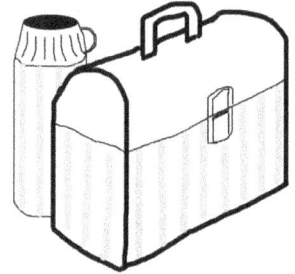

I like to bring healthy cereals and grape or cherry tomatoes. Once in a while I will find a cereal with high protein, low carbs and not a lot of other junk in it. That will do the trick for me. I get the satisfaction of crunching down on a chip-like food. But then again I would probably eat the sole of an old shoe if the research convinced me it would be healthy for me.

"Every patient carries his own doctor inside him. They come to us not knowing that truth. We are at our best when we give the doctor who resides within each patient a chance to go to work." **– Albert Schweitzer**

MAN'S GOT TO KNOW HIS LIMITATIONS

Eliminating certain foods from our diet can make us healthier. A great place to start would be to reduce the amount of sugar we consume each week. Soda has normal sugars and diet soda has bioengineered sugars. Fake sugars have been linked to many health problems like diabetes[81], obesity and bone loss in adolescents[79]. Patients are amazed how much weight they lose just by removing soda from their diet. The calories from sugary drinks can really add up.

With all of your foods, check the labels. Sugar is fine in small amounts but when it sneaks into the majority of our foods it becomes unhealthy. The low calorie or no fat salad dressing you eat is mostly sugar. I mentioned how fat slows your metabolism down. Fat-free ice cream has no fat to slow the rate of sugar absorbed by the body, so you go through the rise in blood sugar levels. This leads to energy levels dropping, tiredness and unnecessary eating. That sugar rollercoaster ride can wreak havoc on your body. You would be better off eating a reasonable portion of regular ice cream.

Desserts, my weakness, are a big problem especially regarding timing. I know I would just as soon eat the six cookies in the pack in one day versus eating chunks of them and making them last. The sooner I get rid of them by demolishing them or tossing them out, the sooner they are no longer a threat. And if you know a food is a problem, don't buy it! Then there is no temptation.

More importantly, families eat dinner and then sometimes move right to the next course. Let the meal digest and wait before you knock back another 350 calories. How many families roll out the dessert tray soon after everyone has waddled their way to a couch? It's too much too soon.

I didn't say no more desserts ever. I suggested waiting, decreasing the portion, or how about yogurt with fresh berries. If you can limit the amount of sugar you eat, the pounds will melt away.

If it's fried then it has saturated fats or they are using an under-researched fat alternative to reduce the amount of saturated fat in a food. Try another way to prepare the food or don't eat that one food all the time. If you like chicken wings for example: don't eat them every night but try having less at one sitting; eat them once a week or two; or, eat breast meat lightly fried in healthier oil with wing sauce.

Maybe you like French fries or potato chips. Thinly slice potatoes or sweet potatoes, brush with a low saturated fat oil and flavor with salt, pepper, dill, garlic, onion or vinegar. Place them in a tray in the oven to bake. Have fun making your own treat. It is also a great learning and family cooking experience.

> *"It is hard enough to remember my opinions, without also remembering my reasons for them!"* – **Friedrich Nietzsche**

HERE'S THE STORY

You pick what you like. I am merely making recommendations so you can find some ideas and take what works and makes sense. It is difficult in this day and age to be so dedicated to changing the entire way you have been raised, or how you buy and prepare food. Congratulations if you are one of the many who have been able to completely overhaul the kitchen and eat organic, raw, undercooked foods.

To the rest of you, it is okay to cheat. We are only human. I don't know how long we each have on this planet, so enjoy life. Try to change a few eating habits to ones that are healthier and hopefully you can enjoy some more time on our rock.

There is a reason our country is one of the most unhealthy in the world. It may be due to the chemicals we add to and put on our foods to keep insects away. So always read labels and wash your vegetables, or better yet, grow your own garden. Pesticides we use have been linked to Autism, Attention Deficit Disorders and Parkinson's. They are in foods and oils we use every day unless you're buying organic.

In 2009 the USDA found seven out of 10 fruits or vegetables had one or more pesticides. Since 2001, they have found more than 200 types of pesticides on food we eat in the US. The CDC tested 5,000 Americans and found pesticides in their blood and urine samples of over 95 percent of them. Holy cannoli!

In Quebec, a May 2011 study from The Department of Obstetrics and Gynecology found that 93 percent of pregnant women who had pesticides found in their bodies, passed these chemicals on to the fetuses 80 percent of the time.

Now it could also be the depleted nutrients in our soils, how we prepare foods, what types of food we eat, or too much animal protein consumed when compared to healthier countries. Perhaps it is what companies use to save money by replacing the more expensive ingredient with genetically altered re-placements.

In general, the fruits and vegetables that you should always buy organic or grow at home include: apples, blueberries, celery, cherries, collard greens, grapes, kale, nectarines, peaches, potatoes, spinach, strawberries and sweet bell peppers. You need to do some research and make better choices. You decide and control what goes into your body. Be informed.

"Those are my principles, and if you don't like them...well, I have others." – **Groucho Marx**

NUTS AND BOLTS

Eat the foods you like, but do so in moderation. Don't always have a steak for dinner and don't eat the entire cow in one sitting.

Try to eat foods from different cultures. Variety is great. You can find some really amazing and healthy dishes like Middle Eastern or Thai food. Many countries have less health problems, so their diets must be worth checking out.

One of the reasons some populations are healthier is because they consume less meats and more plants. For instance, coconut oil has been getting a lot of press because people from tropical regions have less heart disease, but their diet is much different than ours in the U.S.. For years we have been told to avoid tropical oils because of their high saturated fat content.

Proponents say the fats in coconut oil are mostly medium-chain fatty acids and they can be broken down and used by the body. Whereas the long-chain fatty acids found in many plant and animal fats cause more harm. Research on the benefits of coconut oil helping lower cholesterol and weight, increasing energy levels, fighting bacteria and promoting healthy skin are mixed. Like always, use things in moderation, talk to your doctor, do your own research and see how it makes you feel when you try something.

I have been using hemp seeds and hemp protein powder to remove some of the dairy from my diet that I consume in the form of my normal protein shakes, to see how I feel. The chunked up seeds go great in cereal, oatmeal, shakes, peanut butter, etc. If you are eating cottage cheese or yogurt I bet they are good in there too. They add a nutty flavor. These products have high fiber and protein and deserve a chance.

How about exchanging a few of those sodas and fancy coffees, with their 700-calories, for some refreshing water? Water before a meal can help control your appetite and also helps transport food through your digestive system. Not the drinks that have something in front or in back of the name water. Those you can call Junk Water.

One year at a huge body building show I talked with the 8-time Mr. Olympia, Lee Haney. The Olympia title, is like the Super Bowl of bodybuilding. Lee told me Friday night is pizza night with the family. This is one of the greatest body builders of all time, and absolutely one of the nicest people to ever exist. He understands that he can't be that strict all the time. Now he isn't training like he used to be but he still balances the demands of being a father, a businessman and an incredible athlete with the needs of his body. He looks great!

I still have a weakness for chocolate chip cookies, brownies, sushi, birthday cake, ice cream, seafood, a drink and buckwheat pancakes. I just don't eat the whole box of cookies at once or eat these foods all the time. I eat a vast array of diverse foods from different corners of the globe.

Sometimes when I get an urge for a cookie, instead of buying them, I will make them and experiment like a chemist with a plethora of ingredients. I use combinations of whole wheat and/or soy flour to make dark chocolate chip cookies with olive oil, olive oil butter, normal eggs or egg whites, a natural sugar or healthy alternative. Sometimes I add some almond slivers or vanilla protein powder.

I love eating foods with great colors and texture. My wife was shocked by how good my cranberry and almond oatmeal cookies came out with these and other healthier ingredients. I also grabbed some of the left over pumpkin meat from pies and mixed that with extra pomegranate seeds and then added, oat bran, whole wheat flour, some dark chocolate chips, etc. I may need to tweak the concoction a bit but it wasn't bad and it was fun to make.

> *"[The body is] a marvelous machine...a chemical laboratory, a power-house. Every movement, voluntary or involuntary, full of secrets and marvels!"* – **Theodor Herzl**

Exercise

Diet and exercise fads will come and go, but the one thing that remains the same is the fact that they'll keep on coming. Especially if society keeps falling for them. You can't sleep so you turn on the TV because there could be something really boring on to help you doze off. On most nights that would probably be true but tonight something catches your eye, and taps into your insecurities.

They have a piece of equipment and everyone is raving about it. It is easy to use and the pounds melt away. It's fun to use and fortunately it folds up to the size of a matchbook and stores neatly away when it's *"not being used."* The announcer has an intelligent sounding accent and the people exercising in the background throughout the entire commercial are in shape and smiling.

Television keeps pushing these types of equipment or magic drugs, and each year people spend millions for that one machine, sculpting exercise or amazing pill that will make them lose weight.

Part of the problem is society has a belief that if it is on TV then it has to be true. There is a false sense of credibility if it is on television. Some of the commercials are just hilarious regarding items they are selling. With the exercise equipment, the results can be very misleading to the vulnerable public.

To hope to look like the TV model who: trains 2 – 6 hours a day, may be chemically enhanced, has a personal chef, isn't working a normal sedentary job 10 – 12 hours a day, is unreasonable. Sometimes the ads will show *"before"* pictures with someone pushing their stomach out, a woman who is pregnant, or a model before airbrushing and tanning. Ever notice that in the *"after"* pictures, the person stands sideways to look thinner.

I enjoyed the recent ad trying to help women get rid of cellulite. The product must work because the women for the magic cream were jumping around without a care because their legs look smooth and great. Of course, they were probably 18-years-old! Let's really see how effective the cream is by using it on older women who have been working for a living or have a couple of kids.

How much for the stimulation machine? The one I can use that will simulate exercise so I can hang out on my couch and never have to hit the gym? What about the Shape Up shoes that say you can avoid a gym and tone your body by walking. If you started to walk regularly you could tone your legs and lose weight. Do these shoes really make the difference? They will say anything and do anything to push a product. Are we really that gullible?

In fact, most of these advertisements will have a small, practically invisible asterisk next to the comment stating, *"These results are not typical or for best results follow a healthy diet and exercise regularly; or, when you call we are going to try to sell you a bunch of other crap you don't need."* Use caution and listen objectively to the advertisements.

> *"Our own physical body possesses a wisdom,*
> *which we who inhabit the body lack."* **– Henry Miller**

WHAT YOU TALKIN'"BOUT WILLIS?

Now if any product gets you off your duff and gets you moving and burning calories, then it is worth it. You may not see the results they show on TV but if you are willing to make an attempt, then that is a great start. So first you have to set realistic goals for yourself, because the claims they make are so outrageous I don't want you to be disillusioned or disappointed.

Think about the purchase before you make it. Will you use it? Does it seem too good to be true? If it gets you exercising and eating right, then it is worth its price in gold and health.

> *"Too many people confine their exercise to jumping to conclusions, running up bills,*
> *stretching the truth, bending over backward, lying down on the job, sidestepping*
> *responsibility and pushing their luck."* **– Author Unknown**

GOOD NEWS

Since the dawn of man there has always been a quest for eternal life and the fountain of youth. To this day people still search for a magic pill or potion that will keep them young and strong. Amazingly, it was discovered many years ago but only few have actually reaped the benefits.

Can you believe someone finally discovered such a magical creation? Where is it? How much will it cost? Where do I get it? Which mountain do I need to climb? How much would you sacrifice? Who shot J.R.? Do you feel lucky?

The cost does make it obtainable to everyone regardless of sex, race or their medical coverage. It is currently found with greater abundance and ease.

How much do you value a healthy life for you and your loved ones? This medical breakthrough has been found to improve your health and decrease your chance of getting Arthritis, Heart Disease, Alzheimer's, Diabetes, back pain and Cancer to name a few diseases. Just imagine. It is possible to thwart some of life's most dangerous diseases.

It's not a drug, a vitamin or a mineral. It isn't at the four corners of the globe and it doesn't involve surgery. One of the most, if not the most important thing you could ever do for your overall health is, drum roll please … (tada), exercise.

You don't need fancy equipment or fad diet pills. All they do is lighten your wallet.

After a long history of medical experts believing exercise was harmful to the body, they came to realize the benefits of movement are well researched and undeniable. Even us doctors can learn something new every day. Now that we know, we conduct studies to prove we're right.

Most recently, a study by the University of South Carolina was published in *The Journal of the American Medical Association* determining which was more important, being fit or being fat. In the 12 year study of people over 60, people who were fit, or able to walk briskly five times a week for 30 minutes, were more likely to avoid heart problems than inactive, skinny people. It had nothing to do with the person's appearance as in fat or skinny, but in their ability to be active. So simply looking *"marvelous"* is not all it's cracked up to be.

The body was designed to move and this study is a perfect example how exercise can help increase your chance of living. Regardless of your size, being active is imperative to your health.

Dr. Caldwell Esselstyn Jr. has another theory for preventing heart attacks. After studying the diets of the rural Chinese, Central Africans, Papua New Guinea highlanders and more, he found they rarely experience heart attacks in their culture. Their diet is comprised of no dairy, oil, meat, fish or eggs and consists mostly of fruits, grains, legumes and vegetables. He has also seen artery blockages clear up after patients changed to this diet. If you can't go this extreme, make small changes to your diet and see how you feel.

> *"Basic research is what I am doing when I don't know what I am doing."*
> **– Wernher von Braun**

JUST THE FACTS MAM

The cost of healthcare and insurance rates are big problems in the US. Sometimes they are directly affected by insurance company's greed and other times by prices of instruments, supplies and services. To reduce your personal healthcare costs the best thing everyone can do for themselves is exercise and eat right because of all of the benefits. Exercise keeps your body healthy, promotes proper posture and enhances your strength and flexibility, not to mention all of the diseases that can be avoided.

Several reports tried to estimate how much complications due to inactivity and obesity costs our healthcare system. Although the

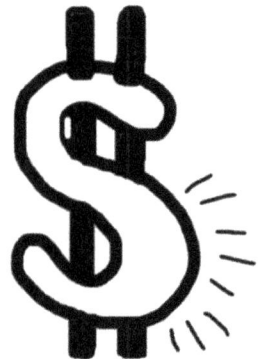

numbers varied, one estimate was more than $20 billion a year.[91] The numbers for future lost production due to permanent health problems make the figures even higher.

In 2000, it was reported that if we could increase the activity level of the people who were considered inactive, this would decrease the likelihood of heart disease, diabetes and obesity, saving nearly $70 Billion in healthcare.[92] Annually!

There is no age limit on the benefits of exercise. Even 90-year-old men and women training 3 times/week for 8 weeks can see their strength increase by 174 percent.[93] Even just training the legs and knees can improve a person's ability to walk faster, climb stairs and have twice the strength than when they started.[94] Can you imagine the sense of freedom and independence these individual test subjects felt?

Do you know someone who might improve, or an elderly care facility that would benefit from incorporating exercise and stretching into their daily activities? This would help: reduce accidents and falls, minimize feelings of helplessness, boost people's ability to do more on their own, and offer a way to maintain health and vitality.

In 1960, The College Alumni Health Study began and monitored their subjects' health, exercise routines and benefits of exercise over 40 plus years. Exercises ranged from weights, golf, gardening and walking. They found the quality of life improved, people lived an extra four years, and it had a dramatic effect on reducing Heart Disease and Stroke.[95]

After reviewing many studies on the benefits of exercise and questioning the validity of this research, the Royal College of Physicians made several recommendations that were published in *The British Medical Journal.* They agreed the research available proved regular exercise contributed to many physiological and psychological benefits and that all healthcare institutions needs to acknowledge this.[96] What's your conclusion?

"It is better to wear out than to rust out." – **Bishop Richard Cumberland**

NOW THAT'S WHAT I'M TALKING ABOUT

The best time to start exercising is not morning or evening, but in your youth. You will have a tendency to develop a routine and stay motivated to continue it into your middle ages. That will enable you to have a more productive and independent senior lifestyle.

All doctors should check to see if their patients participate in any type of exercise program. It should be obligatory for healthcare providers to be knowledgeable and to recommend, if not require, some specific programs or alternatives to help each patient's condition. They should also provide information regarding the correct intensity level, the type of routine, the frequency of participation and sensible precautions, so their patients' aren't counterproductive.

A University of Illinois study conducted by Walter M. Bortz II, M.D. in 2004 found that adding six months of aerobic exercise could help increase your brain function and prohibit the negative things we associate with aging, which are due largely in part to a lack of physical activity.

Research has also shown the surmounting evidence highlighting the importance of diet and exercise in our overall health. Many conditions like weight loss, heart failure, your immune system, Cancers, Osteoporosis, High Blood Pressure, maintaining muscle and bone mass, healthy posture, Arthritis, back pain, higher good cholesterol (HDL) levels, lower bad cholesterol (LDL) levels, poor sleep, Alzheimer's and Diabetes can be prevented or improved with proper nutrition and exercise.

With a stronger frame you can better withstand the likeliness of injuries, perform in sports, enjoy greater strength and flexibility, and have a healthy and well-protected posture. The better you feel about your body the better you feel about yourself. You will be on cloud nine when you see results. Confidence will exude from every pore of your body. You will smile more and hold your head up higher. How do you think that will equate with job performance, other people's perception of you, or even dating?

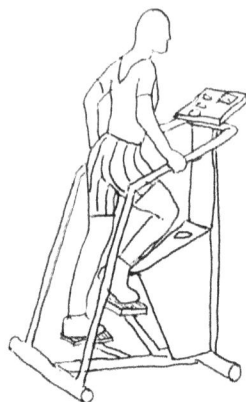

> *"Those who restrain desire, do so because theirs is weak enough to be restrained."*
> **– William Blake**

SO MUCH FOR THAT RUBBER TREE PLANT

Prognosticators said no one could run a mile in under four minutes. It was done. They laughed at George Foreman when he decided to return to the ring until he recaptured his heavyweight title at the young age of 45.

That's what is really cool about the human body. If you run a 240 horsepower engine like it is a 440, it will fail. If you ask the human body to do a similar task that is demanding or beyond its capabilities, it will adapt and become stronger. As long as you have the desire and don't let doubt handcuff your ability to satisfy your goals, you can do anything.

Your body wasn't created with all these neat moving parts because it wanted to sit and let life pass it by. It wants action! The only limitation your body has is its mind. If you set reasonable goals, you can achieve them. Be realistic and regain your health. Don't become a statistic.

"Keep close to Nature's heart... and break clear away, once in awhile, and climb a mountain or spend a week in the woods. Wash your spirit clean. None of Nature's landscapes are ugly so long as they are wild." – **John Muir**

CONVICTIONS OF THE HEART

As we age there are several diseases that are very prevalent and can really rock our world. These are Colon Cancer, Breast or Prostate Cancer and Heart Disease. Always see your doctors and have appropriate screenings if you have a family history of these diseases, notice any changes that seem odd, or if you are over 40, and definitely if you are over 50 years old.

According to The American Heart Association, one in three people have some type of heart disease. It was also reported by the CDC, that approximately 750,000 to a million people will have a heart attack this year. About 25 - 50 percent will die before they even make it to the hospital or the Emergency Department.

A heart attack occurs when blood stops bringing oxygen to a certain part of the body. It is the leading cause of death for both women and men, so understanding the disease, symptoms, prevention and what actions to take may just save a life.

Many conditions are considered a type of heart disease like: atherosclerosis; congenital defects; you may have been born with, such as heart valve issues; infection of the heart and heart rhythm problems, or arrhythmias.

Atherosclerosis is when plaque builds up on the inner walls of the arteries; it narrows them and is similar to squeezing a hose. The smaller the diameter of the hose the harder the water comes out of the other end. Same thing happens to your blood vessels. If any plaque breaks off it can get lodged elsewhere, block blood flow and cause a stroke.

Congestive Heart Failure occurs when not enough blood is being pumped throughout the body so the oxygen needs of your body aren't being met. As the heart becomes less effective at moving blood within the body it may start to accumulate or pool in the legs, arms or internal organs.

An Arrhythmia describes the fact the heart isn't pumping blood with the normal *"thump-thump"* pattern. Like sleep apnea with your breathing, the heart is missing a few beats, pausing momentarily and may even be speeding up periodically.

If there is a heart valve issue, not enough blood is allowed to pass through the valve (stenosis), the valve doesn't close completely (regurgitation) or blood could actually flow backward into the heart's upper chamber (mitral valve prolapse).

Risk Factors for Heart Disease:
*   Family History
*   Smoking
*   Obesity
*   Lack of Exercise, because anyone who can briskly walk 30 minutes a day is healthier than a skinny person who sits in a chair all day
*   High Cholesterol
*   Diabetes
*   Excessive Alcohol or Caffeine use

Common Symptoms of a Heart Attack:
*   Tightness in the center of the chest, tough to catch your breath, person usually has a clenched fist in the center of their chest as a sign of distress
*   Light-headed, wobbly or faint feeling, sweating
*   Pain into the left arm most often, but can also be the right arm or legs
*   Jaw pain
*   May include: abdominal pain; back pain; shoulder pain; indigestion or nausea, confusion
*   Rapid or fluttering pulse
*   Pain can start slowly, worse with activity

If you or someone you know has any of these symptoms, the first thing to do is call 911. If they are responsive, have them sit or lie down, stay with them, wherever they are, and wait for the ambulance to arrive. This will reduce stress and movement and the EMTs can reach you faster, with the necessary equipment to help.

Ask if the person takes meds and if they need to take them. Get the pills and help them take their meds. If the person is unresponsive, call 911 immediately.

Statistically if an adult is on the ground it is probably cardiac arrest. Eighty percent of all heart attacks will occur in the home which is another good reason to become CPR certified.

The following instructions are at the Professional Level. The lay person technique is very similar, with slight differences. Big difference is you won't check for a pulse. If the person isn't breathing you would go right to CPR, as described below.

Look for their chest to rise, listen for breathing and feel the side of their neck for a pulse.

If there is a pulse but no breathing, Perform Rescue Breathing:

- Tip victim's head back, pinch their nose, take a deep breath and breathe normally into the victim's mouth and watch for the chest to rise
- Give 1 breath every 5 seconds to an adult for 2 minutes (about 24 breaths) and recheck (Look, Listen & Feel). Repeat if nothing changes. If they start to breathe, monitor them and wait for help.
- Give 1 breath every 3 seconds to a child or infant for 2 minutes (about 60 breaths) and recheck (Look, Listen & Feel). Repeat if nothing changes. If they start to breath, monitor them and wait for help.

If there is no pulse and they are not breathing, Perform CPR:

- Kneel next to their upper arm on either side
- Center your body over their torso
- Place the heel of one hand over their sternum, located at the center of the chest and between the breasts
- Reinforce that hand with your free hand. For a child you can use 1 or 2 hands but for an infant you would use 2 fingers
- Start chest compressions (at a depth of 1 ½ inches for an infant, 2 inches or less up to age 11 and greater than 2 inches for an adult, 12 yrs and above)
- Compress at a rate of 100 compressions per minute (30 compressions should last about 18 seconds) Five cycles of 30 compressions and 2 breaths should take about 2 minutes.
- With each breath, making sure the chest rises. Otherwise tilt the head back more and try again. Repeat until help arrives.
- To practice your rhythm at home, hum the song "Staying Alive" by the Bee Gees to keep up the pace.
- If the chest does not rise even after the second re-tilt the airway is probably obstructed and you will have to perform the unconscious obstructed airway technique.

For every minute the person does not have any blood pumping oxygen through their body, their chances of survival decrease 10 percent. If you don't know CPR or can't figure out the breathing procedure, just keep pumping the chest! This explanation is a quick review of the procedure. A full class "with hands on" practice will take a couple of hours.

Ways to Keep the Old Ticker Healthy:

- Eat a healthy diet by limiting red meat and saturated fats, decreasing sugar and salt intake, increasing fiber and vegetables.

- Exercise regularly
- See your doctors for regular checkups They can order stress tests, angio grams, ultrasounds to check your arteries and blood work to check your cardiac profile. Healthy Blood pressure is 120 / 80, HDLs should be high, your LDLs, cholesterol and triglycerides should be low.
- Limit alcohol and caffeine intake. A glass of red wine a day has been shown to reduce the risk of heart disease, but it's not an excuse to grow a vineyard and start having wine every night. Moderation is the golden rule.
- Stop smoking. Nicotine constricts your blood vessels and reduces oxygen flow in your blood stream.
- Your doctor may recommend an aspirin a day
- Reduce stress levels
- Maintain a healthy weight for your height
- Take care of your teeth to reduce bacteria and plaque that could make its way to your heart.

Other things you can do to help control your risks of heart disease are: Yoga to stay flexible and reduce stress; Chiropractic to help the body's skeletal system and the nervous system function at its best; Massage to reduce stress and help relax the muscles; Reflexology or Acupuncture to help your organs function properly, reduce pain and tension, improve circulation; a Personal Trainer to stay motivated in the gym; and a Nutritionist to help you eat smarter.

Some vitamins to add to your day:
- CoEnzyme Q10, it helps increase the oxygen carrying capability of the red blood cells so the heart works less. There's been no known interaction of Q10 with any medication. It is found over the counter. 100 – 200 mg/daily
- Niacin and Complex Vitamin B – 1000 – 2000 mg/daily of Niacin
- Fiber Supplements – reduces LDL cholesterol levels
- Plant Sterols – reduces LDL levels
- Red Yeast Rice – lowers LDL. Start at 2400 mg/daily
- Green Tea Extract – 375 mg/daily may help lower LDLs
- Omega 3s – I know a study came out on 9/12 and reportedly found fish oil doesn't help prevent heart disease but I hear junk like that all the time. Eat eggs. Don't eat eggs. Eat eggs. All studies should be scrutinized period. Didn't Hershey's find chocolate is healthy? Maybe in strict moderation.
- We need to raise our Omega 3 levels as a whole, so take the supplements or eat more Flax seed or Chia seeds. 1000 mg/daily
- Garlic, ginger and turmeric – have been found to lower cholesterol
- Vitamin D – reduce cardiovascular risks. 400 – 800 IU/day
- Magnesium and Potassium– low levels have been found to be associated with elevated blood pressure. Eat more fruits, vegetables, whole grains and nuts or take a multivitamin.

"Time is the coin of your life. It is the only coin you have, and only you can determine how it will be spent. Be careful lest you let other people spend it for you." – **Carl Sandburg**

TIME, IS ON YOUR SIDE

The problem is we are too busy. We get up early after a terrible night of sleep, work all day and come home tired. *"There's no time." "I'm too old." "Too tired." "I don't want to get big." "Maybe tomorrow."*

How about the mother who has to keep things running smoothly in the house, or has to care for the household when everyone gets sick? But when she gets sick, the kids go play and the father is out bowling. Stay-at-home Moms and Dads are usually too busy with keeping the family organized to think about exercise, or just too plain tired.

Now granted all of the lovely chores we do at home like vacuuming, raking, doing laundry, playing with the kids do require an expenditure of energy, but they are not a substitute for working out. Especially when you cannot completely focus your efforts on the exercise without someone begging for a sandwich, or a scuffle breaks out between siblings.

We all have to make a decision when we are ready to make a change in ourselves. The longer you wait, the harder it will be. When is your time? You have to make the decision to give yourself some TLC for your health. It needs to become a priority in your life. Your health, is priceless!

For 20 years, Zoe Koplowitz has been participating in the NY City Marathon. No, she's never won it, but her time crossing the line in under 29 hours in 2007 is another example of not making excuses. You see, she has Multiple Sclerosis and Diabetes, and nothing stops her. Now that's inspiring.

If you add 20 minutes of exercise to your day, I promise you that you will feel better about yourself, have more energy and lose weight. I am going to give you a few ideas on how you can add exercise to your day and why it is so important.

Hey if you have even less time, try jumping rope for five minutes or punching a speed bag or weighted bag for one round of three minutes. Sounds easy right? Try it and then let's talk. After you catch your breath.

First off, most people aren't happy with the way they look for ridiculous reasons or standards, or would like to change something about their appearance. When Jennifer Aniston became popular, women flocked to have their hair cut similar to hers. It looked good on her and they wanted to try to capture a bit of that magic for themselves.

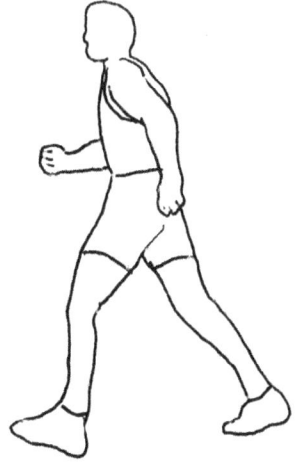

The public is bombarded with pictures of stars who never leave home without *"it."* I'm not talking about their American Express card. I mean the makeup artists, plastic surgeons, teeth whiteners, nutritionists, hair stylists, air brushers, fashion consultants, hired help for their homes and personal trainers to focus on their appearances. They should look flawless with all of that help.

Pro athletes should be in tremendous shape. That's what they do for their livelihoods. They don't punch numbers at a firm and then squeeze in dinner and a soccer game with the family or watch a movie. They are exercising throughout most of their day. They have access to proper nutrition and time to exercise. Someone is always vying for their position so they must be in shape and perform at their very best.

We start to see ourselves in our *"real world mirror"* as having too many faults. Never let the standards someone else or an industry sets determine how you should look. Embrace who you are, be proud of what you have become, strive to be a healthier person and be happy.

It is unreasonable to compare yourselves to famous people or look up to them. Especially the way the younger stars have found their salvation in alcohol and anorexia. They are not people to idolize or be role models for our children. You are.

"To me, old age is always 15 years older than I am." – **Bernard M. Baruch**

IT'S JUST A FLESH WOUND

We all have aches and pains, as we get older. I have a big bucket that continues to get filled with the equipment from sports I used to play. My soccer cleats, soccer balls, softballs, baseball equipment, tennis racquets, skis and poles all remind me of how young and unbreakable my body was.

Now I still will play catch and basketball. I'll try to play any sport depending on how I feel. I know I'm not taking this body with me when I go. I would just as soon like to leave this planet using every ounce of motion I can get out of this model. So I have ice packs in the freezer. I can accept this. The health benefits of regular exercise far out weigh the challenges of a sedentary existence.

A study from the University of Colorado at Boulder looked at 11 men and women of an average age of 80. They spent six months in a supervised exercise program that involved lifting weights and not just going through the motions. They were getting *"pumped up."* At the conclusion of the study researchers found all of the participants showed considerable gains. They noticed improvement in their balance and strength.

This can lead to the elderly being more self-sufficient, as many would like to be, but often only have the mental capacity to do so. Some of the women almost doubled their strength. Wonder Women!

Dr. William Simpson, Professor of Family Medicine at the Medical University of South Carolina says, *"If we stay active, many of the things that supposedly decline with age really don't decline."* More and more research proves this.

For example, Terence Kavanagh, M.D., Director of the Toronto Rehabilitation Center, was the principal researcher of a study that measured the effects of aging on 756 athletes ages 35 – 94, who competed in sports like swimming, rowing, and track and field during the 1985 World Masters Games in Toronto.

Dr. Kavanagh proclaimed, *"We found some people in their late sixties and seventies who had about the same cardiopulmonary fitness as you would expect from sedentary 25-year-olds."* Their hearts were twice as strong as their peers' and they had more lean muscle tissue. Most of these athletes trained for about an hour a day.

Yale University performed a 23-year study of participants age 50 and over and found those who thought positively about getting older lived seven and a half years longer than those who dreaded it.

Another 2008 study from the Washington University School of Medicine tracked 65,000 nurses and found those who were physically active as teens and young adults were 23 percent less likely to develop breast cancer before reaching menopause. Dr. Graham Colditz found the most beneficial time period to make a difference in your future was between the ages of 12 and 22. The more rigorous the routine the better, so start now!!

I could quote you a thousand studies reiterating the proof on the benefits of exercise, but ultimately your mind is the one limitation that has to be convinced. The decision is yours.

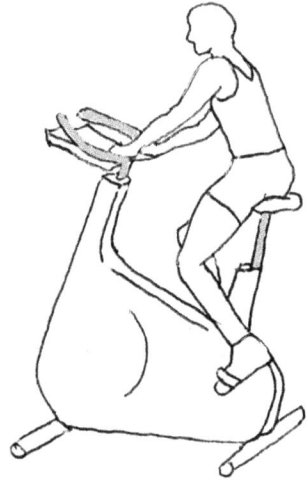

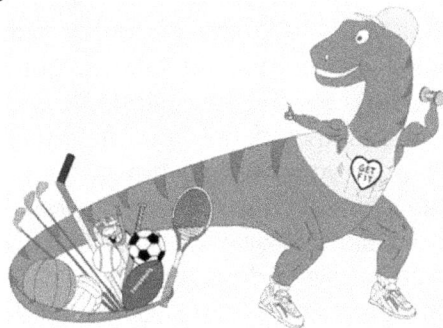

> *"The best and safest thing is to keep a balance in your life, acknowledge the great powers around us and in us. If you can do that, and live that way, you are really a wise man."* – **Euripides**

CAUGHT IN THE BALANCE

Sometimes we are really busy and finding time to workout or lift can be difficult. I have a gym in my house so I have no travel or waiting time. I just need to have the desire to get my can in there and lift hard like I would if there were people around me in the gym setting. There are always distractions beckoning you away from your exercise equipment.

When I used to lift at a gym, I would put the headphones on, crank up the tunes, and get to business. No social time, just work. Throw in a few cute women and I know I lifted more intensely.

At home I have a cat rolling around at my feet or I think of something I need to do and Bingo, I'm distracted. Remember this when you contemplate purchasing a home gym or piece of equipment. You need to be able to focus and have the drive to lift on your own or with your partner.

If buying equipment is what it takes to get you exercising then great. Using your equipment as an expensive coat hanger isn't doing you any good, unless you ran out of closet space. The point is you have to use it.

If you minimize the time in between lifts, and cycle through different muscle groups, you can actually get a component of aerobic exercise because you will be moving fast and breathing harder for oxygen. You can get a great workout in 20 minutes.

> *"Look with favour upon a bold beginning."* – **Virgil**

LET'S TAKE IT FROM THE BEGINNING

Before you start any exercise program consult with your doctor and have a thorough physical. Once you get the *"Go get'em Tiger,"* then you can begin.

A gym can be pretty overwhelming to a rookie. Whether you are going to run or pump iron, there are some steps you can take to get started. If this is all new to you then start slowly. There is no need to run five miles your first day out because that is what you used to run in track 25 years and several pounds ago. Even if you were able to run the distance, you wouldn't be able to walk for ~~a week~~ a couple of days after the run. Start slowly.

Similarly, throwing 200 pounds on the bench when you haven't lifted since high school, is just begging for an injury.

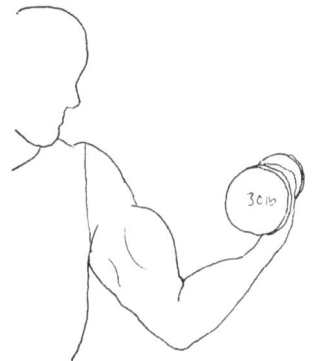

The time frame for a good workout should be around one hour. When you first start out that time should be less. Give yourself plenty of time to warm up and cool down before and after the main exercise. No need to go on the DL (disabled list) this early into your *"Shock and Awe"* health program.

Make sure you have on comfortable clothing. If you are determined to wear your little brother's shirt to look big in the gym or parade around in a tight outfit to showcase your figure, be prepared to be interrupted by people while you try to get a good workout in. When you draw attention to yourself, you will be stared at or asked out.

Some gyms are more about dating than lifting it seems. If you need a date then by all means go that route and the two of you can *"lift together, happily ever after."* Otherwise get some lose clothes so you can move in them and save your sexy body for someone special. If you need to have a new wardrobe, great, but you will still look stupid if you're not busting your butt or you're doing bench presses on a leg extension machine. We will discuss different machines, techniques and strategies for lifting safely and effectively.

Bring a towel to keep your sweat off the equipment and protect you from someone else's. Put the weights back on the rack. My Aunt Rosanne doesn't need to be removing 45-pound plates because you were too lazy. Likewise, make sure when you leave the machine it is back at a height where anyone can use it. If your machine is occupied, wait for the machine, ask if you can work out between their breaks, or try other machines to accomplish the same workout.

Bring lots of water or some kind of sports drink to replenish your body. Learn how to stretch properly. Also you need to get good rest. It is the time needed for your body to repair itself and grow. Continue reading for more information before dusting off your dumbbells and spandex shorts.

> *"Walking is the best possible exercise. Habituate yourself to walk very far."*
> – **Thomas Jefferson**

I MUST BE IN THE FRONT ROW

You could start out by parking farther away from the front door. You also won't get the side of your car dinged up from the inconsiderate people who fling their doors open, or carelessly let the wind take them.

Maybe take the stairs. This simply adds a little exercise to your day and you could encourage co-workers to do the same. They might even stop bringing in desserts and coffee every morning for breakfast. If you car pool or take public transportation, get off a few stops ahead of your destination so you can get some fresh air and exercise if the weather permits.

Given the price of gas, you might want to think about riding your bike to work or walking. You could get some great exercise in, while saving your cash.

"A good listener is usually thinking about something else." – **Kin Hubbard**

YOU LISTEN WELL GRASSHOPPER

I am amazed how many athletes simply don't stretch properly. It leads to problems when they don't and is a reason many of them come in for treatment or wind up on the sidelines. Proper stretching helps your muscles stay long, keeps your body flexible and always able to maintain good posture. It also helps to maximize the effectiveness of your workout.

If your hamstrings are tight, then when you run you will never be able to fully extend your legs and complete a full stride. You cover less distance with each stride and use more time to get there.

In any old man baseball or softball league you can see this as someone tries to advance a base. We joke that they are carrying a piano. If you want to steal a base, you need to explode out from the base and hit full stride, quickly, and not take baby steps. Don't make this mistake and get thrown out.

Before jogging or lifting weights, do some aerobic exercises like walking for 10 or 15 minutes. If you need more time that's fine, but just don't wear yourself out before you can get a good workout in. Warming up before you exercise helps to increase the blood circulating in your body. It then transports more nutrients to your muscles so they have the building blocks to grow. It also helps to prepare the tendons and ligaments for strenuous activity and prevents injuries.

Equally important is stretching during lifting. If you just contract your muscles and never stretch them you are going to wind up with short muscles. First off you have greater range, size and strength with longer muscles. Second, if your muscles are tight and limiting, it will lead to imbalances in your posture and set you up for an injury.

If I am bench pressing, when I am done with one set I go to the wall and stretch. If I am working the triceps, I stretch as soon as I'm done. I need a break anyway and this is a way to lengthen the muscle and give my body time to replenish its energy levels.

Have you ever watched a pro sport where someone isn't stretching before the game? Even the Hulkster grabs the ropes and tugs on them before his patented *"Leg Drop Brother."*

What really amazes me is how many runners don't take the time to stretch after running a considerable distance. Just like with weightlifting, you want to cool down and stretch your muscles because they have been contracting over and over. It will help reduce muscle fatigue, maintain flexibility, encourage quicker recuperation and decrease the chance of injuries. This is the most important time to stretch. Don't miss out.

"The true teacher defends his pupils against his own personal influence." – **Amos Bronson**

HOME SCHOOLED

If you are worried people will see you or don't want to be intimidated; you can always start your exercise program at home. Cable TV has a lot of quality shows that not only make you sweat but teach you a lot about exercising properly, using correct form, protecting your posture, maintaining good nutrition, the importance of stretching and the benefits of your hard work.

I am not talking about infomercials touting their magic equipment or break through diet strategy or whatever else they are selling. I'm referring to shows like Denise Austin, Gilad, Body Shaping, Yoga, etc., and many more that can be found on FitTV or an ESPN channel. Check your local listings because everything you could possibly want is right here. It doesn't get any easier or cheaper. It's like having a private lesson with each instructor.

Most of the instructors are very knowledgeable and are a great source for anyone interested in learning how to exercise smart and safely. The shows are typically on early and can be done before going to work while the family is still asleep or preoccupied. You can then shower up and get ready for your day. Otherwise tape, DVR, or TIVO it.

If you find someone in the fitness industry who motivates you or helps you get results, then maybe you should check out their line of videos or DVDs if they have some. You could also check your local library. Libraries might also order them for you and keep them on file. Your favorite instructor may also have a web site to help you further.

You could see if some of your friends have a disc you could borrow or you could each purchase different DVDs and share. Maybe even work out together for support and motivation. Start a neighborhood exchange.

"Change your thoughts and you change your world." – **Norman Vincent Peale**

WHERE THERE'S A WILL, THERE'S A WEIGHT

Weights cost money but you have some options. You can always walk and jog outside or take it inside a mall. If you want to lift weights, than I have some suggestions for you. Check Craigslist or your local paper for people getting rid of equipment because of moving, disuse, estate sales, etc. The spring cleaning, failed New Year's resolution, *"just get rid of this stuff,"* garage sale is the perfect place to find bargain-priced gym equipment.

You can pick up some great equipment for a fraction of the cost of new. You could also check a used gym equipment store. They will have someone who is knowledgeable on staff who can help you make an informed decision. Like buying a guitar for a beginner, you don't need to buy an expensive piece of equipment. Get a piece of equipment that isn't super cheap and if you like it and are using it regularly, then you are ready to make a bigger purchase.

When I was a teenager, and I was lifting incorrectly, I had a Sears' bench and 110 pound concrete weight set. I hit my arms and chest all the time, and I'll mention something about that in a second. When I got kicked out of the dining room and moved into the basement, the MacGyver in me took over.

I cut holes in the floor joists and ran pulleys and pipes through it. Then I attached ropes and cables to my *"weights."* I filled 5-gallon buckets with rocks, cement and sometimes even added water. There was nothing I couldn't do down there. It may have taken five minutes to make it through the contraption but I'd consider that my warm-up.

You can use cans of food or fill up old milk jugs with liquid, dirt or sand depending on your weight lifting needs. Plop it on a scale if you need to know how much you are lifting. The numbers are not that important. If you are getting tired when you reach the end of you repetitions (reps) for that set, be it 6, 10 or 15 repetitions, then the weight is perfect for you.

You can use surgical tubing or Therabands, which are tubing colored differently depending on their level of difficulty. It's kind of like using elastic or bungee cords. However, bungee cords have metal hooks and can be extremely dangerous if they whack you in the face, so I wouldn't use them.

Onions and potatoes come in five and 10 pound sacks; however I would recommend eating them at some point. So do oranges and grapefruits, which come in sturdy bags with handles. Slip on a pair of gloves and the cords won't hurt your hands.

Don't forget isometric contractions. Making muscle poses and holding them as if you were on stage at the Mr. Olympia Bodybuilding competition, are prime examples of this type of exercise. They used to advertise these routines in the back of magazines after the skinny guy got sand kicked in his face and he lost his girl.

The contracting of your muscles forces nutrient-rich blood into them. This helps build more muscle tissue and the contractions can burn calories too. It's not easy holding those poses on stage. Contestants are always shaking. Well, maybe it's the fear their Speedo is going to break.

> *"Beginning is easy - Continuing is hard."* – **Japanese Proverb**

LET'S GET IT STARTED

Okay so you are ready for the gym. Ask friends where they go. Call around and maybe even get a free pass through a friend or the gym so you can try it out for yourself. I'm not a big fan of the gyms if their policy is when you sign up you can never break the contract unless you are moving a certain distance. What is this a marriage? Find a different gym. That's just nonsense.

Once you have your gym picked out, get a detailed tour of the facility so you know where everything is, including the hot tub and sauna room. Schedule some time to talk with a trainer who can show you how to use each piece of equipment safely and explain which muscles are being worked. Don't watch people to learn. I've seen too many people lifting dumbbells for the biceps yet they were using every muscle in their shoulders and back to assist in the lift. Now who's the dumbbell?

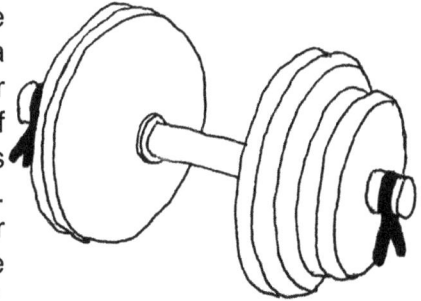

If you would like an entire program, hire a personal trainer to work with you. He or she can help you achieve your goals by better understanding you. The first thing is to find exercises you enjoy. If you like what you are doing then you will probably stick with it. Don't run if you hate running. If you like cycling then do that and get the same results.

Another great thing about having a trainer, or a training partner, is that you have to exercise. At home you can make a million excuses because a certain chore should be done. But at the gym there is no turning back. Consider your trainer or partner as your new form of *"health insurance."*

A trainer should teach you and be there with you, as you are exercising ,to make sure you work hard, prevent you from making common mistakes or to answer any questions. Fire the guy that says walk on this treadmill for 30 minutes and I'll be back. If you are paying him or her, then make sure they are working with you. I think you can catch on to the walking thing on your own after some instruction. You've been doing it for years. If they are preoccupied with their *"crack"* berry or phone, or not focused on you, they are not what you need.

At a gym don't be overwhelmed by the size of the place or the amount of equipment. You can work with all of the individual machines, weights or go right to a smaller circuit of machines to hit each muscle group. With a circuit there is no searching for the right machine or confusion about what exercise to do. You can learn proper form and what muscles you are training as each piece of equipment usually has a diagram of how to perform the exercise, as well as what muscles are being used.

Next up decide if you are more comfortable using cable machines or free weights. Some people feel that using free weights is harder because a lot of stability comes from supporting muscles groups during your lifts, so more energy is expended and more calories are burned.

Free weights allow you to move in your normal biomechanical path. No machine can exactly duplicate your movements because of the variations in each body. You can develop greater power and size with old-fashion iron. The down side is that you need a lot of space for this type of set up whether it is in a gym or in your home. Someone to spot you, or help when you get to the end of your set, is also helpful. In high school I got pinned under 285 lbs. on my chest, alone, in the basement. Twice. Didn't learn the first time as a teenager. I don't recommend it.

Cable machines have been designed to adjust to an individual's height and size but it isn't a perfect fit. Each machine has been designed to focus on one muscle group. This is really good when you want to isolate an area. They also help you maintain proper form and reduce your chance of injury by providing proper support.

I have started to use a dual cable column, called functional training, for my entire routine. It has two towers with separate weight stacks. There are no heavy plates to slide on a bar or drop on your toe. The handles have fully adjustable heights and you can do almost anything on it. For instance, due to my shoulder damage, I can use the cables and I'm not stuck in someone else's designed motion. My arm can work in any angle that does not cause pain, for curls, triceps, benching, rows and more.

Changing resistance is easy because you only have to move a pin in the weight system, called a stack, to select a different weight. During your workout you can cycle through a bunch of different machines. This allows you to move through your workout faster.

However, nothing says rookie like someone banging the plates when you lift. Always lower the weight so it gets close to the start point, but it should never touch. This ensures you are keeping constant tension on the muscles. When the weight goes up, focus on squeezing your muscles tight to get a good *"pump."*

Machines have also tried to achieve the best angles for muscle development from years of research and development. It isn't perfect but there is something to be said about the evolution of equipment with regards to redefining and improving the technology. The old stuff was like ancient torture devices. The new stuff glides smoothly and changing weight is quick and easy.

Companies like Precor, Body Solid, Star Trac, Weider, Nautilus, Paramount, Cybex and others have really made some great improvements. In any case, you should try to use both and make an informed decision about what seems to be best for you. My recommendation would be to work one month with one group of apparatus and then switch to the other.

See what changes you see in yourself and know that by alternating your workout strategy from time to time, you are shocking your muscles. If the muscles get used to a routine and aren't challenged, they will become complacent and not grow. By varying and shocking your muscles they will respond favorably so mix it up every couple of weeks.

It is more than just moving a weight. With either type of equipment, a workout is only as good and productive as the effort you put behind it. Feel the muscles work as you contract them.

"I used to dread getting older because I thought I would not be able to do all the things I wanted to do, but now that I am older I find that I don't want to do them." **– Nancy Astor**

LET'S GET PHYSICAL

There are two types of exercise, Aerobic and Anaerobic. Aerobic exercise involves moderate to intense exercises that last awhile, build up your endurance, and require the use of oxygen. Running, swimming, bicycling, aerobic classes, jogging, walking, jumping rope and basketball are some examples.

Because your legs are used primarily and they are a large muscle group, you will burn more calories than say an exercise that focuses on your arms. Completing regular workouts of 30 – 45 minutes a day can raise your metabolism for 24 – 28 hours. You will burn more calories throughout the next day and beyond.

In the beginning when you first start to exercise, your body depletes any glycogen (a precursor to glucose) stores to make energy. Oxygen helps the body burn fat and converts glucose into energy for the body. It is a slow process, but this is why aerobic activity can help you lose fat. When you exercise for more than 30 minutes you start to put that fat burning process into action.

In addition aerobic exercise helps the heart get in shape and become more efficient at moving blood through the body. The general rule for an effective workout is to train within your Target Heart Range (THR). An easy method to figure this out is to take 220 and subtract your age. Then multiply that number by 60% – 80%. You want to be in this range when you exercise to maximize your results in the shortest amount of time.

For example; 220 – 40 years old = 180. 180 x .60 (or 60%) = 108 Beats Per Minute (BPM). 180 x .80 = 144 BPM. When you are jogging, cross-country

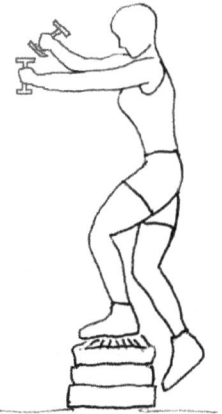

skiing, running, etc., you want to have your heart rate in between these two numbers to get the most out of your hard work.

Another simple rule is to exercise just intensely enough to carry on a conversation, with a little huffing and puffing. If you are able to exchange the neighborhood gossip with your girlfriend, put more effort into the walk, instead of the words. Talk over a juice and fruit smoothie while you stretch afterwards.

Speeding up and slowing down, known as interval training, is another way to boost the efficiency of your workout. I used to go to my high school track and sprint the straight-aways on the quarter mile track and walk the curved ends. This burns more energy. If you run on a treadmill, try sprinting during commercial breaks or for a minute or two, and then go back to your normal pace. You can increase your fat burning potential up to three times. This will also reduce your time on the machine to cover the same distance you normally would because at times you ran or walked faster. Or you can train a little longer.

Think of it as punching the gas at a green light, maintaining the speed limit and stopping at the next light. Then punching it again to the next stop light. You will use up more gas speeding up in your vehicle than if you slowly accelerate your car. The same goes for your body. This time you set the speed limit.

For those people who are convinced they can spot reduce, say their love handles for example, it doesn't work this way. The most successful way to decrease your stomach size and see your abs is to burn more calories than you eat. In addition to that, doing aerobic activities like running and walking has been found to be an effective way to reduce abdominal fat.[97, 98] You may have a great set of abdominals but no one can see them if they have a pudgy layer over them.

> *"The fact that the mind rules the body, is, in spite of its neglect by biology and medicine, the most fundamental fact which we know about the process of life."*
> **– Franz Alexander, M.D.**

HAVE GUNS WILL TRAVEL

Anaerobic exercise is done without the use of oxygen and is associated with explosive exercises done for short durations. Jumping, sprinting and lifting weights are examples. Lifting weights can raise your metabolism for 32 – 48 hours. Combine that with aerobics and you will be a *"lean, mean, fighting machine."*

It is a short duration exercise. You lift for however many repetitions and then stop and wait. This gives your body a chance to recuperate and make more energy for your next lift. I like to lift with opposing muscle groups like biceps / triceps or chest / back. They are called agonist and antagonist muscles, because they work against each other.

I can exhaust my bicep muscles on the front of my arm and go right into a lift for the triceps muscle on the back of my arms. I'm sort of building two muscles for the price of one. When you get a two for one like that you also decrease your time lifting, because you don't have to wait for the muscles to recover before the next lift. Otherwise you do biceps curls and wait, and then do them again. I also get a stretch in the one muscle when I lift with the opposing muscle.

Remember to exhale on the tough part of your lift, when your muscles are contracting. Never lift while you are holding your breath because it increases your pressure on the vertebra, discs and spinal cord, increasing your chances of damaging them.

The key is to focus and have some intensity. If you are just going through the motions you are not forcing your body to improve, you are coasting. Hit the accelerator. Put some muscle into the movement and socialize after your workout.

> *"The trouble with jogging is that, by the time you realize you're not in shape for it, it's too far to walk back."* – **Franklin P. Jones**

A LITTLE GOES A LONG WAY

If 30 – 45 minutes of aerobic exercise can raise your metabolism for 20 plus hours and weights raise it for roughly 30 hours, then you will be burning more calories at rest. Even sitting at your workstation or driving home. More calories burned means more pounds lost.

Remember this when you are exercising because that silly calories burned number isn't what you are looking to accomplish. It doesn't mean you burned off 300 calories and can have a 250-calorie cookie. It means that the workout you just completed is starting to shift your body's engine into a food-burning machine. Do this a few days a week and you will be burning more calories throughout your day.

Eat the wrong foods during the day and your workout will be in vain. Simple sugars, like in a cookie, will only halt everything you just did to raise your metabolism. The sugars slow the metabolism, increase insulin levels and increase the storage of food as fat. So if you are setting a goal, exercise and sensible eating go hand in hand.

If you have no time to do *"real exercise,"* and your chores are calling, they can burn calories too. Pushing the mower, raking the lawn, shoveling snow, landscaping and planting trees will all help burn more calories than sitting on the couch watching The Bold & The Beautiful or The Jerry Springer Show.

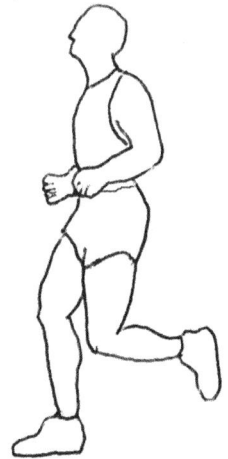

Approximately 300 – 500 calories per hour can be burned depending on your effort and the difficulty of the task. You might be pushing a mower up hill versus flat areas or shoveling dirt with clay and rocks versus soft sand.

Becoming the cleaning tornado can make you sweat too. Vacuuming, laundry, dusting and disinfecting any part of a bathroom will count as a form of exercise. It's not as good as jogging or weight lifting but it is something.

I have patients who tell me that they work hard and can't understand why they aren't losing weight. Doing laundry and dusting all day doesn't burn calories or boost your metabolism like regular physical activity in a gym. Accept no substitutes. Ain't nothing like the real thing baby, but something's better than nothing.

"Lack of activity destroys the good condition of every human being, while movement and methodical physical exercise save it and preserve it." – **Plato**

FORM MEETS FUNCTION

Without concentration there is a greater chance of getting injured by losing sight of good form and failing to maintain proper posture during the lift. The secret is to focus on the muscle lifting the weight. You don't put your mind on cruise control when you work or take care of the kids do you? At least I hope not, so why would you do it now?

This means you aren't merely curling a weight with your arm and lowering it. You are focused on fully contracting the biceps and exhaling as you lift the weight. This motion is known as a Concentric movement. Make a muscle at the top of your contraction. When you slowly lower the weight under control, it is called an Eccentric movement. Using proper form, your body won't sway as a way to cheat by using momentum. The muscle stays under tension the entire time. That's a proper lift. That's the method you should use for the entire body.

When you concentrate on the muscles you can get more out of your workout. If you want, take out a guide to the muscles and learn where they are and how they function. For example, the next time you perform a rowing exercise you will squeeze your rhomboids, the muscle between your shoulder blades, and try to have them touch. That's probably different from what you were doing before, and you will feel it.

Another example is people bench pressing with too much weight. They lift their back off the bench and increase their chance of a back injury. Lighten up.

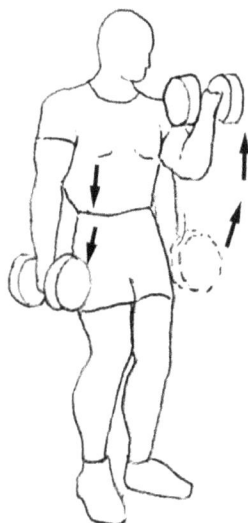

> *"Change your thoughts and you change your world."* – **Norman Vincent Peale**

SPICE IT UP

Variety keeps things fresh. Don't get stagnant with your workout by doing the same routine on the same machine over and over. There are a lot of different exercises for each body part, a hundred machines in the building and a handful of strategies from the beginner level to the all out grunter.

Varying the machines and exercises will change the angle your muscles are worked. It can hit different sections of a muscle group, produce greater gains by shocking the muscles and can help prevent burnout. This helps muscles grow in all regions and will yield better overall results. You might also have an option to lift if your regular machine is being used.

I only have one large gym apparatus in my house now and I am always inventing new ways to use my machine. I have changed the bars I'm using, made six foot cables to be used with individual grips, switched between different handles to do the same exercise and even focused on lifting using my bodyweight. Herschel Walker lifted a lot with his own bodyweight, and sometimes even had someone sitting on his back. He did pushups and other exercises using his bodyweight and he was a *"monster."* My friend Mike just told me about an 80-year old teammate on his softball team. He is in great shape. He does 140 pushups every morning. Sure he breaks it up into simple sets. ONE!

> *"Most people rust out due to lack of challenge. Few people rust out due to overuse."*
> **– Unknown**

THE CHICKS DIG IT

As I was saying before, I worked out my arms and my chest because that is what attracted the ladies. Like my caveman ancestors I wanted to impress my possible suitor but couldn't find a woolly mammoth to slay and bring to her father, so I decided being muscular was my best option.

The problem is I had a weak back and triceps because I ignored them. In fact, when I first hurt my back mixing cement I was told by a chiropractor I needed to do more lifting for my back to establish some balance in my muscles. It was under-developed in relation to my *"guns."* The problem is I couldn't see my back so there was no drive or gratification to work it. Showing off the goods is what drove this 16-year-old boy, and some older boys, to lift weights. We all want to see the fruits of our labor.

I have this great picture in my high school yearbook of me playing soccer. It is from behind, number 12, and

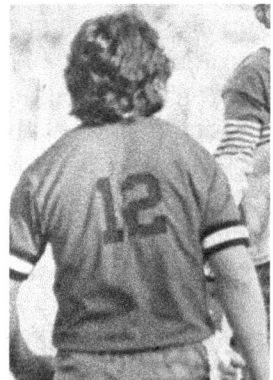

I am getting ready to assist on a play. From the back, my shoulders look like they might touch in the front. My chest muscles are so tight and strong they are pulling the shoulders forward, in and down. And I know what you're thinking as you look at the picture … look at all that *"hair."*

Adults can have similar problems. Just look at the guys grunting with the chicken legs as they bench 500 lbs. Symmetry is more than just looking good; it is essential for great posture, proper biomechanics and a healthier body. You are only as strong as your weakest body part.

If you really want to impress, learn correct techniques before you try working out and remember to train your entire body. I would rather have a garden full of vegetables than one row of magnificent corn.

> *"The body is an instrument, the mind its function,*
> *the witness and reward of its operation."* – **George Santayana**

LET IT BURN

Sometimes when I lift, I may really get in a groove and feel it deep in the muscles. When I add some intensity, the skin feels like it is going to burst over my muscles. That's a great pump. If you don't feel it in the muscle, you're not getting the contraction when you lift the weight. You might be doing something wrong or you're not connecting to the movement.

Think about what you are doing and concentrate. Achieving that pumped feeling will give you greater results in a shorter period. It's like posing or making a muscle when you have fully contracted your muscle. Focusing on the exercise forces more blood and nutrients into the region and will help you get results.

If you are just getting back into lifting don't overdo it. Give your body some time to slowly get back into the swing of things. You will also help your body adapt to the new strains placed upon it and reduce the possibility of injury.

What you definitely don't want to do is swing the weight. You need to lift at a level which you can control your movements. Using momentum is cheating. You are using other muscles to help you complete the lift and aren't getting the maximum benefit of lifting for that body part.

You've seen the guys who do arm curls swinging and pumping the weights, causing their whole bodies to move. They are training their backs and shoulders while moving like pigeons. This is the precursor to an injury. Control the weight.

Something I have noticed even I am guilty of is lifting and moving my head forward. That's a big no-no. Train while keeping good posture. By keeping your ears in line with your shoulders you reduce stress on your neck and strengthen your neck muscles while they hold your neck in its proper position. Now you are strengthening your spine with good posture and this will be beneficial to keeping it healthy.

> *"Although the world is full of suffering, it is full also of the overcoming of it."*
> **– Helen Keller**

NO PAIN, NO GAIN, IS INSANE

If you feel something hurt, then you should stop. You can talk to the trainer for some insight or go see your doctor for an evaluation. Did you warm up properly? Have you been stretching? Is it too much weight? Did you compromise your posture to complete the lift? Did you lose focus? Regardless of the reason, there is no need to push through it if it means you are going to cause serious injury and be left on the sidelines for a while.

Sometimes when I lift I may feel something out of the ordinary, so I stop. I may try it again after some loosening up or try to complete my workout with other exercises. If it doesn't get better and doesn't feel right, then I stop. It will be there tomorrow. The weights that is. Hopefully, not the pain.

If you push an injury you are probably going to make it worse. Listen to your body when it signals something is wrong. Otherwise you could cause permanent damage. If the pain persists, then call your doctor and listen to his or her advice.

> *"The absence of alternatives clears the mind marvelously."* **– Henry Kissinger**

IT'S ALL IN THE WRISTS

There are many different strategies for lifting. It is always good to try different ones so you can find what you like, what fits in your schedule, what gives you the best results or something to mix it up and shock your muscles. Here are a few of the different strategies bodybuilders use to work out their bodies.

The SAID principle stands for Specific Adaptation to Imposed Demands. Because your body has a unique ability to adapt to any physical demand, you need to vary your workouts. Remember we talked about how your body can reset its metabolism. Well, your body also needs constant variations of muscle stimulation in order for it to grow. Now having all of those options makes sense.

Cross-training is a basic concept of this principle. Mixing up running and weight lifting will require your body to adapt to the physical challenges you put on it. Aerobic training like running, with anaerobic training like lifting weights followed up by multiple variations of sports is the best way to get your body to respond to your training routine.

When you move a weight of any size try to use explosive movement to push the weight to the top and then slowly bring the weight back down. For example, if you are bench pressing, push the weight away from your chest quickly, pause, slowly let it return to the starting position and pause before repeating. The reason to move the weight with quick force is to imitate real life situations with sports and force a good contraction in to the muscle.

You could lift heavier weights with a few reps one week, and then use lighter weights and higher reps the next week. When you lift with really heavy weights you aren't completing the typical 10 – 12 repetitions. The weight is too heavy. You are stressing different muscle fibers. One to four repetitions of a heavy weight is a real mass builder. You can take a minute or two break in between sets to allow your body time to replenish your muscles with more lifting energy.

When you switch to the higher repetitions of 12 – 15 and use lighter weights, you are sculpting and defining your body. These are the muscles that will be needed for long-term projects like vacuuming, where as heavy lifting is for that short duration of effort it takes to move a dresser. Together, alternating between weight groups works the muscles completely.

As a general rule you could try to push for 50 – 75 repetitions per muscle. That would be 3 or 4 sets of lifting a weight that strains the muscle enough that you are unable to do more than 15. Otherwise you are just going through the motions, wasting your time and not forcing your muscles to work hard enough. You will not get huge but will end up with toned and stronger muscles. Having greater intensity will result in less time in the gym and more results.

You could superset, in which you complete one set and then decrease the weight, and immediately start another set. You get no break here and it saves time. You will continue to do this until every ounce of energy is drained from your muscles and you are exhausted. Now repeat it. This is a great way to get in and lift, hard and fast. Your workout should be tiring and physically exhaustive, but productive. You can also get a cardiovascular workout by doing this type of routine. Constant effort raises the heart rate and burns additional calories. A bona fide two for one.

I remember thinking everyone in the gym must have thought I was a wimp when I was sweating and straining to curl 5 pounds. That's because I started a lot heavier and then took 5 or 10 pounds off and did as many reps as I could, and then immediately dropped weight again. You can wind up doing 5 or 7 sets back to back. Every fiber in your muscles will be fatigued. You can complete a workout in no time.

A pyramid set is a technique to start lifting with a light weight and increase the weight for each consecutive lift until you reach your peak. Then reverse the program and take weight off as you do each lift until you are back down to the beginning weight. So you could start out doing 10 reps with one weight, take a

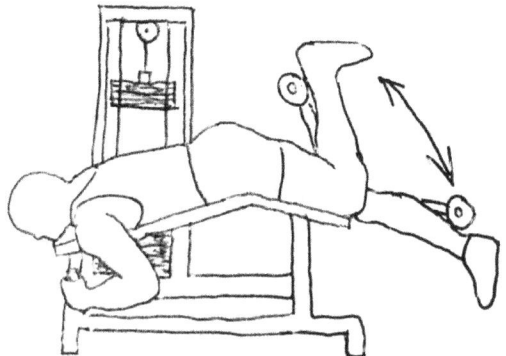

break, then add some weight and go for eight reps. Follow that pattern until you get to 1 or 2 repetitions. Then work your way back down the weights again.

There is no set increment to raise or drop weights. If you truly want to get the most out of your hard work, make sure that when you lift you have no more reps in you before you rest and switch to a different weight.

So for the people pressed for time, supersets and pyramid routines are a great way to totally fatigue your muscles and get out of the gym fast. They are so strenuous that you will also get an aerobic benefit because the body never fully recuperates in between sets.

German volume training is similar to the previous strategies. While doing split routines use a weight that is around 50 - 60 percent of your one rep max. Now perform 10 sets of 10 reps and only take a minute or so break between them. This is for the larger muscle groups: chest, back, shoulders and legs. Only lift 3 sets for smaller muscles like: calfs, abs, biceps and triceps. Take a day off between workout sessions.

Other strategies are the 10-second rep. You lift the weight quickly to the peak position in around 1 second, contract the muscle and hold for 2 seconds, now slowly return to the start position over 3 seconds and then hold the weight for 4 seconds before attempting another lift. It helps to focus on the eccentric or negative action of a lift, so you control the weight as it comes back down to the starting point. This technique keeps your muscle fibers under tension longer than when you go through the motions quickly. Longer tension can lead to bigger gains.

You won't be able to do your normal repetitions with your regular weight because your muscles will be under constant stress and they will tire out. Another real benefit results from pausing at the bottom. You have no chance to use momentum to start the lift. This can help strengthen weak spots, like the lowest part of an arm curl, and help you achieve greater success in the gym. If you don't want to count out the 10 seconds, just slow down and approximate the hesitations.

Slower movement allows you to decrease the weight and save your joints while still getting a great burn in your muscle fibers. There is a lot of research that points to the eccentric movement or lowering of the weight to be a truly effective muscle builder. Many bodybuilders feel this is the most important, muscle building part of a lift. Don't discount using lighter weights, slowing down and protecting your body.

Because many of the everyday chores and demands life throws at us require us to perform them with one arm or the other, you can lift weights using one arm or leg. Most of us have a dominant side. That side typically becomes stronger, more developed and can cause postural distortions.

Lifting independently from the other arm or leg will build a more powerful and symmetrical body. Using your arms or legs together when you lift, allows the body to overcompensate and cheat for its lagging muscles so you can lift more. The strategy of lifting independently really emphasizes the individual muscle, and allows greater range of motion that leads to deeper contractions, and great results.

Using dumbbells or a functional training machine, which has two individual cables and complete freedom of motion, allows you to isolate and strengthen a weaker side of your body. If you balance out the strength of each side comparatively you will have superior strength overall. You remove the weakest link in your armor.

There are many choices when it comes to lifting weights. Choose the one that's right for you or switch back and forth to keep shocking your muscles into achieving growth and results. That is what the P90X Fitness program you see on TV is all about. It preaches varying your workout to shock your muscles and keep them from reaching a state of complacency.

> *"So many new ideas are at first strange and horrible, though ultimately valuable that a very heavy responsibility rests upon those who would prevent their dissemination."* – **J. B. S. Haldane**

IT ISN'T LOGICAL CAPTAIN

I did this calculation for a friend and it is mind blowing. Let's say between your arm curls and squats you lift 100 pounds on average. Now let's say you do 10 repetitions and 10 sets. That's 100 pounds x 10 reps = 1,000 pounds. Averaging your number of sets per workout to 10, that is 1,000 pounds x 10 sets = 10,000 pounds.

I lift 5 days a week by working different body parts, called a split routine. So 5 days x 10,000 pounds = 50,000 pounds. If you work out 50 weeks a year that would mean 50 weeks x 50,000 pounds = 2.5 million pounds. If you have lifted for 20 years, that is 20 years x 2.5 million pounds = 50 million pounds. If you average 50 pounds per lift, with 10 reps and 10 set workout, 3 times a week schedule, then you would have lifted 5,000 pounds a day, 15,000 pounds a week, 750,000 pounds a year and 15 million pounds over 20 years.

That is a lot of weight and stress to put on your joints. No wonder my shoulders hurt. Throw in some sports injuries, shoveling snow, chopping firewood and building stonewalls and it's pretty obvious how the body gets beat up. More reason to lighten up, try going slowly or at least lift smart.

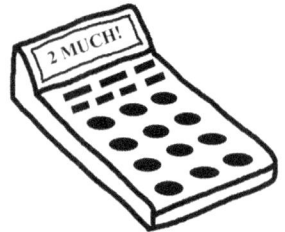

"The strongest man in the world is he who stands alone." – **Henrik Ibsen**

HEY MR. BIG STUFF

Women are afraid of lifting weights because they think they will get big and bulky and look like Wonder Woman. I have a neighbor who used to compete and when she lifts she does respond quickly, but she gets lean and defined. Most women wish they had her problem and genetics, but most of us aren't that lucky.

You need to have high levels of testosterone to build muscle. That's why people cheat and take steroids. Now they can create the unnatural, unhealthy, consequence-filled body they could DIE for. Males typically have higher levels of testosterone so they respond more quickly when lifting. Training your legs involves more large muscles than any other body part and is a natural way to raise your natural testosterone levels for better growth.

It takes weeks and months to actually put on muscle mass naturally. Remember muscle burns more calories than fat and no one becomes huge overnight by lifting weights. It takes years of training hard and dedicated dietary sacrifices, so don't be afraid of getting defined muscles. Your goal should be that the back of your arms may become sculpted and firm or that the definition in your calves is turning heads. This is toning the body. It is beauty without bulk.

In order to gain a lot of muscle weight, there is a whole structured diet you need to follow. I will discuss this in two more sections and yes, carbs are important and vital to your success. Many guys are still the same size after years of lifting weights because they don't follow these nutritional demands. So ladies, no excuses.

"Get knowledge of the spine, for this is the requisite for many diseases."
– **Hippocrates**

THIS IS HOW WE DO IT

If you are looking to tone and sculpt your body, then you will use lower weights and higher repetitions (reps). Increasing your cardio will also help to shed a few pounds of fat covering the lean body that waits to emerge. Toning up requires you to do 12 – 15 reps per set. At a gym they may have a cycle of exercises you can run through a few times to get a great and effective full body workout.

If you are doing 3 sets of curls and at the end of the third set you could still do more, do yourself a favor and increase the weight. You don't want to just go through the motions do you? Why else would you have on that form-fitting Under Armour gear?

To achieve results from your hard work you need to use enough resistance to fatigue the muscle. If the sets are completed like this; 15 reps, then 13 reps, then 12 reps, that is perfect. You don't want to lift anymore if it means you have to use your body to cheat and forfeit form.

For the normal person who wants to get a little bigger and increase strength, you will lift heavier weights. Your reps will range from 8 – 12 per set and you may be doing 4 – 8 sets per body part. Focus on exhausting the muscle and feeling it with each contraction.

You might work the upper body one day and the lower body the following day, split up by cardio and repeated. Another strategy is to do a split routine so you can focus on each muscle group separately. Remember they need a break to recuperate because you are focusing on them.

Concentrating on a specific group of muscles will damage the muscle fibers, which is why they need time to repair and get stronger and bigger. Make sure you rest them. Some of us have been giving our muscles a couple of years to rest. I think it's okay to start your next rep now.

I like to adjust my lifting for the sports I play. If I'm training for baseball, I will take the high cable from the pulley system and slowly swing it like a bat to work the exact muscles I need for an explosive swing. You could do that for throwing or serving a tennis ball too. I have drilled holes in a baseball and inserted hooks or ropes so I can attach it to the high cable of my home gym. Now I can grip a baseball and go through the throwing motion with some resistance.

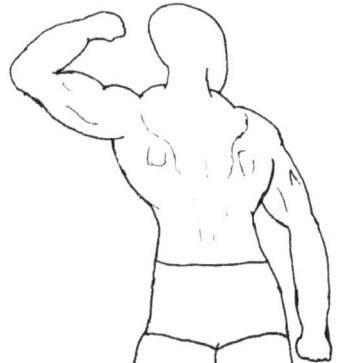

I have even altered a bat to attach the same way. That's why baseball players use weighted bats or put a metal donut on the end of their bat. Using weighted resistance can improve your golf swing as well. In fact, you don't have to be extreme like me. Just the fact that you are in the gym strengthening your muscles is a sure way to improve your sport and well-being. It would be frightening to see what kind of numbers Ted Williams or Babe Ruth would have put up if they were training regularly.

Okay big boys. If you want to get really big and strong then this is your section. You want to lift heavy weights for low repetitions. Completing 1 – 6 reps are for strength and mass. You want to overload the muscles so they are forced to grow. Like a professional bodybuilder, you also need to give your muscles 4 – 5 days to rest so they can repair and rebuild.

Muscle repair can take as long as 7 – 10 days. The swelling in the muscle tissue occurs during and immediately after lifting. The cleanup crew removes the damaged tissue and leads to the formation of free radicals. We know from the vitamin section that increasing your antioxidant levels can help remove these harmful critters from our body faster. Working different body parts can allow you to keep lifting while other muscles are recuperating, or do some cardio.

Another way to see if you have fully recovered is to wait until the muscles you are planning on working out have recovered from the previous workout. They shouldn't be sore and they should have their normal range of motion again.

You are probably going to be doing split routines. This allows you to completely blast your chest one day, your back the next, your legs another day, rest or cardio, your arms and then your shoulders and rest or cardio. That is a tough week but this allows you to completely hit all of your muscles and make them grow. Your training partner can help you complete lifts when you are exhausted by adding a little assistance. That will help your muscles push past any sticking points in your training regimen.

In the old days Arnold and his training partners Franco Columbo and Frank Zane used to work chest in the AM and the back in the PM. If you have the time and dedication, you could hit the gym twice a day. If you have a job, once a day may be all the time you can afford.

Remember that your arms are involved with chest exercises so mixing in a lower body day, abdominal or cardio day will help them rest before you lift. If your arms are still tired and tight from your chest workout, when you attempt to work the arms you will not be as productive, because they are still fatigued. That goes for other exercises as well. Either work your back and shoulders on the same day or put a few days in between their workouts.

You should do 10 – 20 sets per large muscle group and 8 – 14 for smaller groups. You need to be taking in water and carbohydrates to keep the body fueled. Eat often and eat plenty of good nutrition to help keep enough energy in the system. For you teenagers that raid the fridge when you get out of school, nobody gets big and strong eating Ding Dongs and Ho-Hos.

If you train really hard you will raise the caloric demands of your body. You need to feed the machine to make it bigger and stronger. If you don't have enough nutrition then your body will eventually break down muscle tissue. As I have said before, this is why some guys never get bigger after years of lifting.

Research suggests that there is a window of opportunity to take in large amounts of simple carbohydrates during and especially within 5 minutes of finishing your workout. It doesn't matter what form it is in either, but sports drinks, energy drinks and fruit juice would be ideal. Liquids are better absorbed in the body because the surface area is smaller. When you eat you have to breakdown food into small enough pieces so your body can utilize it.

This will help replenish the carbohydrates stored in the body, while storing some in the bank for your next workout. Then within the next hour you should eat or drink a good amount of protein to provide the building blocks to allow the muscles to repair and grow. Consumer Reports found many popular protein powders contain dangerous heavy metals like Arsenic, Cadmium, Mercury and Lead, so do some research and choose wisely. Skim milk, Greek yogurt, cottage cheese, walnuts, almonds, egg whites and tuna fish are just a few examples of higher protein foods to replenish your body's needs.

Serious bodybuilders consume up to 6,000 calories a day to pack on muscle and drink casein protein shakes before bed to preserve it. They can always lean up by altering their workouts and diet, once they have accumulated the additional poundage. Good luck and get ready to shop for some new clothes.

> *"It is better to deserve honors and not have them, than to have them and not to deserve them."* – **Mark Twain**

DO THE RIGHT THING

The sporting world is constantly reporting on athletes from various sports using drugs as a means to get an upper hand on their opponents. There was even an incident when Nascar drivers were guilty of using illegal fuels in their vehicles. I believe they consider this cheating too. Kind of like a cowboy having an ace up his sleeve to win big at the saloon. It is frowned upon and often met with an untimely death.

Sadly, and too often, so are the athletes who feel they need to use steroids to be competitive and succeed. Athletes' drive for winning is at all costs. They want to be the best for themselves, for financial reasons and the fame. But there is a price much greater than being on a cereal box.

Even Hollywood stars and musical performers are resorting to improving their bodies through unnatural means. When someone has a change in their body and it happens too quickly, it should raise a red flag.

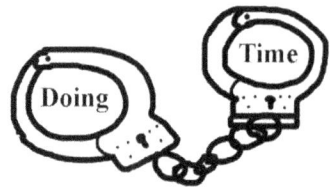

Current news coverage reports how baseball teams are riddled with steroid use, but they are not alone. Any sport is susceptible to athletes looking for an edge. The worlds of martial arts, boxing, football, track and field, cycling, pro wrestling and bodybuilding also have problems.

To help maintain a fair competition and for the health of the athletes, many countries have organizations to test and punish athletes for using drugs. Stiffer penalties have been adopted to discourage cheating. At the same time, distributors and athletes are constantly searching for ways to confuse test results or have drugs that are designed to be undetectable at the current time.

Cheaters try to stay one step ahead of the laws and rules of fair competition. How many years did we have to hear the denials before finally hearing the truth from Floyd Landis and Marion Jones, regarding their steroid use? Lance Armstrong was next and has been stripped of his titles because of steroid use.

Kids look to many of these top athletes as role models. Warranted or not, kids see these competitors as larger than life entities who can do no wrong. Sometimes parents are around less than they should be, or can be, and athletes are all a child has to look up to. Charles Barkley was once in a commercial and stated, *"Athletes aren't role models for your children, you are."*

I am from a divorced family and my role models and influences were Elvis Presley, Thurman Munson and John Wayne. I was from a different era so my only quirks are my left leg shakes, I play to win, and I say *"pilgrim"* a lot.

With the lure of a professional career, big money, parents' expectations, popularity in the high school or college setting or a scholarship, our youth is being drawn to taking shortcuts. Studies suggest that there is an increasing prevalence of boys and girls using steroids in high school and middle school. With boys, five - 12 percent are using steroids. The numbers are less with girls.

Steroids in the hands of a physician are a different story. Doctors can use steroids to help people recover, regain their health and decrease their pain. When good things are used for purposes other than what they were originally intended, is when problems, including abuse, arise.

> *"What lies behind us and what lies before us are tiny matters compared to what lies within us."* – **Ralph Waldo Emerson**

A COLD, HARD LOOK

Athletes trying to gain an unnatural advantage on their competition utilize Anabolic Steroids and substances to help promote increased steroid production, known as precursors. These hormones can lead to muscle and bone growth by increasing protein synthesis. They also stop the destruction of muscle tissue by cortisol, during stressful times. The body will grow and become stronger but there is a consequence for these actions. Common names of steroids in the news are Testosterone, Androstenedione and HGH (human growth hormone).

Some general side effects of these drugs are Heart Disease, Liver Disease, enlarged heart, impotence, Osteoporosis, birth defects, acne, baldness, a bad temper and mood swings. Male specific side effects are Gynecomastia, or development of breasts, reduced sexual functioning or infertility and testicular atrophy.

Female side-effects can include a deepening of the voice, increased body hair, changes in the physical appearance and less frequent menstrual cycles due to acquiring more male characteristics.

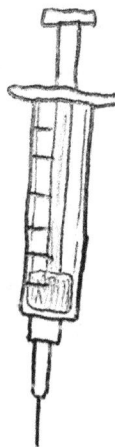

Some athletes resort to blood doping, which puts more red blood cells in the body so more oxygen can be carried throughout the body. This is a common reason for cheating in aerobic events like cycling and track due to the athlete's need for oxygen. With more blood cells carrying oxygen your body is less likely to get fatigued and you can finish strong.

How do athletes feel when they are found guilty of cheating? Sometimes it is only their personal medals and accolades that are stripped away. Other times when they play for a team or win a track event with three others, everyone loses their medals. Now they have to face up to their teammates for taking away their dreams as well. We all watched Lance Armstrong be stripped of his titles.

Any form of enhanced performance is known as cheating in my opinion. Don't take a shortcut to improve your performance and ability. Improve what you have or what you can do, naturally and safely. It's called: hard work, dedication, commitment, heart, perseverance and respect. Sounds a lot like a good relationship with someone special. Maybe even your conscience?

> *"Someone must teach new things, someone must take the abuse, someone must be ostracized, someone must be called a fraud or a quack. Then out of all of it comes the new truth to become a part of us....Thus we receive new facts to make up our proud possession of knowledge."*
> **– Fred Hart (Founder, National Health Federation)**

PLYO-WHAT?

Plyometrics is an exercise method that uses explosive movements to increase strength or speed. The principle is to stretch the muscle and then contract it quickly to produce elastic energy, like a rubber band.

If you pull a rubber band back, hold it and release it, you will not get as much distance as you will when it is pulled back the same distance and released quickly. Try it for yourself. That's elastic energy! Using that energy to assist you to generate more force or strength is the goal. Capturing that brief moment of energy, and contracting the muscle just as it is stretched, is called the Stretch Shortening Cycle.

Being able to convert strength into speed is the goal. It's based on trying to develop maximum force in the shortest amount of time. Having strong legs that can squat 500 pounds will not have the ability to elevate a basketball player as quickly as a player who quickly pushes up 250 pounds as soon as it is lowered, to simulate jumping.

Performing a pushup and then forcing your body up and high enough to clap your hands is another example. Just when you lower the chest and the muscle is stretched, explosively push back up.

One of the more common exercises seen for jumping is using one or more boxes and jumping up and down quickly. The heights can be different, but when you land and come all the way down, you have to explode off the ground up to the next box height. Training involves light weights or multiple repetitions of using bodyweight for resistance.

I've seen sprinters running while they drag a small parachute, or a tire, and then release the resistance to push the speed limits further. Looks crazy but the pros rely on it to improve their performance.

Before you decide to surprise your Wednesday night basketball crew by dazzling them with your dunking abilities, make sure you have the strength, flexibility, balance, coordination and good instruction in the form of a book, video or trainer, before attempting these types of maneuvers.

"In matters of style, swim with the current; in matters of principle, stand like a rock."
– Thomas Jefferson

TAKING THE PLUNGE

One of the greatest exercises to help develop or strengthen the body on the inside and the outside is swimming. Just ask Johnny Weismuller, who used to play Tarzan when I was a kid. Granted he splashed more than he swam but he was in great shape. Hey, he was also swimming toward alligators while he was splashing. I would have been more apt to splash, than swim toward them too. Maybe they would turn around.

One of the great things about swimming or exercising in water is that the water provides a gravity-reduced environment. It's like being a little weightless. That means if you have pain when you are standing, the water can decrease the amount of stress to the spine and impact to your joints. This will allow you to exercise in some form.

Even if you're not swimming you can walk or do water aerobics. This is a way to do all the exercises you would normally do using the water for added resistance. You can lean against the side of the pool and do some gentle leg kicks or bends. There are all sorts of fins, paddles and specialized gear, like pool weights, in the form of foam gloves or water-filled weights, to use as added resistance to build strength and muscle.

The pool can also be a saving grace before, during and after pregnancy. The buoyancy of the water can allow you to move and release some of the tension in your body from carrying the little bundle of joy.

The art of swimming involves both your cardiovascular system and muscles. With each stroke you are reaching and then contracting. It's almost like doing Pilates and resistance training simultaneously. You get greater flexibility and range of motion in your joints. By using the major muscle groups of the arms and legs you are burning more calories because more muscles are involved with the exercise.

You can burn anywhere from 300 – 800 calories per hour depending on the intensity of your swim and which style you use. You do need some weight bearing exercise to help prevent osteoporosis and maintain bone integrity.

Two cautions. One is for the person who constantly swims freestyle and keeps turning their head to one side. If you are a competitor, try to alternate breathing from either side for practice laps. This is a way to give the overworked side a break during practice sessions and maybe strengthen the rarely used side to balance out the spine. You could even use a snorkel so you don't have to turn the head in either direction. This way no one gets twisted the wrong way. Favor the side that is comfortable for intense training and competitions. Otherwise you will overdevelop one side of your neck and upper back and create a problem.

Secondly, a recent study found that kids who swam in enclosed pools had a higher incidence of asthma and other health problems from breathing in the chlorine, when compared to children who swam in open air or outdoor facilities. More studies are being conducted but in general it may be better to swim in open air to avoid breathing in the chemicals from the chlorine or pool.

"Courage is being scared to death - but saddling up anyway." – **John Wayne**

EVERYBODY WAS KUNG FU FIGHTING

The Martial Arts have been around for centuries. They are a discipline employing mental focus, inner and outer strength, self-confidence, combat and agility. There are many different schools of Martial arts. Some concentrate more on punching while others incorporate only kicking, variations of both, or even weapons and submission holds.

Each has different ranks depending on how far your training goes and what level of competency you achieve. It is a great exercise for people of all ages, but getting clearance from your doctor is never a bad idea before starting any new routine.

It can help the flexibility of the elderly, self-confidence of a child, reassurance of a woman who works in a bad neighborhood or a competitor who strives to learn and understand more about his sport.

It includes aerobic training, muscle building exercises, balance, quickness, movement and inner peace. There are classes offered everywhere. Find which discipline might be right for you.

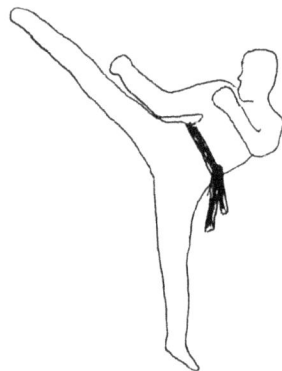

> *"Destiny is no matter of chance. It is a matter of choice. It is not a thing to be waited for, it is a thing to be achieved."* – **William Jennings Bryan**

Other Options

There are many options if you don't want to be lifting a weight or spinning in a gym. If any routine or program you try wants you to bend or contort in a way that causes pain, stop. If it looks dangerous or it might aggravate an injury you know you have, then do something else for a minute or two and then continue with the routine. They have plenty of other moves that are beneficial to your health. I remember putting my feet over my head while I was on my back, and the classic doing a bridge exercise on my head for wrestling. Two moves I didn't like then and will never do again.

You could try exercises like Taebo, the dance routine workouts, Richard Simmons or Jazzercise. It doesn't matter what you decide to use as long as you try something. Here are two that you should try if you are interested in slower and lower impact types of exercises.

> *"Stretching his hand out to catch the stars, he forgets the flowers at his feet."*
> – **Jeremy Bentham**

PILATES

This is a series of movements that combines strength, efficient motion, flexibility, balance and agility in an environment focusing on a healthy mind, good posture and graceful movement. It helps define muscles without bulk to develop a longer and leaner physique.

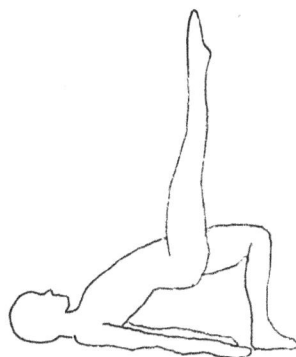

There is no preset body type needed to participate. You can proceed at your own pace and incorporate the ideas into your workout as you go. There are many different routines to prevent you from becoming bored. If you have any discomfort with any movement, then try to use different exercises or modify your position.

Benefits associated with Pilates besides the aforementioned, are also improving your circulation and lung capacity. Having a strong core with greater strength and flexibility, your mind more in tune with your training, greater perception of balance and a healthier body are some of the additional benefits.

All of these traits can be useful in keeping you feeling young, independent, sharp, better coordinated and injury free.

> *"Always aim at complete harmony of thought and word and deed. Always aim at purifying your thoughts and everything will be well."* – **Mahatma Gandhi**

YOGA

Some people envision contortionist positions of the body when they think about yoga, which hardly seem beneficial or relaxing. However it can be because it is actually a combination of many principles to focus on uniting your mind, body and spirit. Through exercise, breathing and meditation; true harmony, peace and less stress can be achieved. It will keep your body flexible as well as your mind.

There are several different schools of training. Some are easy and gentle while others are more difficult and aggressive. There are eight limbs, or teachings of yoga that guide and help us understand different components of inner peace and enlightenment. They include everything from concentration and meditation, breathing, withdrawal of senses, and postures.

Some of the mental teachings of yoga help give meaning to one's life and show purpose for existence. It helps us to act appropriately with regards to moral and ethical situations. It is about respecting yourself, others and life in general. The old adage treat others as you wish to be treated comes to mind. Some instruction may be more about reading and learning, than stretching alone.

Most people engage in the exercise and stretching portion of yoga for better flexibility, strength and overall health. Whether you are a beginner or an expert, this is a great exercise for any age. Go at your own pace. You too may find that yoga may be part of the secret to reducing stress and clearer thinking.

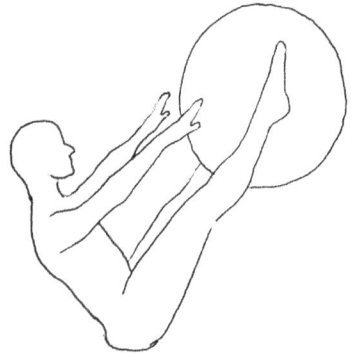

> *"Remember that what you believe will depend very much on what you are."*
> – **Noah Porter**

REMEMBER

Before starting any exercise routine, discuss any health concerns with your doctor. If you have any problems during any exercise, stop what you are doing and please consult a healthcare professional immediately. Your friends are not trained to diagnose your pain. Go to a doctor. Not someone who slept at a Holiday inn.

Remember the weight you might be trying to lose doesn't come on overnight and it is not going to come off overnight either. So grab your spouse or a friend and take a walk, play tennis, go dancing and have fun. Start slowly and incorporate some fitness into your life and enjoy greater health and increased energy. Grab the kids and go to the park or join them in a game of kickball. You'll feel like a new person and you will owe it all to yourself.

There are lots of websites to show you how to lift. Unfortunately a lot of them are also selling you all kinds of stuff and making outrageous claims about items they sell. Some that I found to be pretty good for demonstrating a variety of exercises for each muscle group are: www.betterbodz.com/exercise_main.html, www.bodybuilding.com/fun/exercises.html, and www.shapefit.com/training.html. With any website, don't get sucked into all of the items for sale.

You can select any body part and there will be around 10 exercise variations for you to choose from. When you click any of them there will be a video demonstration of how to perform the exercise correctly. The video can be really helpful. Other websites may also offer great video demonstrations if you need assistance. There are always instructional DVDs for sale as well.

conSequences

impoTence

enlargEd heart

biRth defects

osteopOrosis

organ faIlure

blooD clots

diSease

"You can either hold yourself up to the unrealistic standards of others, or ignore them and concentrate on being happy with yourself as you are." – **J. Jacques**

Basic Workout

In this section I am going to give a brief description of what each muscle does, help you understand the muscle itself and show several variations of exercises you can do. Having good strength and balance of all of your muscles improves your posture, protects your spine and will keep you healthier and more mobile over the years.

▪ Warm up before exercising and always cool down and stretch afterwards.

▪ With exercises you always want to exhale as you lift the weight and the muscle contracts. Then inhale as you lower the weight. Otherwise you will create too much internal pressure and can really injure yourself.

▪ Give yourself a minute or two in between lifts no matter what lifting strategy you are following or whether you are lifting light or heavy weights.

▪ Starting position is usually with your hands or feet about shoulder's width apart. With lying down exercises don't arch your back. Maintain good posture and form with each exercise.

▪ Concentrate on the muscle you are using. Control the weight when you lift. If you bring a weight or cable down too far you will hear a clanging of the weights. This is a great indicator that you are allowing the weight to control your movement and that you are not keeping the tension on the muscles. Everyone around you is going to have a headache.

▪ Go slowly. Don't swing, allowing momentum to do the work for you. You are really cheating, yourself and your muscles.

▪ Don't do too much and get discouraged. Start slowly and build up muscle, confidence and experience. It takes time to get out of shape and longer to get back into great shape. Be patient and faithful to your regimen.

▪ Discontinue exercise if you have pain and consult with your doctor.

Biceps

This muscle is comprised of two muscle groups on the front of your upper arm. It flexes your forearm toward your shoulder and is recognized as the strength muscle. If someone asks you to make a muscle, this is where the spotlight shines. Bicep curls are a well-known exercise for this muscle group.

Triceps

Located on the back of your arm, this muscle is made up of three muscle groups. People refer to this area as the wiggly part of the arm as we age, or the part that gets jiggy when we wave. When the triceps muscle gets big, your arm will really show some size. The muscle straightens your arm at the elbow, like pushing yourself up from a chair with your hands. Triceps extension works this area of the arm.

Chest

The pectoral muscles are comprised of two muscle groups that are thick and fan shaped. There is the larger group, known as the pec major, and the smaller pec minor, which connect the sternum, or breastbone, to the shoulder and upper arms. They are the muscles that are used when you do a pushup or a bench press.

Back

There are several muscles lumped into this section including the trapezius, rhomboid and latissimus dorsi (the wings).

⊠ The Trapezius muscle is shaped like a kite. It starts at your neck, goes out toward your shoulders and then tapers in toward your lower spine. There are three muscle groups known as the upper, middle and lower trapezius. The upper group brings your shoulders toward your ears like you are saying, *"I don't know."* It gives that thick neck look. Doing shrugs build this muscle. The middle pulls the shoulder blades, or scapula, together. The lower trap brings the shoulder blades downward. Doing a row type of exercise can help develop this muscle group.

⊠ The Rhomboid muscles also have major and minor components. They are located between the inside edge of your shoulder blades and the spine. They retract the scapula and keep it against the ribs. Doing rows will strengthen the mid back.

⊠ The Latissimus muscle is a large, flat muscle on the back. It's main function is to bring each shoulder down and back, and to your side. This muscle gives the wide, wing-like appearance from your waist to your shoulders. Rows, chin-ups or pulling a weight down to your chest or into your abdominal region from overhead strengthens the latissimus muscle.

Shoulders

Broad, thick shoulders develop by exercising the three deltoid muscles. The deltoid is a triangular muscle made up of the anterior, middle and posterior deltoid muscles. With your elbow and upper arm parallel to the floor, arms out to the side, they help to bring your shoulder forward, upward and backward, respectively. Deltoid raises and overhead press are great for this region.

Legs

The legs have a few major muscle groups to discuss in this section. The front of the thigh is called the quadriceps and has three components. The hamstring is in the back of your leg and has two muscle groups. The adductors are on the inside of the leg where you get a pulled groin. On the outside of your leg you have the abductors. In the lower leg are the gastroc and soleus muscles, which make up the calf. Together they help stabilize and support the knee.

⊠ Quadriceps

The front of your leg is comprised of four muscles that are large due the workload they have. These muscles keep you upright and propel you forward when moving. If you sit and contract your thigh, you will extend your leg and knee joint so your lower leg is parallel to your upper leg. This is a leg extension exercise. Squats or leg press are also great to strengthen the entire upper leg.

⊠ Hamstring

This is also a large muscle group and is the counter balance to the quads. They are like the biceps muscle of your leg. Their action is extension of the hip but mostly to flex your heel to your buttock. They play an important role in core strengthening and balance. Standing, lying on your stomach, or prone, and curling a weight to your buttock, known as a hamstring curl, is a great way to isolate this group.

⊠ Adductors

These are the muscles on the inside of your leg. They bring the leg back to your midline or *"add"* to it, as in ADD-uct. Any movement that brings the leg inward against resistance will build this muscle group.

⊠ Abductors

Located on the outside of your thigh, these muscles move your leg away from your midline. Movements that bring your leg outward against resistance strengthen this muscle group.

⊠ Gastroc

This is the major muscle of the calf area and is attached to the heel by the Achilles tendon. It functions to flex the knees but predominantly to point the toe or extend it. This is also known as plantar flexion because the bottom of your foot is called the plantar surface. Calf raises where you lower your body and raise it again develop these muscles.

⊠ Soleus

Behind the gastroc is the soleus muscle, which also flexes the ankle and is attached by the Achilles tendon. Same exercises for the gastroc will also build the soleus muscle.

Abs

The abdominals include many muscles. The more common ones are the upper and lower abdominals and the external and internal obliques along the side of the waist. They are balanced by the low back muscles and are instrumental in keeping your back strong.

Abdominals

Upper and lower abs approximate the upper torso to the pelvic region. There are many variations and we will cover some specific and easy to learn core exercises later. When you are trying to strengthen these muscles, remember to maintain tension on the stomach through the entire movement.

Obliques

They flex forward the upper midsection and laterally flex the spine. Baseball and golf get some of their power from this region. These are trained by working the abs and adding a twist when you come up.

Proper Abdominal Technique

Everyone wants great abs. When I was a kid we had to do sit ups for gym class and were tested for a minute's time. We at least had our knees bent for the ab test. Before my time, people were instructed to keep their legs straight when doing sit ups and that must have injured a few backs along the way. Since then, many variations have been developed.

A recent study conducted by San Diego University found the old reliable knees bent sit up is pretty much worthless. Current belief is that the bicycle movement is best. Supposedly it is 250 percent better at hitting these muscles.

The hanging leg raise looks like it works wonders. This is the maneuver where people suspend themselves by their arms and raise their legs up. The problem is too many people swing their legs for momentum or don't control the descent of their legs.

You will always get the most out of an exercise if it is done slowly and with full concentration of the muscles being used. Likewise, the abs are being trained when you bring your knees to your chest and raise them above your waistline.

When you allow the legs to drop below your waist toward the ground, you are activating your hip flexor muscles and increasing low back pressure. This can cause low back pain by creating excessive hyperextension in the back. Form is key. Knowledge is requisite. Use control.

The hip flexors are also over trained when doing incline sit-ups with your feet locked under a bar. Try to do them in a position that you have to use your abs to complete the motion without holding on with your legs in any way. Two more old standbys that can be forgotten are the straight leg raise and straight leg sit-up. They don't work the abs and impart too much pressure on the discs.

Once your shoulder blades have come up off the floor, don't let them touch again until you are done doing repetitions. This will keep the abs tight. If you're not sure, tap your stomach while you are exercising and see if they are tight all the way through the movement. Also if you must twist when you contract your abs and elevate your body, come up first and then add a twist. Twisting as you come up creates more stress to the low back, than the obliques.

Speaking of twisting, there are people who try to decrease their love handles by using a machine that does waist twisting or they use a bar. Done slowly and to a limited range these could be okay, but many people load up the weights, or they turn completely.

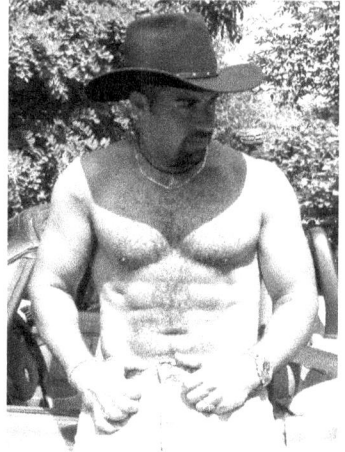

Just like lifting a box and turning with your feet planted, it compresses the spine and then shears the disc. You only have about five degrees of rotation in each lumbar vertebra. Too much weight and forced motion compresses the disc and can cause a major problem. This makes me cringe. This move can be done standing as well. Although standing reduces the stress on your discs, you should still use caution when performing an exercise like this. Be careful not to twist too far and don't twist at the knee.

The other love handle exercise is to stand with two dumbbells. I don't really need to make a joke here do I? Anyway, you bend from side to side to hit the obliques. Each time you lower and rise you are working the sides of your waist. However, you can make the muscle larger by training it and wind up with a thick waist.

Aerobics are the best way to lose your handles, especially in combination with an abdominal routine, reducing your calories or changing your eating habits. Go that route.

When you start doing abdominal exercises you also need to think about hand placement. Don't place your hands behind your neck because if they are there you may start pulling with them and hurt your neck. Pretend there is an orange under your chin so you don't keep bending your neck and exercising it, more than your stomach. Look at the ceiling. I'm not interested in having you train your neck.

Some people like to train abs on the ball. This does allow you to get a fuller range of motion but the key is to go slowly. Perform a strong contraction when you come up to gain the most benefit from the movement. Your feet can stabile you so the ball isn't rolling around. Use your hands to maintain balance while on your back and do reverse abs by bringing your lower half up, much like a hanging knee raise.

There is some controversy over being able to train the upper abs with one move and lower abs with another because the muscle is continuous. You should focus more effort on each exercise as the best way to train your abs completely.

With that said, if you want to attempt to compartmentalize, work your lower section first as it will fatigue quicker than the upper region. Because the upper abs are used for lower abdominal work and are stronger, they can withstand another set of repetitions specifically designed for them like the bicycle.

The newest craze is the dancing abs routines. If you are standing and bringing up your knee to the waist, that will activate some abdominal muscles. When you add contracting your stomach, bending your upper body to the knees and moving your arms you will get some aerobic calorie burning to boot.

The more calories you burn, the leaner you will get. Your clothes will also stay cleaner because you're not on the floor.

Extensor Muscles

If you have strong abs in front you must train the muscles in the back, which balance the core. The erector spinae muscles run vertically along both sides of the spine and are the muscles responsible for keeping you in an upright position. They also support and protect the spine when we lift and move. They are also vital in keeping a healthy midsection. Using a machine or lying on the floor and arching backward can develop better strength in these muscles.

Proper Technique

Extension exercises can help certain types of disc problems and also develop strong back muscles. The extension machine requires you to load your spine and then bend really far backwards. This can compress the spine and the discs. I prefer to use body weight or little resistance for this exercise.

The machine I use is the Roman chair. Your lower body is locked into the machine, as you lie perpendicular to the floor. Bend at the waist and lower your upper body to the floor, pause and bring your body back up. You can safely extend to about 5 degrees beyond the starting position. This is a big difference from bending like you would in the extension machine and it is a lot safer. If you feel like you need more resistance then grab a 10 pound weight or plate and hold it to your chest through the entire movement.

If you have a physiogymnic ball (a blue exercise ball) or a kid's big ball, you can lock your toes under a couch and put your waist over the ball. Now bend forward and bring your back up again. You can even try grabbing the couch with your hands, placing your stomach on the ball and then raising your legs. Same exercise. Don't overextend your back though. I don't care what they do in stretch classes or Broadway shows, listen to your body.

Neck

Many muscles are involved in controlling the movement of the head because it is a 10 pound weight sitting on top of a perch. Basically we have six main movements in the neck. These are bending your head forwards, backwards, turning right or left and bringing your ear toward your shoulder on either side. Keeping the muscles that support the neck strong can help prevent injuries to the body during sports or car accidents. Men typically have less damage to their necks after a car accident because they have more muscle mass supporting their heads.

"The most important work you and I will ever do will be within the walls of our own homes."
— **Harold B. Lee**

The Home Workout
LOWER ABDOMINAL

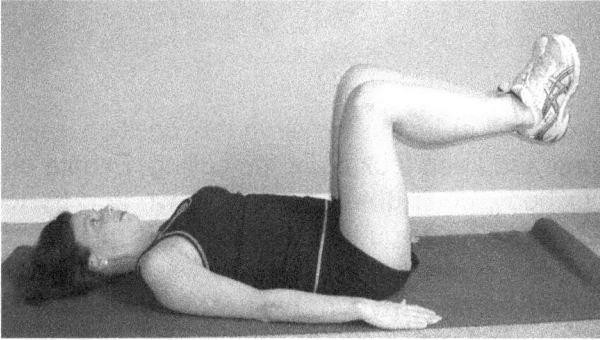

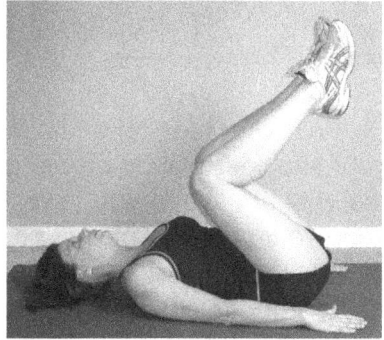

Start with your legs bent at a 90 degree angle. Exhale as you raise them toward your chest. Your buttocks will rise slightly off the floor. When you go to repeat the maneuver, do not let your muscles fully relax. Try to keep your bottom from touching the floor until you are done. Keep the knees at 90 degrees to focus on your abs.

A lot of people use a ball to do abdominal exercises. One variation is to put the ball between your knees and do the exact same movement here. It forces inner thigh contraction and abdominal work. You could do this, and add weight, by placing a couch pillow there.

The other is to place the ball under your feet. Straighten your legs and roll the ball. Then roll the ball back toward you as you bring your knees to your chest. This adds some resistance to your ab workout too.

UPPER ABDOMINAL

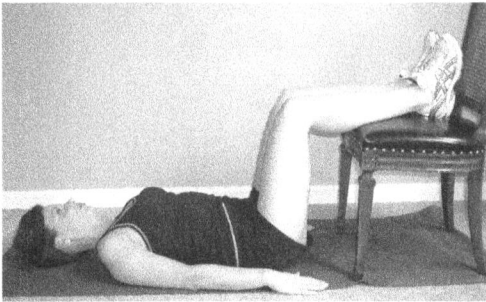

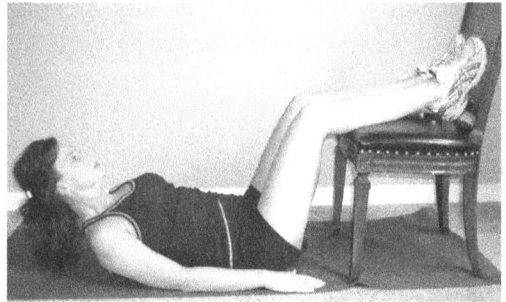

With your legs on a chair, couch, ball or just in the air in this position, raise your shoulder blades off the ground and keep looking at the ceiling. Exhale on the way up. When you lower your body, don't go all the way down and try to keep your shoulder blades off the ground until you take a break. This maintains tension on the abs. Then repeat.

For greater resistance place your hands on your chest or on the sides of your head, but be careful not to pull your head. If you wanted to you could also place a weight on your chest. The reason not to tuck your feet under the couch is you will cheat and use your hip flexors as well. You can feel this where your leg and pelvis join in the front of your body.

TOTAL ABDOMINAL

The bicycle maneuver is being rated as one of the best moves for your abs because you are doing more movement and affecting more muscles. Lie face up and slowly bring your elbows, one at a time and with control, to your respective opposite knee. Exhale as you approximate the elbow and knee each time.

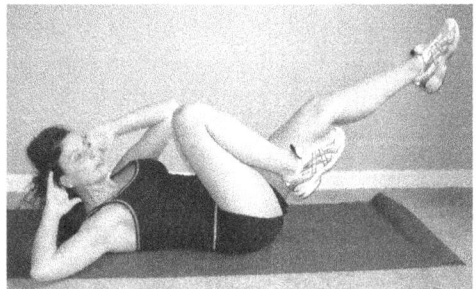

Go slowly and feel the muscles work or you might pass out from breathing to fast and rushing through the motion. Too fast and you might even tip over. Same rules apply to keep constant tension on the abs. When you straighten the leg each time, do so in a pedaling motion and at around a 30 – 45 degree angle. Don't relax them until you have finished your routine.

If you notice any low back discomfort, this exercise may not be for you. When the legs are out straight it can be too much pressure in the low back. There are many abdominal exercises. Choose the one that works for you. It's not what routine you do, it's that you do the routine.

ABDUCTOR (outer thigh)

Lie on your side and raise the upper leg toward the ceiling. Hold the contraction for a second and lower your leg but don't relax it completely. You could throw on some ankle weights or heavy boots to make it harder.

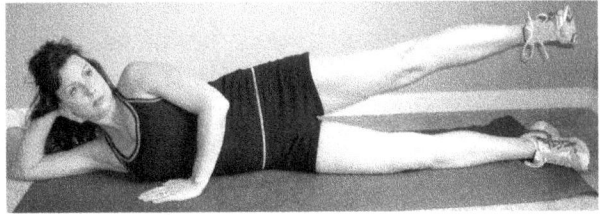

ADDUCTOR (inner thigh)

Lying on your side, raise your bottom leg off the floor. Bring it up a few inches. Lower slightly and then bring it up and contract it again. Switch sides. The non-lifting leg can be bent as shown or on the floor next to the leg working.

This is the same exercise except you are using the upper leg as resistance for greater results. You can also use a ball and hold it between your legs. Then you tighten the inner thigh as you contract and work the outer thigh, raising the legs up.

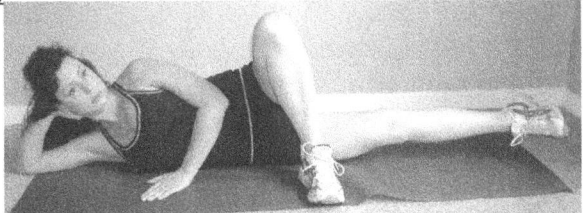

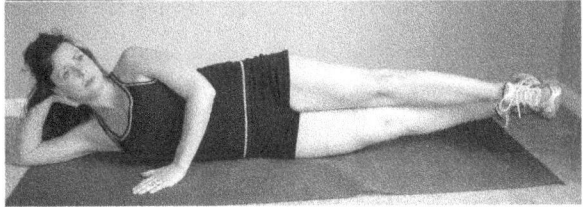

BICEP CURL

This can be done with weights or bands. Have the knees slightly bent to protect your back. Slowly raise the weight and exhale as you do so. Contract or make a muscle when you reach the peak. Next lower the weight with control and don't let the weight lower your arms. This keeps tension in your arms.

You can also reverse your hand position by taking a palms down grip or even rotate it and turn your hands 90 degrees so the thumb and pointer finger face up. Repeat the same movements and you will hit the biceps at different angles.

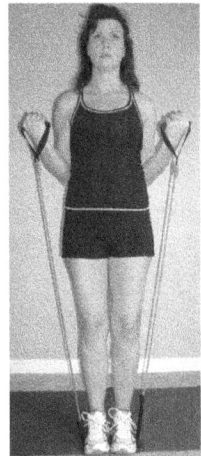

BUTTOCKS (glutes)

Get on the floor on your hands and knees as if to do a cat stretch (this position is covered in the stretching section if you are unfamiliar with it) or as if you were getting ready to play horse with a child. Then raise one leg and straighten or extend it while you push your foot toward the ceiling. Hold for a second and lower it, but don't rest it on the floor. Now repeat.

CHIN UP

This move can be humbling. If you can't lift your own weight, stand on a box and either use one leg or both to help bring you to the finish position, which is with your chin at the level of the bar. Exhale at the top and slowly lower your body. Try to always keep some tension on your arms and don't straighten them completely.

If you are using your legs as an assist when you go up, see if you can handle your body weight when you lower yourself. This will help build more muscle and maximize your efforts.

The reverse grip also works the biceps and may be easier. It can be a great place to start if the normal version of a chin up is too difficult.

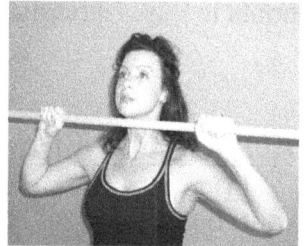

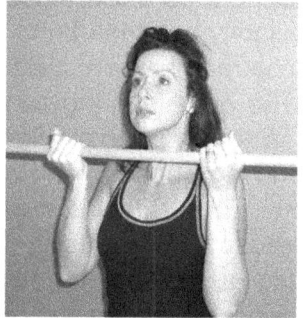

EXTENSION EXERCISE

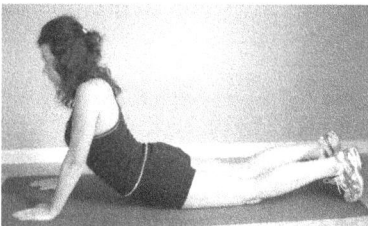

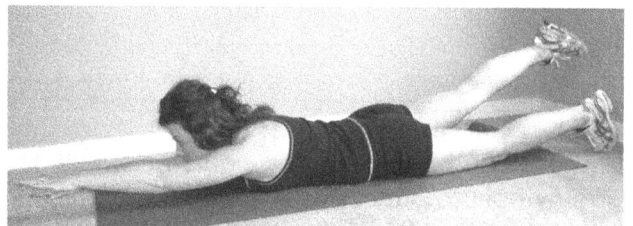

This picture above shows a stretch for the abs and a move that can alleviate some disc problems. A plank position requires you to strengthen the low back. For this, assume the pushup position but rest your body on your elbows and forearms. Try to keep your waist and legs straight, and off the floor.

An additional set of moves would be to lie flat on your stomach with your arms overhead like you are Superman, or Superwoman, and raise one arm and hold it off of the ground for a few seconds and set it back down. Then raise the other side. If that is okay, you can raise both and hold for a few seconds. Next you can try lifting one leg up, then both legs, try opposite arm and legs or even both arms and legs. Sometimes I pretend to swim so all of my limbs are off the floor and I'm flailing around like I'm crazy or need to be thrown back in the water. Well actually I do it slowly, but both arms and legs are off the floor, which increases the difficulty level.

LUNGE

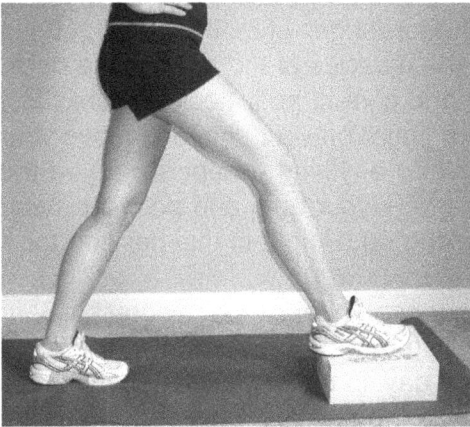

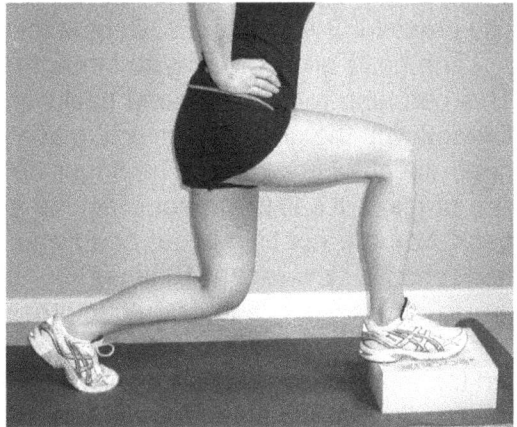

A lunge can be done with or without weights. It can also be performed with or without a step or box, which increases the difficulty. So if you have no weights then try to use a box or phonebook to make it harder. Step forward and only bend the knee to 90 degrees. If you have to, reposition your back leg to achieve the correct position. Anymore than a 90 degree bend will compress the knee joint and could cause damage to it.

A **REVERSE LUNGE** is done by placing the top of your back foot, where your shoe laces are, on a chair behind you and bending the front leg. You still strive to keep the knee of the forward leg over the ankle and lower the body to do so. This adds some resistance to the move by adding more of your own bodyweight.

NECK

Start with your head in a neutral position. Place your hand on the front of your head and push your head into it like you are bending your head forward, but don't move your head from the neutral position. Use about 10 percent of your maximum effort. It creates an isometric contraction and strengthens the muscles.

Next put one hand on the back of your head and press in that direction, but keep the head straight. You will complete the series by placing one hand on the side of your head as if to tip your ear to the shoulder. Then try turning your head into your hand but always keep your head in a stationary position.

The next variation is to actually put your head in any of the six ranges of motion and then keep it there. Your hand then presses against your head trying to get it back to a straight position. For example tilt your head to one side about half way and then take the hand of the same side and press against your head as if you are trying to return your head to the neutral position. Keep it there as you press for 3 – 5 seconds. Repeat for all other ranges of motion.

The head glide is a way to strengthen the muscles of the back of the neck. This can help retract the head backwards and correct poor neck posture. Just to show you the glide movement, place your finger on your chin and move your head directly backwards. The finger doesn't do anything except show you the line of glide. It's like someone behind you grabs your ears and pulls the head back. You are not tilting your head and looking up. Hold it in this position for a few seconds, and repeat 10 times.

To add resistance to it you can press your head against the headrest in your car or place your hand behind your head. Use only 10 percent of your force. I did too much once and had a sore neck for a day. In the car it can occupy some of your time at the light. You could also lie on the bed and press back into the mattress.

To really strengthen the neck, lie on your stomach and lift your head straight up off the pillow and hold it for a few seconds. Now you are lifting the weight of your head and building muscle strength much like curling a dumbbell with your arm. You could hang your head off the bed and do the same thing.

PUSHUP

As a beginner, you can do these against a wall or eventually against a desk as you get stronger to increase the weight you are lifting. When you get to the floor position you have more body weight and may need to do them from your knees.

When you get strong enough to do them on just your hands and feet, try to keep your back straight throughout the entire movement. Stop with your chest a few inches above the

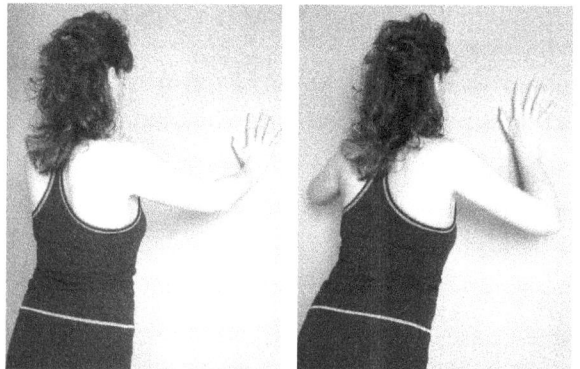

ground for a few seconds and exhale as you push back up.

For the really advanced, push your body up quickly and try to clap and then resume at the start position. If that wasn't enough slap on a back pack and load it up for more weight.

Possibly the backpack your kids are lugging to school. You could use the same backpack for lunges, calf raises and other exercises as well to make your workout more difficult.

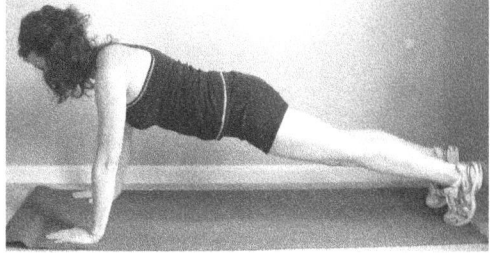

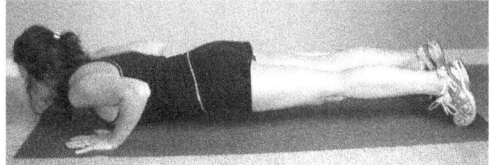

TRICEP DIP

Use a sturdy chair and place you palms on the seat. Lower you body until your elbows are at 90 degrees. Exhale as you push your body back up. If you need to cheat use your legs to help. As you get stronger, place your feet on a desk or chair. This will increase the weight you have to lift.

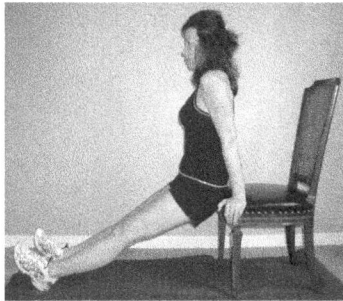

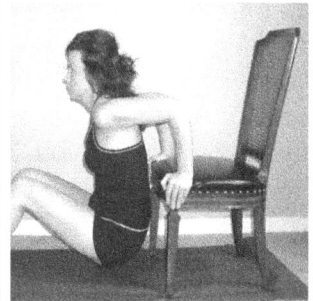

SQUAT

Your feet should be shoulder width apart and when you squat try to lower yourself until your knees reach the 90 degree mark. Then push back up and exhale as you do so. You can use a chair or a ball to limit how low you go. You could also hold on to a doorknob or put a ball behind your back to perform this exercise using good form.

Make a conscious effort to maintain perfect form and posture. Never round the back. Start with light weights you can easily handle so you can perfect your form. If you have bad knees don't drop too low with the weight because you will damage the knee joint. Look straight ahead and don't lock out, or completely straighten your knees when you stand back up.

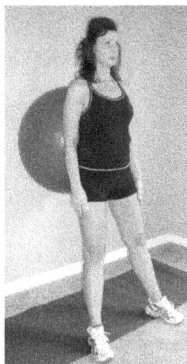

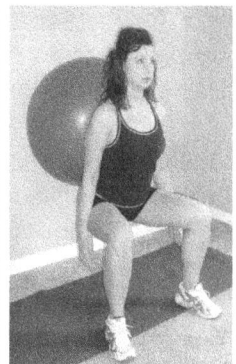

"America believes in education: the average professor earns more money in a year than a professional athlete earns in a whole week." – **Evan Esar**

The Gym Workout
HANGING KNEE RAISE

Sometimes people will do hanging raises off of a chin up bar. You can be limited by your arm strength because you have to hold your bodyweight off the ground. They have designed slings for your elbows to reduce that problem. The only other problem is swinging. Leave that for the playground. Control your movements so the focus is on your stomach. Other machines, like the one shown, have a backrest to stabilize your back when you do this exercise.

With this example we start at a 90 degree position and contract as we curl the abs before returning to the start position. Exhale as you bring your knees up toward the ceiling. Hold for a second and then slowly lower your legs to just before the start position. Hold and then repeat. The legs are only lowered to be parallel to the floor to show how to focus on the abs and limit back discomfort.

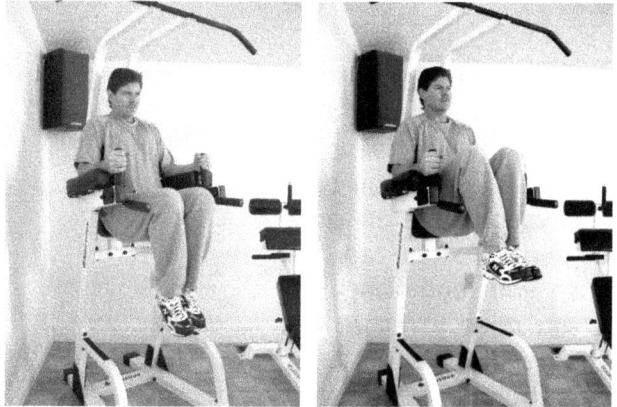

When you drop the legs down toward the ground you have a tendency to use momentum to raise your legs. If you want to let the legs down, do so slowly and maintain control. At the bottom position, hold the legs there for a second, keeping tension on your muscles, before raising them above your waist again. This prevents momentum and injury.

If you like to let the legs all the way down be aware this can increase the tension on your lower back and also waste a lot of energy. When the legs drop below the waistline you start to activate the hip flexors. When you bring your feet up from the floor to get to the start position shown here, you focus much of your effort on your hip flexors and not the abs.

As you get stronger you can try either of these positions with your legs straight out instead of with your knees bent. You can also bring your legs up and add a little twist as if to make one knee reach the opposite side. You still have to hold it there if you make it.

AB INCLINE SITUP

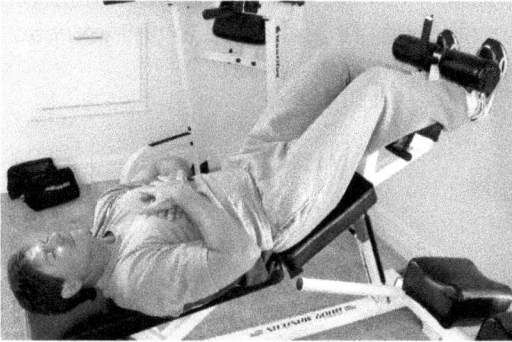

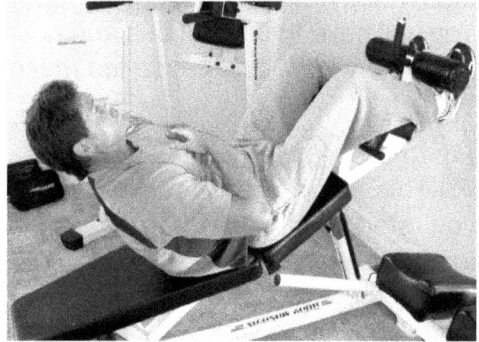

You start lying on your back with your knees bent. Exhale as you bring your shoulder blades off the bench. Keep your eyes and head facing the ceiling or pretend to have a grapefruit tucked in between your chin and your chest. You don't need your head bobbing back and forth through the exercise. It's an ab exercise not a neck exercise.

You can add a little twist at the top, but twisting and coming up at the same time may cause increased stress to the low back. Either way, be careful. These movements can also be done simply on any floor. Just prop your legs up at 90 degrees on a chair, a couch or hold them in the air for a greater challenge. For more resistance place a weight on your chest and hold it.

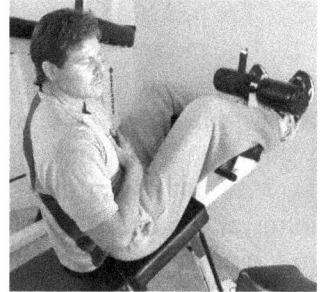

SEATED AB CRUNCH

Don't use too much weight so the weight pulls you back off the seat up or backwards. Move your shoulder blades away from the backrest so you are holding the weight. Now slowly bring you shoulders to your knees and don't pull the weight with your arms. Exhale as you go through the motion.

Then hold for a second or two and control the weight as you return to the starting position. Don't let your stomach muscles relax. Your shoulder blades shouldn't touch the backrest and the weight won't pull you backward.

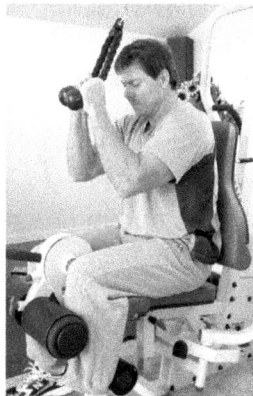

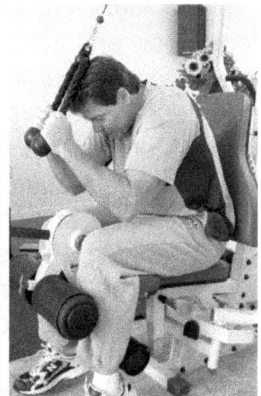

Sometimes you may see people at the gym kneeling in front of some gym equipment and pulling the weight down similar to this. It's just another variation. You still have to be cautious and not allow the weight and cable to pull you back up. Otherwise it may cause too much pressure in your low back.

ABDUCTORS (outer thigh)

This machine has you start with your legs together and the pads are placed on the outside of your legs. Push your legs away from each other and hold. Return to the start position, but maintain tension on your muscles and repeat.

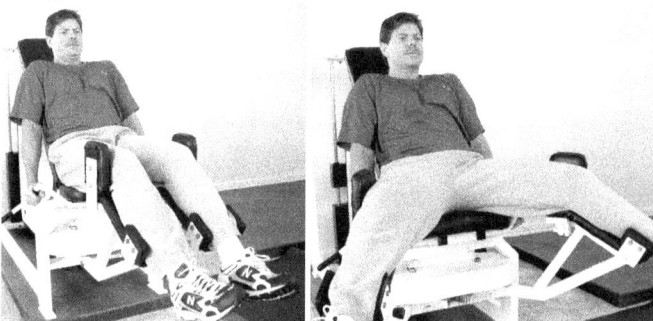

The machine should never have the weights clang when you lift. If they do, that means you let the muscles relax and rested for a moment. The other version would be to attach an ankle strap to your, ankle of course, and attach a low cable to it while you are standing. Now hold on to the machine and move your leg in any direction.

You can even go from one side to the other, by turning around to hit both inner and outer thigh and then switch legs to maximize your time. Facing the machine and moving the foot backwards can target the buttocks or glutes.

ADDUCTORS (inner thigh)

This time you start with your legs apart and the pads will be on the inside of your legs. Now bring your legs together, hold and slowly move them apart again.

There is a standing version of this exercise and the one above for your leg. These offer less stress to the hip joint because you are moving the hip at a more natural and safer angle in relation to the hip joint itself. You hold on to the railing and set the dial for comfort. Then one leg at a time, you move the leg like a pendulum swings. Always control the movement. There is a little greater range of motion with this exercise.

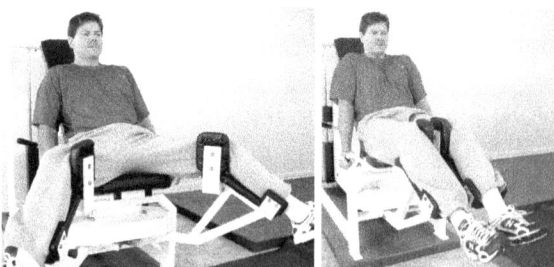

BICEP CURL

Have the knees slightly bent to protect your back. The motion is the same whether you are using free weights or a cable.

Slowly raise the weight and exhale as you do so. Keep your elbows in close to your sides. Contract or make a muscle when you reach the peak. Next lower the weight with control and don't let the weight lower your arms. This keeps tension in your arms.

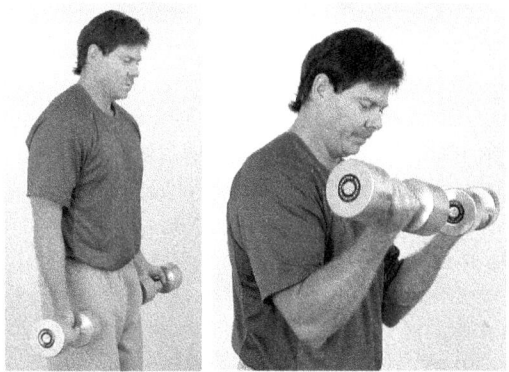

Sometimes I lie on the floor and do curls. I use a bar attached to the lower stack of weights. This allows me to support my back and eliminate any chance for rocking my body or using momentum. You could put your back against the wall to decrease the likeliness of swaying or for greater stability.

The straight bar used for curling locks both shoulders into a slightly externally rotated position. Again this is the critical information I never learned when I first started lifting. Normally your palms face a little bit toward your midline but a straight bar keeps the palms up. This is another reason to use dumbbells. Each arm can work independently and develop on its own.

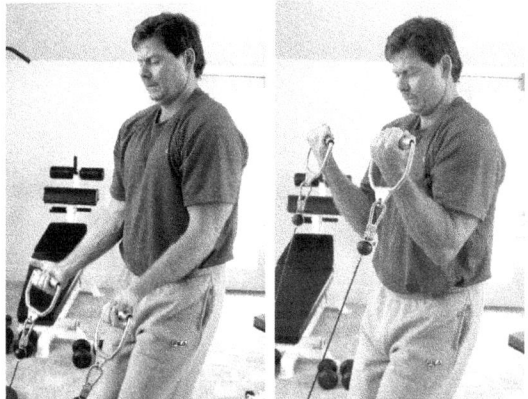

There are single hand cables, EZ bars, which are bent for your wrists and the hands' normal angle, and even rotating handles to adjust to each individual's normal wrist and arm angles.

CALF RAISE

Using weights on top of your knees, holding a dumbbell in your hands or using your own bodyweight, the motion is the same. Rest the balls of your feet on a surface and push up as if you are standing on your toes. Hold, and then let your heels lower below what your feet are on. This not only stretches your muscle and tendons, it allows you to work the calf through its entire range of motion.

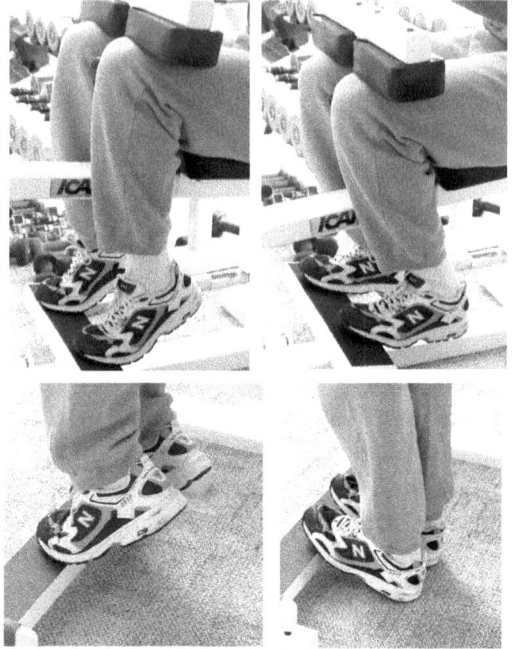

CHEST OR BENCH PRESS

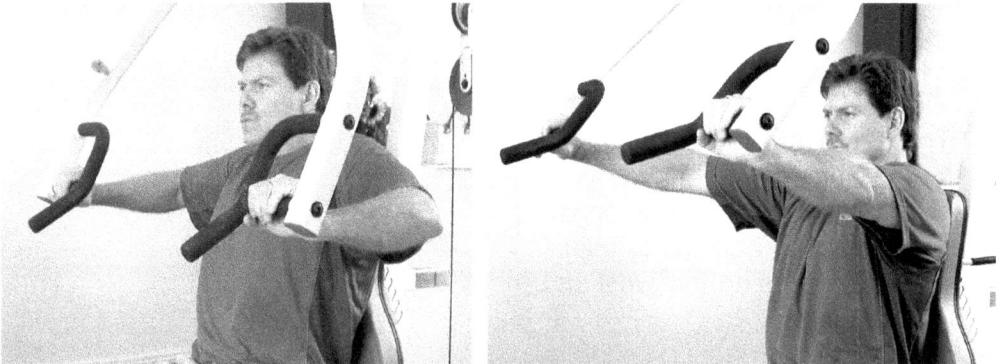

Whether you are lying on your back or sitting up, grip the bar with your hands about shoulders width apart. If you take a wider grip it puts more stress on the outer chest fibers, while a closer grip will focus on the inner fibers. Grip too closely and you will be working the triceps. If you are lying on a bench for any exercise, keep your feet flat on the floor. Some people like to put their feet on the bench but be careful. Never arch your back to complete a lift unless you want to get injured. Your head, shoulders and pelvis should all stay in contact with the bench.

Push the weight away and focus on contracting the chest. Lower the weight. There is some controversy as to how far you should lower the bar or your hands. If you are using a bar, stop when your elbows reach 90 degrees. When you go beyond that the shoulder is straining to pop out forward and will cause irreversible shoulder damage. Trust me. I have the aches to prove it.

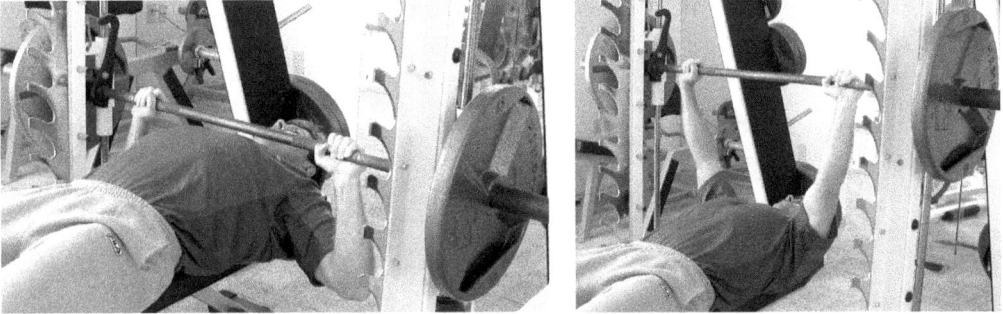

If you are using dumbbells or cables then you can let your elbows lower a little more because you aren't locked into a position by a bar. You have greater individual range of motion for each side. The dumbbells may be able to come down to your shoulder, but listen to your body for further instructions.

CHEST INCLINE PRESS

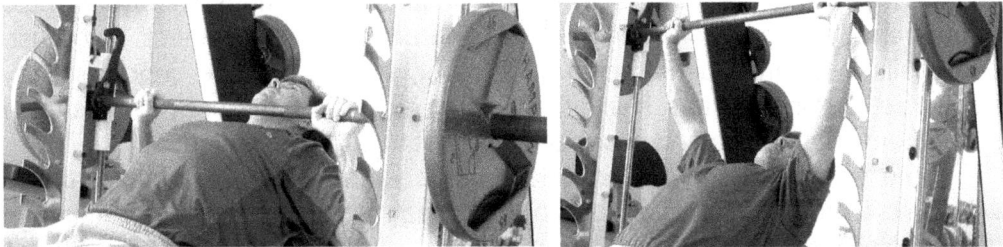

Same rules apply here. You can use a bar, dumbbells or cables. The bench is raised to around 30 degrees. Any more than 45 degrees will focus the lift on your shoulders and not on the upper chest where it should be.

DECLINE BENCH PRESS

Lower the head of the bench to about 30 degrees. Now the move will focus on your lower chest. To vary lifts, you can turn your hands so the palms are also facing each other when using cables or dumbbells.

CHEST FLY

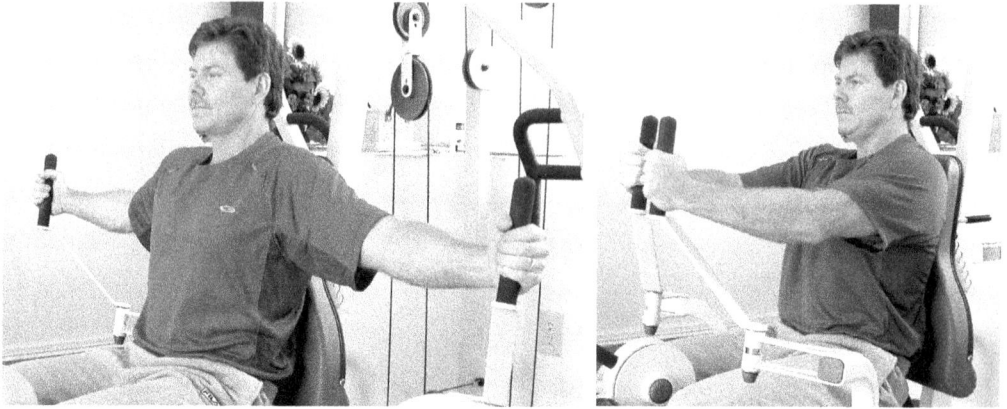

This exercise can be done on a bench with dumbbells, standing using cables, or while sitting. In the machine version shown, your arms will be out to the side and they should be slightly bent at the elbow. Contract your chest muscles as you bring the weight in front of your body and maintain that slight elbow bend. Hold for a second and release until you feel a nice stretch. Then repeat.

The chest fly can also be done on an incline bench to target higher up in the pecs and on a decline bench for lower pec development. Keep the angle of the bench low, around 30 degrees, so you are working the chest. If you use dumbbells, have the palms facing each other, sit down on the bench and lay back. Your starting position is with the weights elevated in front of you. Then you lower them to your side and squeeze the chest to bring the weight up.

Some fly machines have foot attachments you press down so the handles will come forward. Otherwise you have to reach far back to start and this can strain the shoulder joints.

CHIN UPS

Grip the bar about shoulder width apart or slightly wider. If you can't lift your own weight, there are machines that can assist you or stand on a box and either use one leg or both, to help bring your chin to the level of the bar. Exhale at the top and 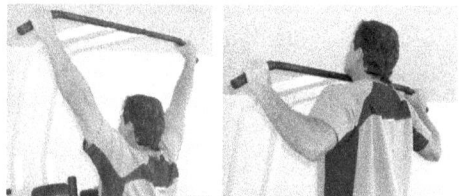 slowly lower your body. If you are using your legs as an assist when you go up, attempt to handle your body weight when you lower yourself. This will help build more muscle and maximize your efforts. Use an underhand grip to work biceps and the back.

ELLIPTICAL TRAINER

This machine decreases the impact on your body and tries to imitate the motion of our legs when we move. It has handles that move as well to burn more calories by involving more muscles. Using aerobic equipment for 10 minutes is a great precursor to any workout. It helps lubricate the joints and warm up the muscles.

For a cardio workout, a good 30 – 60 minutes is fine. Make sure you warm up before reaching your designated speed, and also cool down after. So maybe a lap to warm up and a lap to cool down will do your body good.

On any machine that has arm movements, make sure you also stretch out your upper body. When your arms are doing a lot of row-like movements your midback and shoulders can get tight. You could be doing hundreds of these every time you workout.

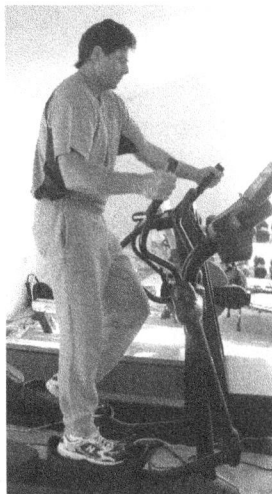

HAMSTRING CURL (back of the leg)

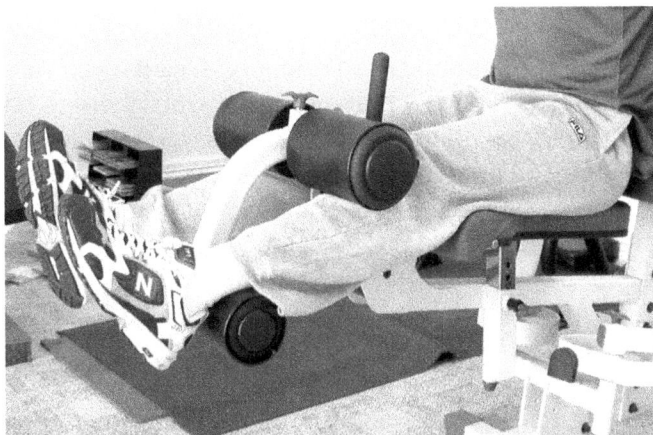

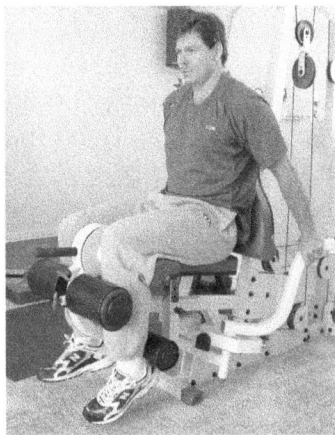

In a sitting position the legs will be straight and a pad will be under the back of your ankle. Pull your heels into the machine. This exercise can also be performed in a standing position, or prone on your stomach position.

The danger of using the prone hamstring curls is that people have a tendency to arch their backs up when lifting gets more difficult and this can lead to an injury. If you can, peak the bench at your waist to inhibit this arching movement.

LAT PULLDOWN

There are several different handles you can use with this exercise. I recommend using several to keep it fresh. Also see which seems to give you the best workout. Most machines have you sit and face them. Your knees will have a pad or bar across the top to prevent your body from rising off the seat.

Reach up and take a grip about shoulder width apart. If you can't reach the bar, stand up and grab it and bring it down so you can assume your start position. When you pull the weight down, exhale and lean back slightly, as you pull the bar to your chest.

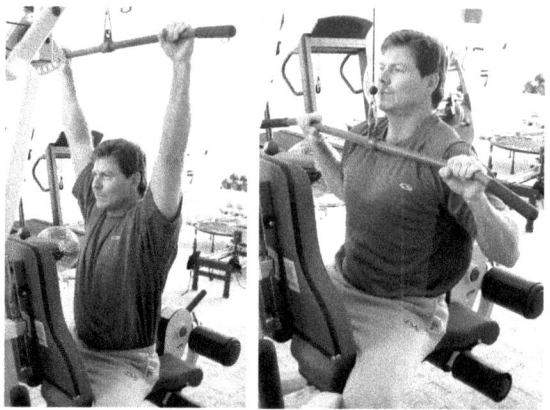

There is less stress to your shoulders and the lats move through a greater range of motion, which can increase the muscle's growth. Hold and then slowly lower to just before the weights bang together, and repeat. You can also use an underhand grip and bring the bar to your lower rib cage. Variation is the spice of life.

Pull downs behind the head are another bad motion. Unless you are training for competition and feel this is going to make or break you, there is no reason to do it. If you must do it, try using individual handles versus the bar. Handles would give your shoulder joints some freedom. The bar locks you in a position that can rotate your shoulder joints and make them vulnerable or wear unnaturally, especially if you have forward instability or other shoulder pains.

The bar can sometimes be pulled down with too much force and start pounding the back of the upper spine. Not good. I had a patient Bill who broke the spinous process off the back of one of his neck vertebra, known as Clay Shoveler's Fracture, because he brought the weight down too forcefully.

Using slow controlled movements would be better if this is an exercise you really want to do. Try not to continually flex your head forward as you attempt to bring the bar down with a behind the neck pulldown. You will strain your neck, reversing the natural curve and may cause real damage over time.

LEG EXTENSION

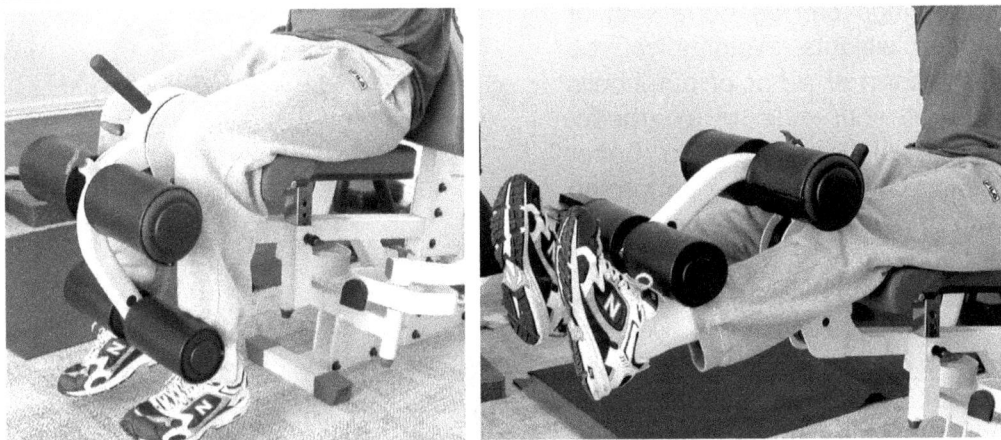

This exercise works the thigh. In a sitting position pads will rest against your lower leg above the ankle. Exhale as you tighten your thighs and raise the weight. Hold for a second and lower the legs, being sure to not let the weight stack touch when you do so.

By turning your toes outward you can direct more stress to the inside (medial) of your upper thigh muscles (quads). This is a great exercise if you have patellar (kneecap) tracking or Chondromalacia. In this case, the movement is only the last 15 degrees of contraction. If you turn your toes inward you can better develop the lateral (outside) of the quads.

Now the bad news. There has been a lot of controversy as to the safety of this movement. The leg extension machine causes the 4 quad muscles to fire at slightly different times. This unevenly stresses the kneecap and can cause damage to the tendon below the kneecap, called the infrapatellar tendon. This is what former President Bill Clinton injured when he took a wrong step.

I have also heard some expert trainers complain that too much weight on your lower leg bone can prevent its normal motion when the knee straightens, therefore causing more damage to it than good. Many professionals believe that the first 1/3 of the movement, in which the weight is first moved, is the dangerous portion.

Looking at the picture where the legs are bent is the starting position. Once the weight is brought up, your legs are straight like in the next picture, then lower your legs 2/3 the way, and repeat so the legs are straight again. Don't bring the legs back to the starting position until you are done.

I would say use common sense. If it seems to make things hurt, don't do it. If you already are nursing a knee injury, use caution. There are plenty of other alternative machines to try or vary because you aren't married to one machine. Do leg press, squats or lunges.

LUNGE

A lunge can be done with or without weights. Weights can be in the form of a bar or dumbbells held at your side or overhead. Do whichever gives you better balance. It can also be performed with or without a step or box, which engages your core muscles and increases the difficulty.

So if you have no weights, then try to use a box to make it harder. Step forward and only bend the knee to 90 degrees. If you have to, reposition your back leg. Anymore than 90 degrees will compress the knee joint and could cause damage to it.

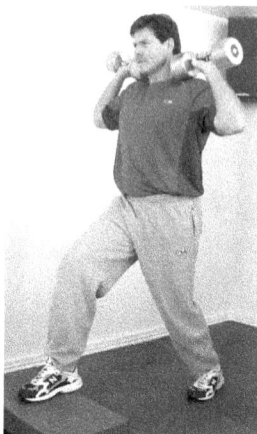

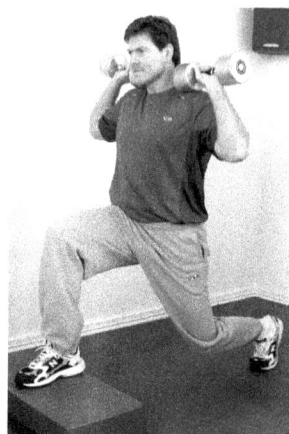

PREACHER CURL

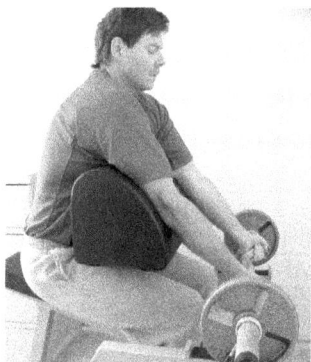

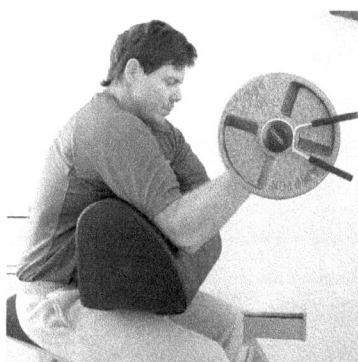

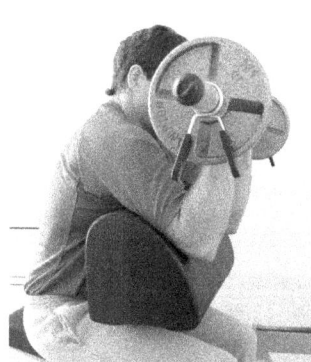

The preacher curl is designed to isolate the biceps but you must use strict form. Never let the weight hyperextend your elbows. Set the seat so your armpits fit over the pad and keep your chest close to it as well. Take a grip about shoulder width or wherever feels comfortable. Lean forward a little when you lower the weight, as this will keep the tension on your biceps. Then curl your hands toward your chin. You may also use dumbbells or a cable for this exercise.

RHOMBOID ROW (midback)

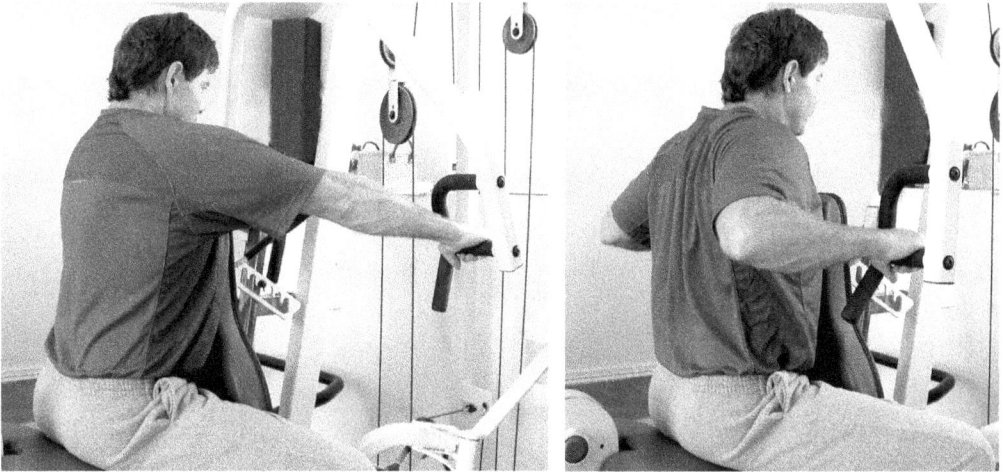

There are many variations for this type of exercise. Some people like to use machines, while others prefer cables, dumbbells and bars. Either way, make sure that when you pull the weight straight back, that you squeeze your shoulder blades together like your squishing an orange to get the most out of your hard work.

On a machine your chest may be against a pad as you face the machine. With a cable machine you have free range of motion. When you pull the weight back you can lean a little backwards to get an extra contraction. As you let the weight move forward allow your back to stretch.

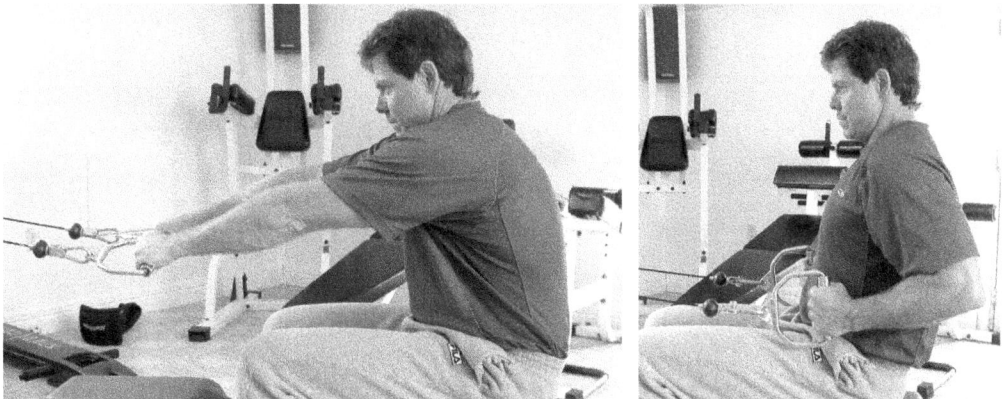

If you use a dumbbell and work one arm at a time, place the opposite knee on a chair and keep your back straight. If you need to, hold on to something for balance. When you bring the weight up, keep the elbow close to the side and perform the motion as if you're starting a lawn mower.

ROMAN CHAIR

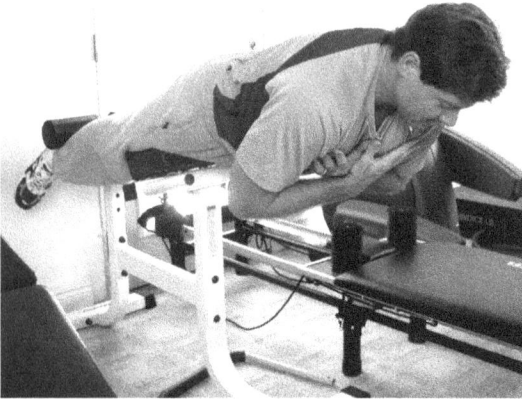

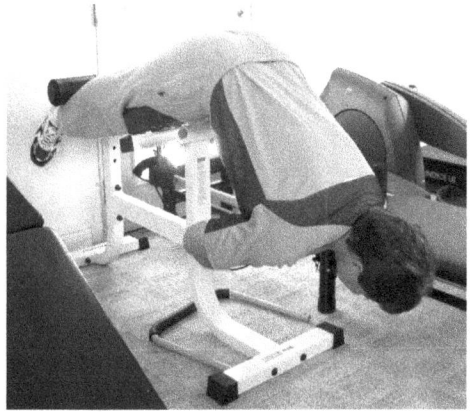

This machine helps strengthen the low back muscles. Using a ball or machine, you lock your feet against something to hold your body still. Then lean forward to the ground. Lift yourself back up and be careful not to rise higher than 5 degrees beyond being straight with the rest of your body. Hyperextending causes injury to the low back, so use proper form.

If you need greater resistance you can hold a gym plate or weight against your chest and cross your arms when you hold it.

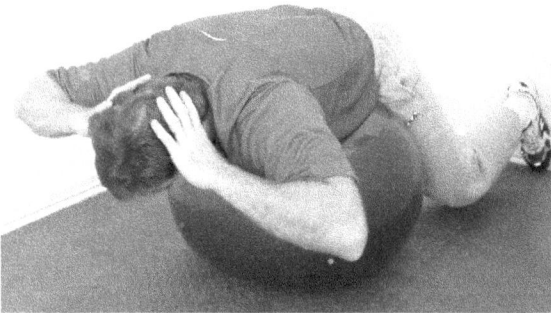

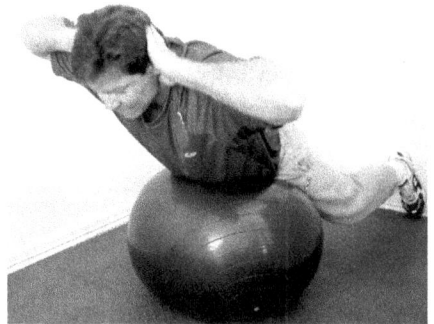

SHOULDER PRESS

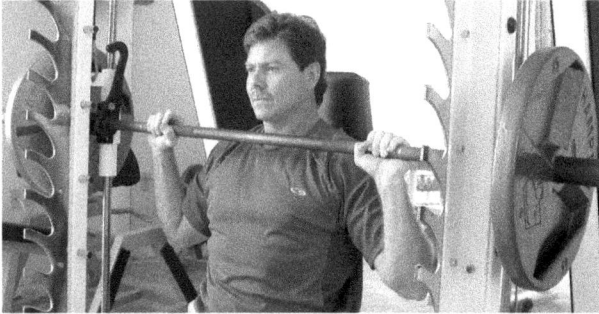

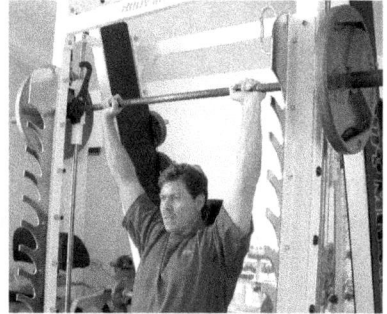

There are several machines that can be used for this exercise. The Smith machine has a bar with hooks that can lock with the turn of your wrists if you get stuck. It is also great for bench press and squats for that reason. Take a grip around shoulder width apart and exhale as you push the weight overhead. Hold, and then slowly bring it down to a comfortable level, wait, and push it back up.

The problem with this exercise is if you are sitting, the weight compresses your disks. The bar also limits the range of motion of your shoulders to what the machine allows. Using dumbbells will give each shoulder individual freedom to move in a comfortable range of motion.

Another way to do this is by using a bar or dumbbells and lifting the weight while you are standing with your knees slightly bent. This reduces the stress to your low back but you must use good form. When you use dumbbells each arm benefits from doing the work independently.

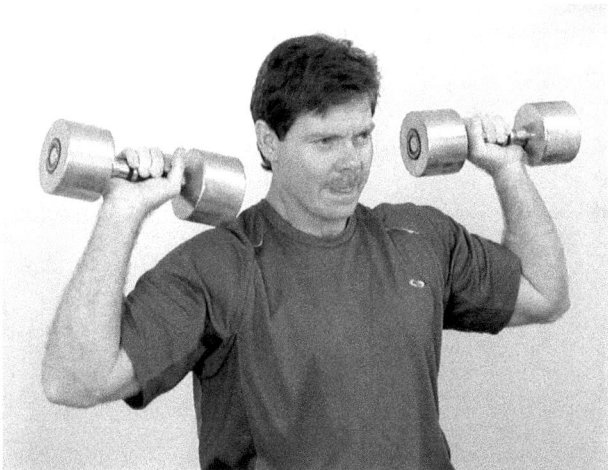

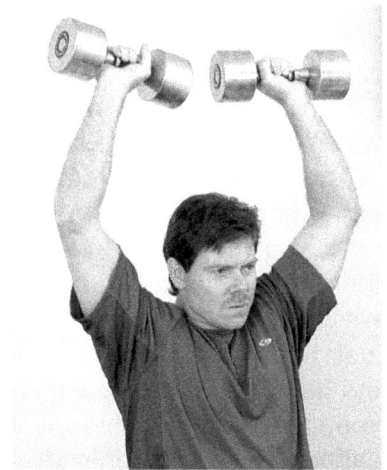

SHRUG

Take a hold of two dumbbells and place them at your sides. Now raise your shoulders toward your ears as if to say *"I don't know"* and hold them there for a second. When you lower the weight you can let the dumbbells stretch your shoulder muscles, or traps, which run from upper neck to your shoulder. You can also do this type of exercise with a straight bar.

The lower and middle trapezius muscles get a good deal of work performing rows for the midback. Use dumbbells or a bar and squeeze the shoulder blades together to feel the burn.

An example of another version using weights would be to take two handles that are attached to a low pulley and stack of weights. Facing the weights, open your arms wide as if to hug someone and hold it for a second. Use light weights or rubber tubing when you do this exercise.

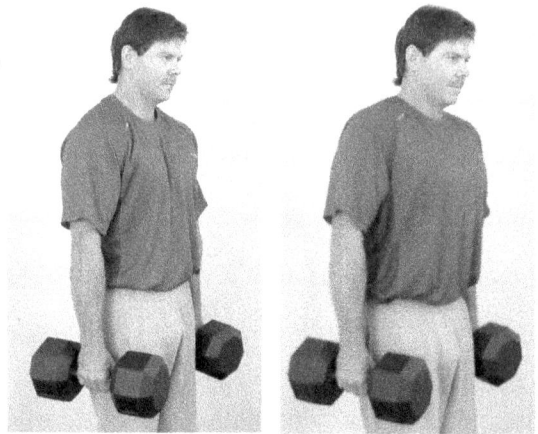

SQUAT

Start with your feet about shoulder's width apart and point the toes slightly outward. Using a ball or a chair is a great way to prevent you from over compressing your knees with this exercise. It is a gentle reminder that you are low enough. When you lower the weight and your bottom just touches the seat, you've gone low enough without the risk of causing damage to the knee or back. Now straighten back up. Touch and go!

There are squat machines, which are great for the solo lifter in case you get too tired. Some have bars to rest the weight on if you run out of steam and then there's the Smith machine, which has a hook system. You just turn your hands and lock the bar. The machines also help keep you stable so there is less chance for swaying or injury.

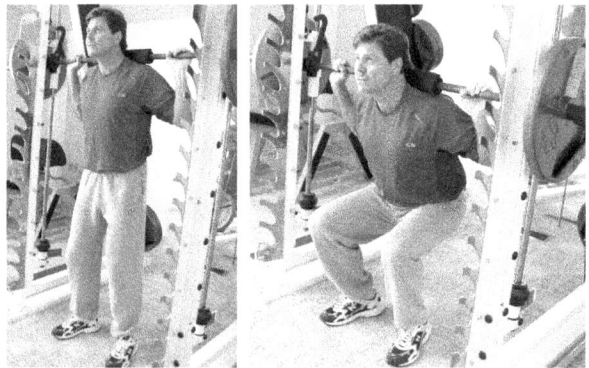

With a bar, I like to take a foam pad or a towel and place it around the bar while it rests on my neck and shoulders. This helps to evenly distribute the weight of the bar on your body and helps to protect your spine from damage. That weight can really start to hurt after a while. They also make plastic and foam contraptions that rest on this area with a groove for the bar to rest in. You can also use dumbbells at your side to do the same exercise. Then no weight is compressing your spine.

Inhale on the way down and stop when your thighs are parallel to the floor. Rest a second and exhale as you push up. This is a great exercise for your entire lower body. Because it works the largest muscle group, the quads, it will stimulate an increase in testosterone in the body for growth in all of your muscles. This is a natural way to increase your secretion of growth hormones without cheating.

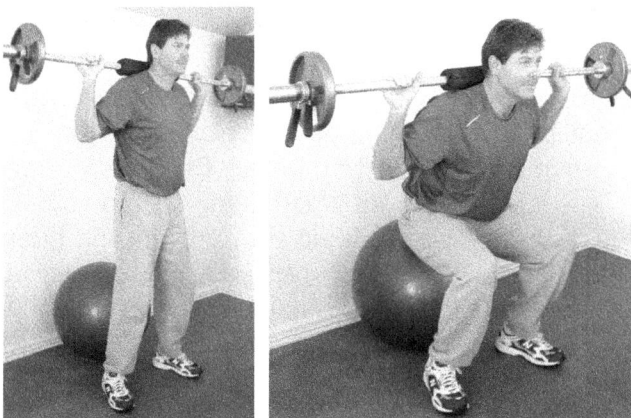

There are other leg press machines, which can support your back while the legs do the work. You sit and hold onto some handles and your feet control the weight. Lower the weight and then push it back up. Again don't go too low. It can round your back and compress the knee joint too much. But with care it can be a great exercise to add to your arsenal as you vary your leg routine.

TREADMILL

This is the old standard if you have terrible weather or want to workout in the privacy of your home. If you have a bad knee or back, try walking first. Some treadmills have cushioning to help reduce the impact, but if you have a bad lumbar disc that flares up once in a while, you may notice the constant pounding causes pain just like the road. In that case try different sneakers or walking on grass.

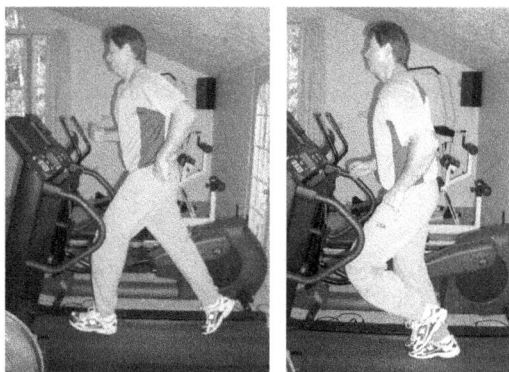

Another thing I noticed is a treadmill pushes your feet backwards and increases extension forces to the low back. This is important. If you find relief from low back pain by doing flexion exercises, then the treadmill may increase your pain. A recumbent bike would be more beneficial for you.

For your aerobic workout, start at 20 minutes and work up to 45 minutes to an hour. The faster the machine goes the harder you will have to work, which will equate to more calories burned. Remember, burning 300 calories isn't accurate and it doesn't mean you can eat a 200 calorie cookie and still be ahead. It means you are resetting your resting metabolic rate so the body will burn more calories throughout the day. If you switch between running and walking you will achieve better results.

Similar to this is the stair master, elliptical machine or Jacob's Ladder. All are great for working out or as a great warm up before you lift weights. I recommend warming up for 10 or 15 minutes. Don't tire yourself out before you try to lift.
It is a great way to get blood pumping into your muscles, delivering nutrients to the muscles and can help with growth and strength development. A light set with weights using high reps will also qualify as a good warm up for your muscles prior to more strenuous lifting.

TRICEP PRESSDOWN

You can use a cable for this exercise or one of the triceps machines. With the cable machine shown, you can be facing the weights or turn around and have your back toward the weight stack. Try to keep your elbows in close to your side and maintain a slight bend in the knees. Your feet will be about shoulders' width apart.

With your elbows at around 90 degrees, exhale as you push the weight down and straighten your arms. Your elbows should work like a hinge as the arms move downward. Hold for a second and then slowly return to the starting position. Always keep the tension on your muscles through the entire motion.

When you use a triceps machine, try to adjust the set up so your elbows are in alignment with the hinge mechanism of the machine. Also the elbows should not be pressing against any pads so they can move freely. The back of the arms, yes.

The tricep exercise is the movement that I have to constantly remind myself to keep my head back and not stick it out like a duck. You can always check the

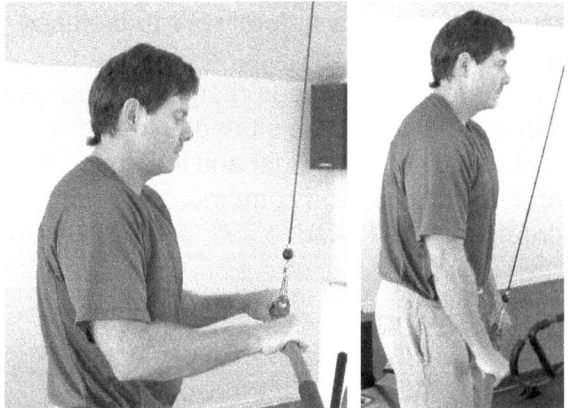

mirror for your form and not your hair.

This next version of the press down uses a rope with individual handles. This allows you to turn your wrist outward a little at the bottom of the movement and get a better contraction in the muscles. You can separate the fists when you push down about a foot or so, instead of keeping them in the midline. This will add some more isolation and a deeper contraction of the muscle fibers.

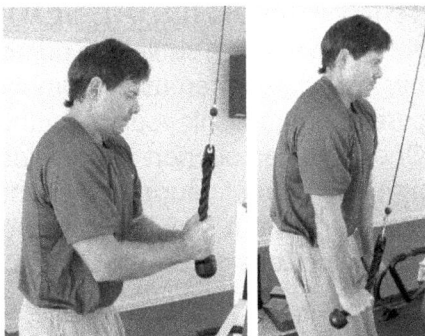

TRICEP DIP

This is another way to hit the back of your arms. Facing the equipment, take a grip and raise your body upright. Try to keep your body straight through the lift and your elbows close to your sides and facing backwards. Lower your body, hold and exhale as you press back up and lock out your arms. Hold and repeat. To focus more on your chest muscles, lean forward.

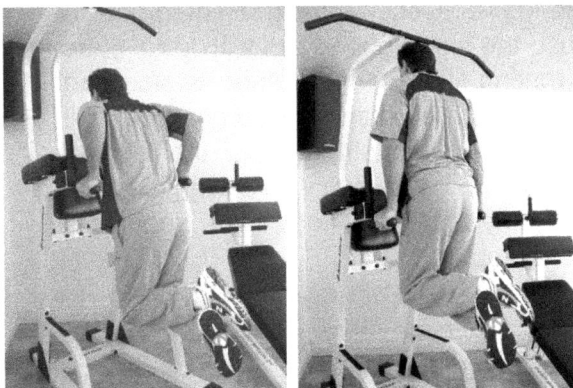

TRICEP ROPE OVERHEAD PRESS

With your back facing the machine start with your elbows in the 90 degree position again. Now force the weight away from your body with a hinge-like motion at your elbow.

When you bring your wrists back toward your head you can allow them to go further back to stretch the triceps some. Then repeat your exercise. With this exercise you can keep your fists close together or separate them a little at the end to add more contraction to the muscles.

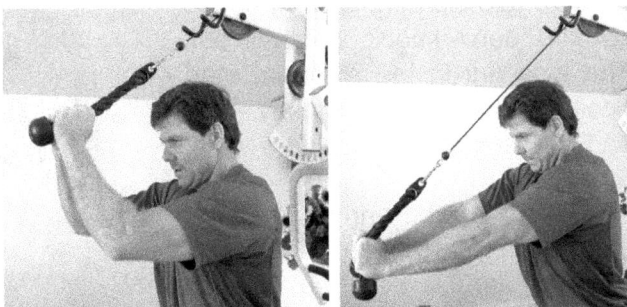

TRICEP INDIVIDUAL SEATED PRESS

You can use a cable or a dumbbell for this exercise. When using dumbbells, be careful not to clunk yourself in the head. One hand can support the outside of the arm exercising to support the elbow and prevent it from moving outward. That keeps the tension on the triceps. Lower the weight and exhale as you push it back up.

You can also use a bar and work both arms at the same time. This is called a French press. Remember to use the same good form with your arms working like a hinge. Either version can be performed sitting on the bench, a ball with your back straight and the feet on the floor, or standing with a slight bend in the knees and the feet about shoulders width apart.

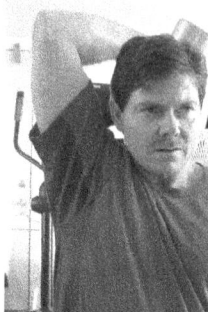

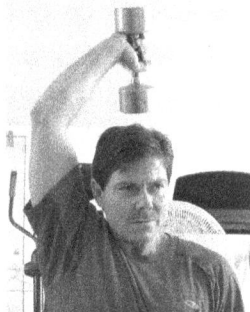

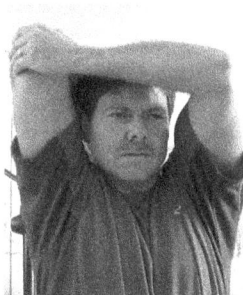

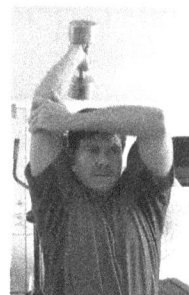

UPRIGHT ROW

Using a bar, dumbbell or cable, the movement is to bring your fist up to your chin and stop at collar-bone or clavicle height. Do it slowly so you don't knock yourself out. The legs are in the standard start position, with knees slightly bent and the feet about shoulders width apart.

Exhale as you bring the weight up and get those elbows up high around ear level. You should feel this in your upper back and shoulders. If you have a shoulder injury or instability, this could aggravate it. I love this exercise but I have to use caution because it can make my shoulders hurt more.

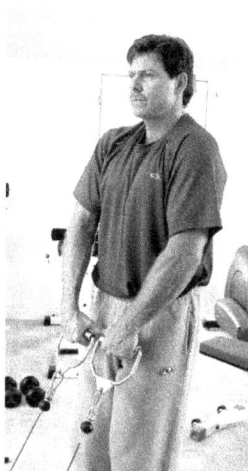

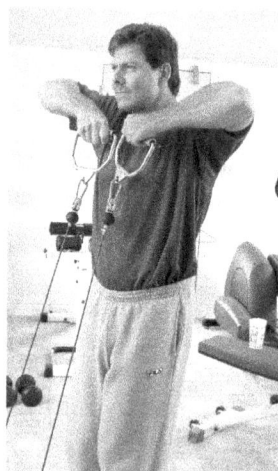

> *"When we got into office, the thing that surprised me the most was that things were as bad as we'd been saying they were."* – **John F. Kennedy**

Office Workout

Maybe you don't have time to throw the weights around regularly or there is a huge project, which is making it difficult to get to the gym. How about the line for your equipment or the constant conversationalists? You're sure there is no convenient gym in a lower floor of the building or one close by? Some pieces of spare equipment from your house or a used gym shop would be great. Go rummage through the basement, your neighbor's garage (kidding) or a Salvation Army if you need to. As Yukon Cornelius said in Rudolf the Red-Nosed Reindeer, *"Nothing!"* Okay. Let's be creative then.

Your office can be an authentic gym Mecca with a little ingenuity. Of course this little workout is supposed to be done on a break or during your lunchtime so you don't get fired. So if you don't own a set of dumbbells to leave in the office, no resistant bands or cords, then a bucket of paint from the maintenance room would do the trick because this is about improvising. An example would be using rubber bands as resistance to strengthen your fingers.

For simplicity and to look somewhat professional in this book I am using a dumbbell for some of these exercises but you can replace that with a book, a well-sealed jug or paint can filled with water, sand, or pebbles. Anything you do at home or in the gym you can find a way to duplicate the exercise at your office. Okay, now let's get to work, so to speak.

ABDOMINAL RAISE

Actually I'm really sitting but this incorporates several muscle groups. Make sure the chair isn't going to recline. Place your hands on the arm rests and lift your butt off the seat. Your entire upper body is working to hold you up off the seat of the chair, including the lower trapezius muscle. Start with the knees bent at 90 degrees and then curl them toward your chest. Hold and slowly return them to the starting position, and hold them there.

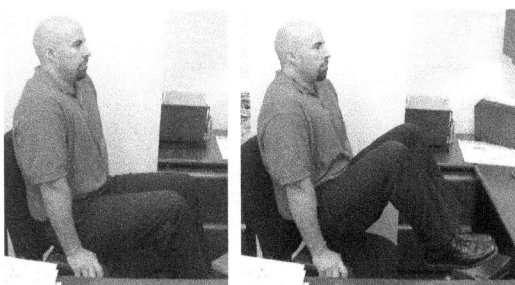

Try to keep your neck straight and eyes forward. Sure you could lie on the floor and do some abs but I'm trying to keep you clean and wrinkle free.

BICEP CONCENTRATION CURL

By placing your hand behind the lower part of the arm making the lift, you prevent it from moving or swinging to cheat when you raise the weight. Bring the weight up and exhale. Contract for a second and lower the weight to the point where there is still tension in your arm. Hold it there and then repeat.

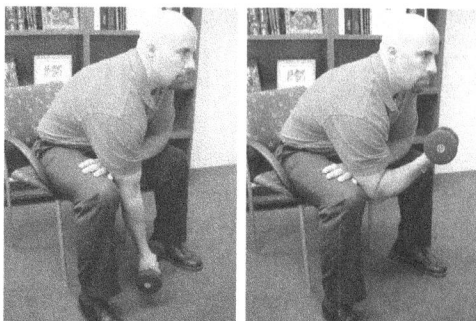

CALF RAISE

Place a book on the floor and put the balls of your feet on it. Use the wall for support and lower your heel to the floor to get a full stretch. Then press up until you are on your toes and squeeze hard for greater results. This is great for the calf region. If you need to increase your efforts you can raise the height of the book or place one foot over the other heel for added difficulty and resistance.

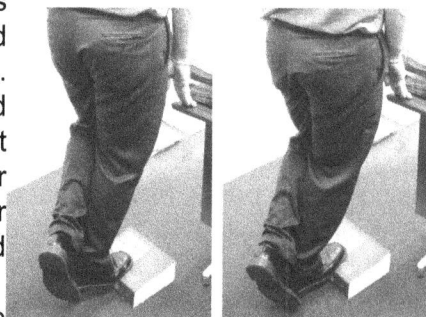

If there is a stairway close by, it would be even easier and sturdier than a book on the floor. Use the handrail or wall for stability.

Again, keep the ball of the foot on the tread of the stair and let the heel drop below the top of the stair. Then go back up onto your toes. If it's too easy, again use one leg at a time.

CHIN-UPS

Putting a chin-up bar would be useful in a closet or inconspicuous area. Chin-ups with palms towards you and arms in close work the biceps muscle more than the back. Palms away and widening the grip works the back and lats.

If you really wanted to do some without the bar, lie on your back under your desk, have the knees bent, feet on the floor and grab the edge of your desk. Now pull yourself up.

DELTOIDS

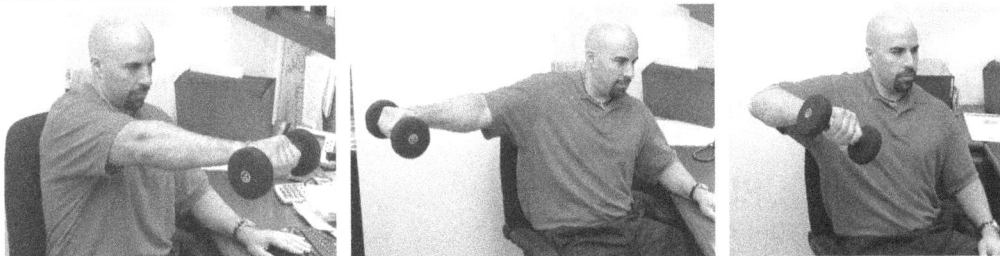

For a front deltoid raise, start with the dumbbell at your side. Bring your arm forward and raise your hand in front of you until it is even with your shoulders. Your palm should be facing the floor when you hold it there for a second, before lowering it back down.

With a side raise, the dumbbell will be at your side. Raise your arm up laterally or away from you like you're pouring out milk, except do it slowly, and hold it for a second and lower. This can be done with your arm straight or bent. I think I was typing emails while I did this.

EXTENSION EXERCISE

Just lean back. If you are doing extension exercises and it is helping a back problem, this is real easy to do to get some relief. Otherwise to really get down and dirty, lie on the floor and go through your extension routine. You may want to bring a yoga mat so you don't ruin your work clothes.

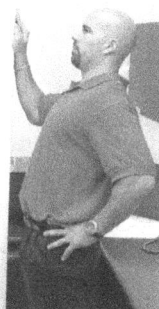

LUNGE

You can do lunges just by stepping forward with one foot in front of you and bending the knee until the upper leg and lower leg are at 90 degrees. You need to try to keep the knee over your ankle to reduce knee stress. A 2003 University of Memphis study found that bad form would lead to 28 percent more stress on the knee. However, if you lean forward at the hip you will increase stress there by almost 1,000 percent. Strive for great form.

To do this exercise properly, take a step back and bend that knee toward the floor while maintaining a straight upper back. Then return to the standing position with your feet together in a normal stance. Repeat with the same leg

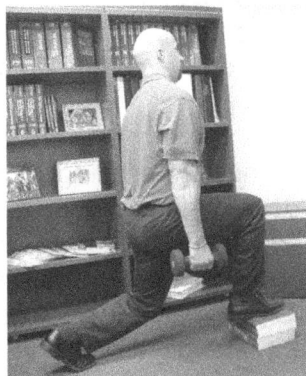

or vary from one side to the other. For more difficulty you can perform these by placing your foot on a few phone books or hold weight in your hands.

If you wanted to hide your leg routine from your co-workers, pick up a set of ankle weights. Strap those babies on and they are cleverly concealed. With each step you take you will be burning extra calories and toning up.

PREACHER CURL

The back of your computer chair is perfect to rest the back of your arms against while you do some curls. This helps focus the lift on your biceps muscles. Sink in to the armpits to better support the body.

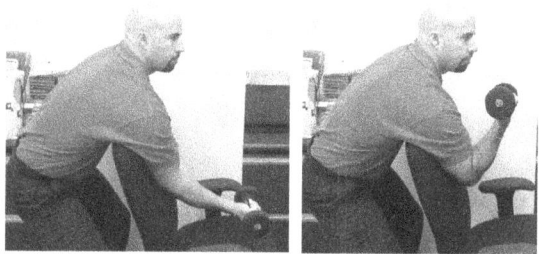

PUSHUPS

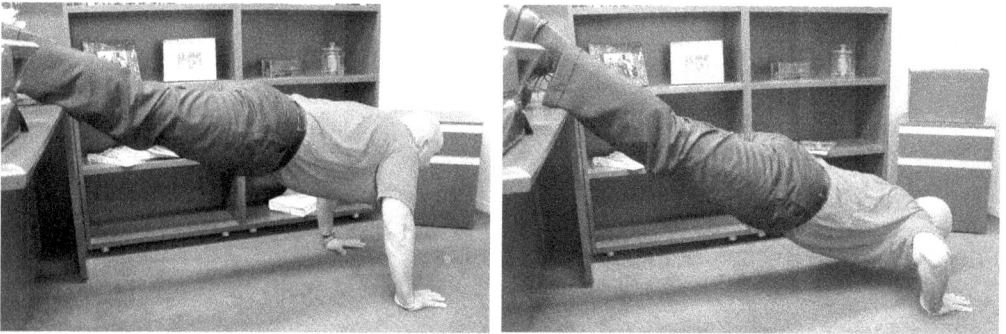

You can do the old-fashioned pushup with your feet on the floor. Place your hands about shoulders width apart and lower your chest to a few inches from the floor. Hold and then push back up.

Try some variations like bringing your hand in close together for an inner chest and triceps workout or go really wide for the outer chest. Beginners can do chest presses against the wall, against your desk or from your knees when you're on the floor.

Advanced pushups can be done with your hands elevated, perhaps on a book or on a set of the handles that are sold specifically for pushups, for a deeper stretch of the muscle fibers. Another muscle builder would be to put your feet on a desk so there is more weight towards your arms making the pushups harder to do. If you want explosive power, push up off the floor and clap your hands. That trains your muscles differently than typical pushups.

To make the pushup a real shoulder builder, you need to do an inverted pushup. Take off your shoes. Now get close to a wall and place your hands on the floor. Next try to get your feet up on to the wall so you are doing a handstand. If you don't need the wall for balance then maybe you should join the circus. Anyway, with your hands around shoulders width apart and about a foot or so from the wall, let your body down and then push yourself back up. It is basically a shoulder press, only upside down with a slightly less vertical position.

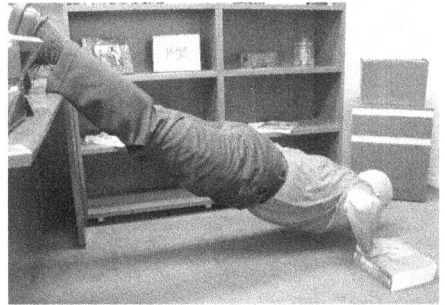

RHOMBOID ROW

Place your left knee on a chair and place your left hand on the backrest of the chair. The right leg can be slightly bent but keep your back straight and at a 45 degree angle to the ground.

Use your right hand to grab the weight and pull it toward you, with your arm close to your side like you're starting a lawn mower. When your arm bends to 90 degrees, hold, lower the weight and repeat. Then switch sides of course.

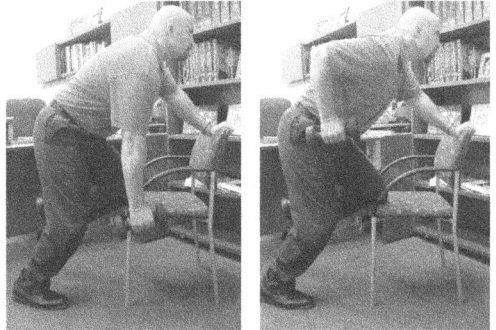

SHOULDER PRESS, ONE ARM

Just take the weight and press it up. You can start with your palms facing in or facing in front of you. Pushing anything in the office over your head multiple times, while sitting or standing, will work the shoulders like a shoulder press.

For a more advanced exercise, take your shoes off. Assume a handstand position against the wall so your stomach is facing the wall and you are vertical. Try to lower your body and push back up as if you are doing pushups. This places more stress on the deltoid, or shoulder region, as well as some upper chest. You can always move your hands away from the wall to vary the angle so it's easier.

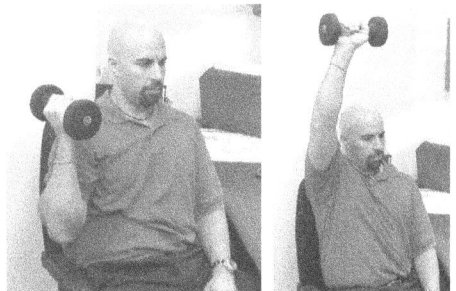

TRICEPS

Place your palms on the edge of your armrests or the seat and then prop your heels on your desk. As you get ready to perform a triceps dip, make sure the chair isn't going to roll away. Lower your bottom by bending your elbows to around the 90 degree mark, then press back up with your arms. Straighten your arms and contract, or squeeze the back of your arms hard to feel the burn. If the desk puts too much weight into your arms then lower your legs to a stool or keep them on the floor so it is easier.

You can also do a triceps extension with one arm at a time using a dumbbell. Keep the elbow close to your ear and bring the weight up and down without bonking your head. Unless you have hair to hide the dent. I don't.

To be less of a gymnast you could do isometric exercises at the office. Watch a bodybuilding show and remember how they pose. Run through your own version and have fun. Making muscles and holding them burns calories. It also forces blood and nutrients into the muscles and can make them grow.

You can use a towel or a rope and contract against the resistance as you hold the other end in your hand or underneath your foot. You can even tie one end off on a door knob. Now you can duplicate many of the exercises you would do in the gym with just a simple towel for resistance. You could also use your body to help with your isometric contractions routine.

Like for the triceps, bend your left arm to 90 degrees with your elbow at your side. Your palm can face up or down. Now put your right hand on the bottom of your forearm and press upward. At the same time press your left forearm down toward the floor.

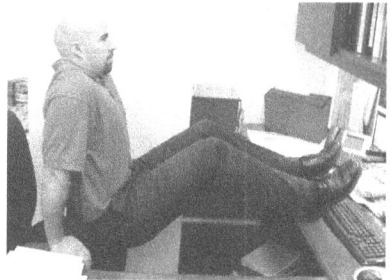

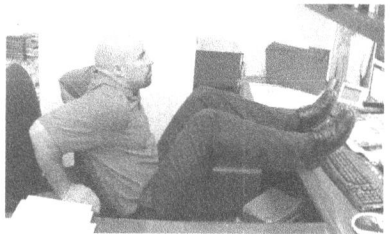

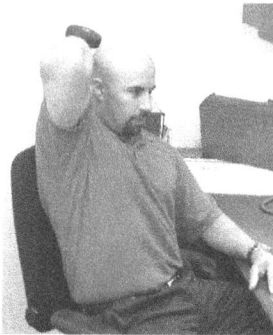

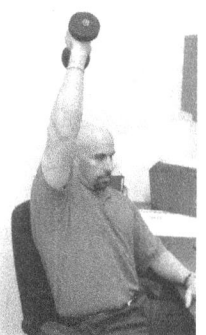

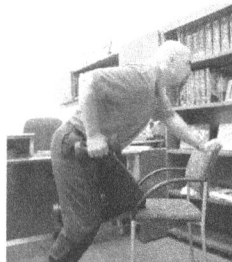

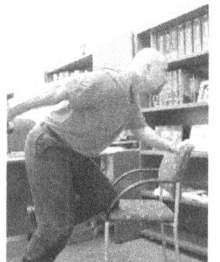

UPRIGHT ROW

Start with the weight between the knees and bring it up to your chin. Elbows should be pointed upward a little.

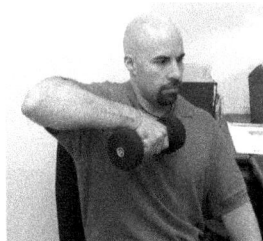

WALL SQUAT

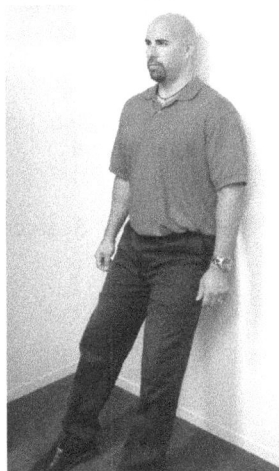

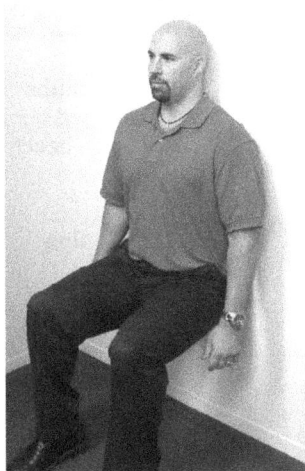

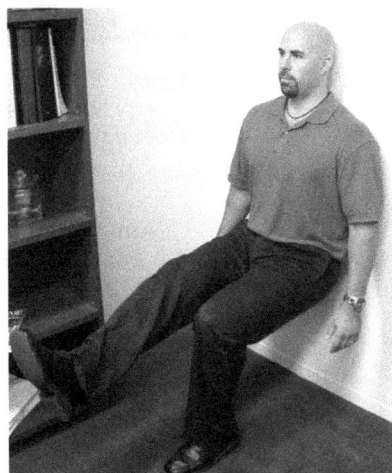

For your legs, simply place your back against the wall. Place your feet out in front of you. Slide your back down and keep your knees over the front of your ankles. When your thighs are parallel to the floor and the knees are at 90 degrees, this position places less stress on the knee joints then if you were to go beyond this point. Now you press back up.

If you find this too easy then try it with one leg. Place the unused leg out so your core has to tighten to hold it. Or cross your leg and lay it over the other leg for added resistance and really increase your strength, balance and coordination.

Another version would be to hold the doorknob when the door is open. Keep the same form with your knees at 90 degrees and your back should be straight.

This exercise can help strengthen the exact muscles you would be using when you lift something up using your legs and not your back. It may even help prevent or protect you from an injury because your legs will be strong enough to complete the task.

If you want a reminder for your knees and back, place a chair behind you. When you get low enough, your buttocks should lightly touch the chair's seat. This will prevent you from over compressing the knee joint.

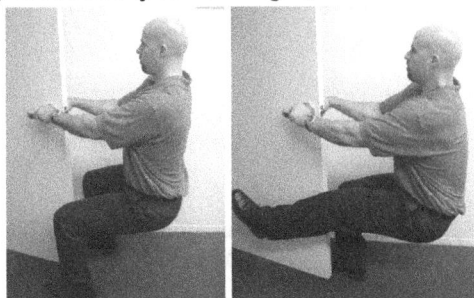

SUMMARY OF EXERCISES

You can do any version of these exercises wherever you are. Mix it up.

MUSCLE being used	At the OFFICE	Using Your Body Weight	At the GYM *can use reverse grip
CHEST	**Pushups** vary hand positions, feet up on bench, clap, one arm	**Dip Pushups** vary hand positions, feet up on bench	**Bench Press** incline, decline, and neutral
BACK	**1 Arm Bent Over Row** with jug or weight	**Chin Ups**	**Lat Pulldown* Seated Rows**
SHOULDERS	**Deltoid Raise** with jug or weight **Shoulder Press** with jug or weight	**Vertical Pushup**	**Shrug Upright Row Seated Press**
BICEPS	**Concentration Curls** with jug or weight	**Chin Ups** palms up	**Curls** w/cables*, hammer, dumbbells*, EZ or straight bar*
TRICEPS	**Kickback** w/wt **Overhead Press** w/ jug or wt	**Chair Dip**	**Press Down* Triceps Extension***
LEGS	**1 or 2 Leg Squat Calf Raise** on phone book or stair	**Wall Squat** 1 Leg or 2 **AB/AD-ductor** floor exercise	**Leg Extension Leg Press Squat Hamstring Curl**
ABDOMINAL	**AB-Raise** in chair **Crunch** on the floor	**Crunches** w/ Ball, incline, reverse, bicycle	**Crunches** w/ wt, using cables **Hanging Knee Raises**
LOW BACK	**Extension Exercises** on the floor or standing	**Extension Exercises** on the floor	**Roman Chair Extension Exercises** w/Ball
Quick all over body burn	**Isometrics**	**Isometrics**	**Isometrics**

"Underneath this flabby exterior is an enormous lack of character." – **Oscar Levant**

Car Workout

I drive a lot and it can seem like wasted time. Oh who am I kidding, it is a waste of time. Sometimes I might bring an audio book to enrich my mind, talk to friends, crank some tunes or do some exercise. What? He really has lost it. Nope. Actually, there are some things you can do while stuck in a car to help your physique and burn some extra calories.

There is a simple rule. The more muscles you use the more calories you burn. I have a routine I like to keep in mind so I can justify some of the questionable munchies, along with the good ones, on my trips.

Do not try anything in this section until you are in a safe area with minimal traffic or have enough of a buffer between cars. It is bad enough so many people drive like they are the only ones pressed for time, they own the road, or have a need to pull out in front of you when there is no one behind you. I probably avoid three accidents each time I am behind the wheel by dodging stupid moves like that. Too many people drive too fast for the conditions. So before you try anything, make sure you have good command of the art of driving, respect for your fellow drivers and a good idea of where they are in relation to your vehicle.

First off, cruise control is very helpful. It frees up your legs. Make sure you are not in bumper car traffic before attempting these exercises and keep your eyes on the road at all times. Safety comes first. Grab your dumbbell set and let's get started. I'm kidding.

Because people who sit too long can tighten their backs or increase the leg pain caused by varicose veins, of course taking breaks is one way around these problems. I put my feet against the floor board and stand at an angle to straighten my spine. You can even bend the legs to get the blood flowing but don't hit the emergency brake pedal. If your pain is bad, just take a few extra breaks to stretch.

Okay, let's start with the legs. I like to crank tunes so I like to play air drums. My legs will often pretend to be working the bass drum and high hat with the skill of professional drummer. Picking up of the entire leg or just the heel and moving it up and down can be tiring and effective. It can also stave off muscle tightness and help your blood flow.

The proper way to breathe is to let your stomach out when you inhale and pull the stomach in to exhale. Well in the car or even at your desk at work, take a few breaths and when you exhale try to squeeze your stomach in as far and as hard as you can. Hold it a second and repeat when you think of it. This will tighten the midsection too. Pelvic tilts might feel pretty good too. Especially for the back.

The safest exercise to do while driving is an isometric routine in which you just hold your muscles in a tightened state. They are easy to do in the car. Just make a muscle. For example, pretend to squeeze the wheel together from the sides to tighten the chest like the Incredible Hulk.

Using one arm, make a muscle pose for biceps and straighten the arms and tighten up the back of your arms for a little triceps burn. Hold it for a couple of seconds or you can even go back and forth making a muscle and then straightening the arm. Then switch sides. You could also push your knees outward or inward against the car or your hands for some thigh sculpting.

Because driving is stressful, I have noticed I was elevating my shoulders, especially in bad weather. A simple stretch to do at a stop sign is just to tip your head, right ear to right shoulder or vice versa, to alleviate some shoulder tension. Squeeze your shoulder blades together for a pec stretch, midback burn and better posture. Whatever routine you try, a few extra reps and calories burned can help your figure and make you forget about the long drive ahead.

> *"A mind once stretched by a new idea never regains its original dimension."*
> **– Oliver Wendell Holmes Jr.**

Stretching and Flexibility

HOW LOW CAN YOU GO?

Just like people take their health for granted, they also ignore the importance of stretching regularly and staying flexible. Flexibility can be defined as being able to move your joints through their full range of motion without restrictions or limitations.

There are several factors for why some people are more flexible than others. In general women are more flexible than men. We also lose flexibility as we age unless we maintain our bodies properly. A common factor for age related limitations is physical inactivity. If you don't move, you lose your groove.

If you have decreased flexibility it can be due to: years of work that caused muscles to become overdeveloped and tight; scar tissue that formed in joints and muscle fibers; trauma associated with a car accident; or from a tackle in football or fall, in which the spine was pulled out of its normal alignment.

You could also be at a disadvantage genetically. Conditions like scoliosis, a short leg or other postural distortions in your body like abnormal lordosis can also be a source of inflexibility.

Without proper flexibility and stretching, your body loses some of its ability to function as it was designed. When you use only 80 percent of your normal range of movement for your muscles, they can't operate at their peak. As a result your muscles and tendons will shorten and tighten and this can lead to injury. In addition, this tight area can affect many other muscles that adapt as they support the body.

Two of my friends who popped their Achilles tendons had chronically tight calf muscles that were forced to contract suddenly after these regions had adapted to being short, tight and comfortable functioning in a limited range of motion. The result was torn tendons. Have you ever tried tuning a guitar when the strings are cold? Each string will not tune as easily as when it is warm, and will probably break.

Many elderly people could do themselves a world of good if they would start a stretching routine. Their inactivity is a reason they have terrible flexibility. Some may be hindered by injury or disease, but almost everyone could benefit from some light exercises and stretching.

Even those huge bodybuilders can do splits on stage because they know their muscles can get bigger and stronger if they are exercised and stretched throughout their full range of motion.

I am reminded of my youth when so many teenagers come into my office with back pain and terrible flexibility. No wonder they have problems. The fact is sitting around all day at the computer, in class, in front of a game console or TV, contributes to tightening the hamstrings in everyone. This can lead to an imbalance in core muscles and is the source of common back pains.

Is there enough emphasis at school on the importance of stretching? Do gym classes and after school sports have good stretching programs for our kids nowadays? Do they have an appreciation for and an understanding of the benefits of flexibility? Success in the sports kid play is dependent on more than just lifting weights. Check your kids' flexibility. Can they touch their toes with their knees slightly bent?

One of the reasons my back went out when I was 27 was because my hamstrings were tight. If I tried to touch my toes I bet I reached mid-shin on a good day. My lower back was so tight it had pulled my pelvic region like a wedgie and tightened my hamstrings. Not to mention I didn't stretch them like I did the front of my legs. That's why balancing the core muscles in terms of strength and flexibility is so important to stabilize the low back and avoid pain.

To re-establish balance in my core I had to stretch my hamstrings constantly throughout my other training. I would stretch at my office, in the shower, out with friends, and anywhere. In six months my fingers were at the ground and my back felt good. I was able to return to baseball and only took time off if I needed to rest my aging body; not due to injury. It takes time to see results like losing weight does. Don't get discouraged. Gains take time, but good things like flexibility are worth the wait.

"To reach something good it is very useful to have gone astray, and thus acquire experience."
– Saint Teresa of Avila

HOW LONG, HAS THIS BEEN GOING ON

Most individuals do not stretch correctly, and this happens at all levels of athletic ability. There are some simple rules for stretching techniques to give you a better understanding of their purpose and benefits.

How long should you hold each stretch? I tell patients to try for 15 seconds minimally. I'm ahead of the game if I can get patients to even participate in their healthcare. When you start to work up to stretching 10 times per side, the time spent stretching can be equal to a commercial break or two during a TV show. And that's a great time to do them, when you're not thinking about them.

For the best results, thirty seconds is the amount of time that minimal muscle fiber stretching and elongating occurs, but 60 seconds is optimal according to MRI research. If you have the time and dedication, then good for you, and I mean it! If you can't make the time, anything you do will be helpful.

If you are stretching and it feels like a sharp pain instead of a stretch-like pain, then discontinue what you were doing and see your doctor. There could be more going on than just a stubborn, tight group of muscles. Always check with your doctor whenever you have a question about your health.

When you stretch a muscle, it is like a rubber band with one exception. The rubber band will lengthen and immediately return to its original size due to an elastic principle. Muscles will also lengthen, slowly returning to their original size with a gradual motion similar to tar. This is known as viscoelasticity.

When patients are trying to regain their health I recommend they stretch 1 – 3 times a day. The more they stretch the more they will help themselves. If you are healthy then just add this form of exercise to your regime. Because flexibility is closely related to balance, posture and muscular coordination, always making the time to stretch can help decrease muscle stiffness, decrease your risk of injury and help improve your game.

I always tell patients to warm up before they exercise to get blood flowing and loosen the muscle fibers. Some studies found that warming up and then stretching is the only way to decrease the chance of injuries associated with exercise. Take 5 – 10 minutes to walk or jog to get warm. Then go through your stretching routine. Now that you're loose, go run, lift or walk.

When you are done lifting and contracting your muscles or running 5 miles, you need to relax the muscles that you have just been contracting for the last hour. This is the most important time to stretch. If you don't, over time the muscles will get tighter and tighter. They will decrease your ability to fully extend your muscles, limiting overall motion and the results you will get from your future training.

Stretching after exercise will also reduce the amount of soreness you experience the next day, known as Delayed Onset Muscle Soreness (DOMS). Did you ever workout hard or run one day and then feel like you aged 35 years two days later? That's DOMS.

"Science is organized knowledge. Wisdom is organized life." – **Immanuel Kant**

BLINDED ME WITH SCIENCE

A noted researcher Vladimir Janda, MD, DSc and some colleagues classified all of our muscles into two categories in relation to our posture. Postural muscles are more involved with holding correct posture while phasic muscles respond to the postural muscles, to keep things balanced.

The muscles are also known as agonist and antagonists, muscles that work against one another. Examples are your triceps and biceps, hamstrings and quads, cats and dogs, or democrats and republicans.

The triceps, hamstrings, erector spinae (low back), pectorals (chest), upper trapezius, sternocleidomastoid or SCM (from your collar bone to behind your ear) and subocciptal muscles (highest part of the back of the neck and under the skull) are part of the postural group. These agonistic muscles tend to be overused. They are mostly comprised of slow twitch fibers and can work hard for a long duration and usually do. Over time they become extremely tight and short. They are the muscles that typically need extra attention from your massage therapist.

The phasic muscles like the abdominals, glutes, lower and middle trapezius, rhomboids and deltoids are examples of fast twitch fibers that tire out faster and can become weak quickly. Due to this inability to respond to the postural muscles they work against, they must be strengthened. That is why many people have low back pain. The low back or erector muscles are tight and the abdominals are weak. That is the basis for the core workout.

When your hamstring is tight it can be considered the agonist. It will neurologically inhibit information trying to get to the thigh muscles, or the quads (the antagonist), and limit the contraction and how far the opposing muscle can move through its normal range of motion. Both of these actions are known as Sherrington's Law of Reciprocal Inhibition.

It's kind of like Newton's 3rd Law, for every action there is an equal and opposite reaction. In this case it means that a tight muscle will negatively affect the opposing muscle from working normally, and from receiving the right instructions to function properly. The moral to this story is to stretch all of your muscles, not just the tight ones.

It is better to keep them all happy and loose then have them running around antagonizing each other.

> *"Prepare yourself for the world, as the athletes used to do for their exercise; oil your mind and your manners, to give them the necessary suppleness and flexibility; strength alone will not do."* – **Earl of Chesterfield**

I DID IT MY WAY

There are many ways to stretch. Use whichever technique is right for you. Some people respond to different stimulus so don't think you have to do one version or the other. You may find using several stretching methods help you accomplish your goal; much like changing your weightlifting routine can push your muscles to new gains.

In general you shouldn't bounce when you stretch. This form of stretch, known as Ballistic stretching, will cause a stretch reflex in the muscles. The nervous system will try to protect the body from an overstretch injury by triggering the very muscle you are stretching, to tighten even more.

Much like tapping the tendon below your kneecap causes your thigh to contract and kick the leg out, it is a protection method used by your body to reduce injury to the muscle while maintaining tension. Do that bouncing stretch over and over and you can understand how this will create a chronically, tight muscle.

When you stretch, hold for 60 seconds for maximum long-term benefits of changing the muscle's length. The muscle must be in the stretched position long enough for the muscle fibers, or the neurological system, to adapt to the lengthened position.

However, some sports like karate and ballet do use this technique. Momentum is used to push their bodies further than they could go by stretching slowly. It is kind of like being able to go where no joint has gone before. You are forcing your body to go just a little beyond its normal limitations to gain greater range of motion in the long run. I would only recommend this form of stretching for the elite athlete or someone under the supervision of an experienced trainer. There are better ways for you and me.

Another protective response by the body to excessive muscle stretching is known as the Inverse Myotactic Reflex. Your muscles are attached to your bones by tendons. At the unification of the tendon and the muscle fibers, there is something called the Golgi Tendon Organ (GTO).

If a muscle that contracts too intensely or a stretch to the tendon may cause damage. The GTOs can override the system and relax the muscle so injury to the tendon or muscle won't occur. This is another reason to be careful if you are going to bounce your stretches.

What's great about these mechanisms is that they are prime examples of how your body is trying to protect itself at all times. That's why it's a good idea to take care for the body that looks out for you.

I ask patients to show me how they stretch at home and about half of them bob up and down. Stretches should be done slowly or by holding a specific position, known as a Static stretch. When you reach the end of your range of motion and feel the muscles stretching, you simply stay there between 15 – 60 seconds. This form of stretching is a safe and slow method for lengthening muscles.

Active stretching is using one muscle to stretch the opposing muscle. An example would be straightening your leg and feeling a stretch in the back of the leg. As the quadriceps, or thigh muscles contract, your hamstring is elongated and stretched. This is called Reciprocal Inhibition and is helpful when improving your flexibility with movement.

A Passive stretch is when the muscles are relaxed and you use a prop, or someone else, to help make the stretch happen. It can loosen a persistently tight muscle. If while on your back you wrap a towel around your foot and pull your leg straight and back it will stretch the back of your leg. If you decide to work with a partner, make sure they don't push you beyond your capabilities. Just because they can do a split doesn't mean you can right now or should ever attempt to.

Several techniques for assisted stretching incorporate breathing to achieve greater flexibility. If you take a deep breath and exhale as you perform a stretch it can help you relax and permit the muscles to lengthen more.

Proprioceptive Neuromuscular Facilitation (PNF) increases the speed at which the muscle, its tendons and nerves communicate with each other to understand and sense what is going on regarding their position (bent or straight). We'll stick with PNF for now. Initially PNF is used for rehabbing injured muscles so they get back up to speed with the rest of the body. Kind of a *"use it or lose it"* principle.

In an athlete or someone with chronically tight muscles, it is great for targeting trouble spots or stubborn muscles that don't want to loosen up and lengthen. It is also commonly used to increase the flexibility, strength and range of motion of the muscles.

Two of the more common variations of this technique are Contract-Relax Technique (Hold-Relax) and Contract-Relax-Contract Technique (Hold-Relax-Contract). In order to accomplish these stretches you need a good partner to help you.

For example, Contract-Relax Technique of the hamstring is performed like this. You lie on your back and elevate your right leg until you feel a light stretch in the back of your leg. You then place your right heel on your partner's right shoulder. Now start with light resistance, and over a time period of 6 – 15 seconds, increase pressure down into the shoulder by doing an isometric contraction, all while taking a breath in.

Gently increase to your maximal pressure, as long as it does not cause pain. The amount of downward pressure you use should be limited by your physical condition and whether or not you are recovering from an injury.

Your partner should talk to you about what they need you to do as far as the force of contraction, when to relax and proper breathing. After 6 – 15 seconds, exhale and relax your leg muscles. Now have your partner step toward your head to increase your stretch. Hold 30 seconds and then switch sides and repeat.

The Contract-Relax-Contract Method is performed like the Contract-Relax Technique, however when you exhale, you contract your quadriceps muscle as your partner steps forward to apply the stretch. This contracts one side of your leg while the other side is stretched.

Another effective stretch is Post Isometric Relaxation (PIR), which uses breathing and sight to assist the stretch. To stretch the hamstring, use the set up like the previous stretches mentioned. The leg is elevated and held just at the point of feeling the stretch and before any pain. You would press your leg down into your partner's shoulder for 5 – 10 seconds with about 10 percent of your maximal effort as you breathe in.

At the end of this time your partner instructs you to breathe out. As you exhale you also look in the direction of your stretch. In this case you look overhead because this is the direction your leg is going. Your partner performs a stretch similar to the other ones described by stepping forward, or toward your head.

Once this position is held for a few seconds, repeat the stretch, as this becomes the new starting point. Repeat 2 – 4 times. You should try to actively attain this fuller range of motion with some aerobic exercises. Enjoy your newfound motion. These stretches are sometimes not the most pleasant, but they are extremely effective.

Another strategy for stretching is Post Facilitation Stretch (PFS). This is similar to the PNF methods except when you relax the muscle, the stretch is performed differently. The muscle is contracted into your partner's shoulder for 7 – 10 seconds. After you exhale and relax, your partner rapidly moves forward to stretch the muscle quickly. It is held there for 20 seconds and this procedure is repeated 3 – 5 times, without ever releasing the gains you have made.

"A good exercise for the heart is to bend down and help another up." – **Anonymous**

Stretches For The Body

If you have any discomfort with any movement, don't do it and seek professional care. If these pictures and descriptions don't adequately explain how to stretch your body, try the web sites previously mentioned or just search for books, TV shows or other Internet sites that may help you.

ACHILLES TENDON (above the back of your heel)

Place the ball of your foot against a wall or any other vertical object and lean forward. You should feel a stretch in the tendon running from the back of the shoe upward.

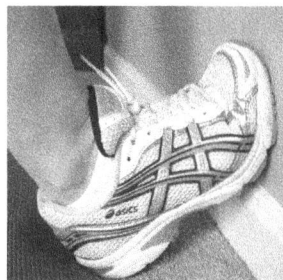

BICEP STRETCH

The upper arm is difficult to stretch. Try putting your arm out to the side with your thumbs up. *"Aaaaay,"* as The Fonz would say. Now turn your wrists so your thumbs point down and palms facing behind you. Hold a towel in your hands in this position while they are behind your back.

Let the cloth slip through your hands until you are at a comfortable distance apart or around shoulders width. Now pull the towel with one hand and that will cause a stretch in the other arm.

Another option would be to use a doorway. Lodge the top of your hand, or both hands, against the side of an open door. With the arms out to the side and your elbows almost straight, move your body forward.

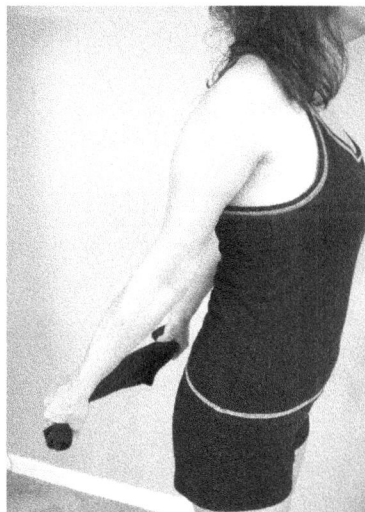

The stretch will be mild compared to some of the other ones you've done before. You could also use a wall.

CALF STRETCH

Place one hand against the wall and the other behind your back. Put one foot forward and one back so the ball of the foot is touching. As you lean toward the wall press the heel of your back foot into the floor. For an increased stretch, place your front foot behind and over the back of the ankle of your back foot. You can also lean further forward to increase the intensity.

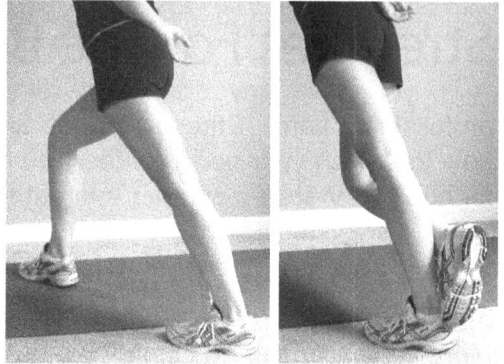

CHEST STRETCH

Reach your hands behind your back and interlock your hands or fingers. Now rotate the shoulders back while you push your chest forward and try to touch your shoulder blades together. You can also put your hands on the frame or sides of an open doorway. With your elbows bent, lean forward and allow your body to move through the doorway. You could do this in the corner of a room as well. I know, *"nobody puts Baby in the corner."*

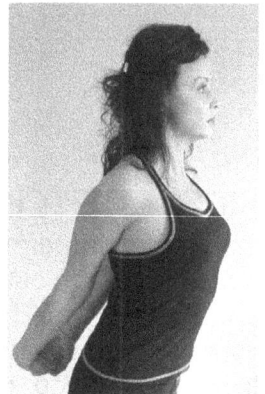

FINGER STRETCH

Assume the prayer position with your hands. Push the fingers on one hand backward and then repeat for the other side. We constantly grip things and the fingers and forearms get overused and receive very little attention.

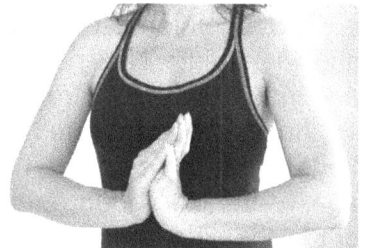

FOREARM STRETCH

Bend your left arm to 90 degrees and keep your elbow against your side. Take your right hand palms facing up and press the hand and fingers down toward the ground. You can bend them away from your body for a little more intensity.

You can also place your hands together like you're praying and lower your forearms so they are parallel to the floor. This is similar to the picture above. Now push one direction and then the other with your fingers.

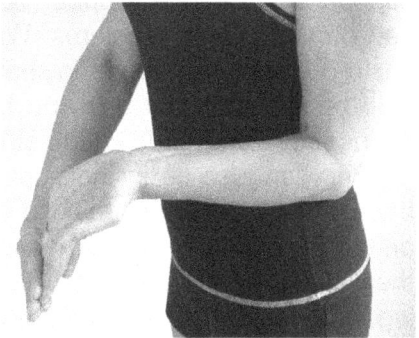

GROIN STRETCH

Sit on the floor and bring the soles of your feet together, while your knees are as far apart as possible. It is sometimes referred to as Indian style of sitting. Now grab your feet with both hands, push your knees down with your elbows and lean forward. You can also just place your hands on your upper thighs, above the knees, and press down.

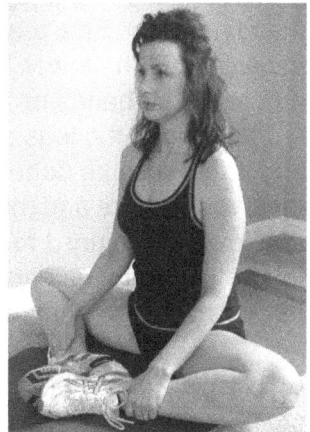

HAMSTRING STRETCH

Place a foot on a chair and lean forward with the elevated leg slightly bent at the knee. This maneuver is sometimes called a runner's or hurdler's stretch. The hamstring muscle can also be stretched while standing. Spread your legs about shoulders width apart and keep a slight bend in the knees. Now bend forward while reaching forward to touch your toes.

When you lean forward you can grab your pant legs or calves to help guide you to a better stretch. In football they would have us grab the grass and pull down.

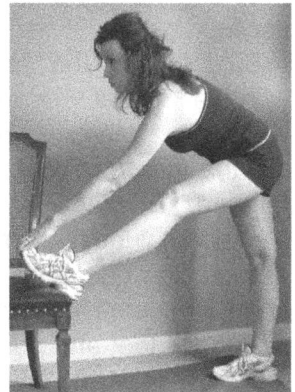

I like to place my hands on my knees for support as I lower my upper body because I have had previous back problems. When you reach your desired stretch and have finished, use your arms to help bring your body back up by pressing on your knees, therefore reducing the stress to the back.

You can also lie in the supine position, on your back, and bend both knees. Be sure to have the feet on the floor. Now bring one leg toward the chest and then straighten the leg. Again you can grab a pant leg, or put a towel around the foot, and bring the leg higher up.

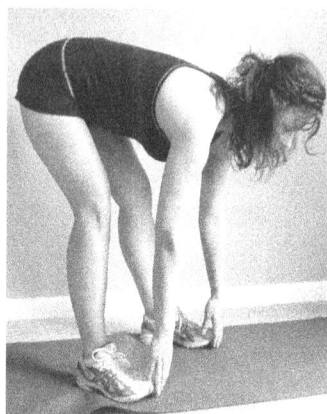

Recently I watched in shock as two women on national TV touted their exercise routine for the stars as a great program. In horror, I witnessed them perform the straight-legged toe-touch, which I thought became extinct with the dinosaurs. The toe touch causes a simultaneous stretch in the back of the legs and the lower back. This can cause an injury. Bend the knees slightly and rest your hands on your knees for support.

Also when the legs are straight, each time you bring your body upright again and the lift may be done improperly by using the back muscles. That doubles the force to the discs and muscles each time you raise your body up. It the precursor to a low back injury. I recommend a forward stretch all the time because it helps to stretch the hamstrings and open the spaces between your vertebrae in your back, but you need to use a little caution.

HIP FLEXOR STRETCH (front of thigh above your pants pocket)

Kneel on the floor like you are watching a kid's soccer game. One foot should be on the ground with the knee at 90 degrees while the other knee is on the ground. Just lean forward. This position can also be attained by standing and placing one knee on a chair, or something else, and then leaning forward. To add to the stretch, grab your back foot and pull it up. If you can't reach your foot, place the top of your foot on a chair and lower your body.

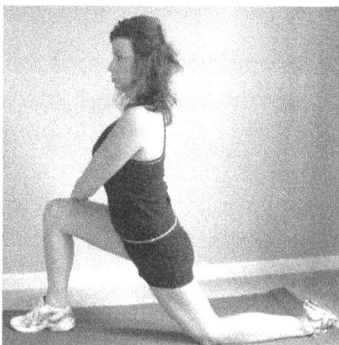

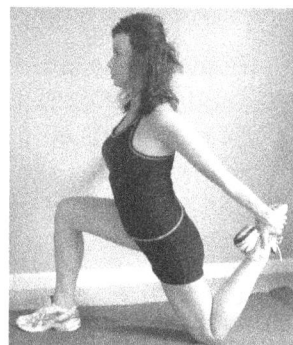

LOW BACK STRETCHES

Some people have back pain and have to pick which direction feels more comfortable to them. The choices are flexion or extension. These stretches can help or hurt your back depending on your health status. If a doctor has recommended you do flexion exercises for your pain then stick with them. Don't worry about what Suzy from the office tells you her boyfriend's sister's neighbor's uncle, who works for Kevin Bacon (six degrees of separation), does for his. If you are in relatively good health and have no pains then try both of them.

It may come as a shock, but your shoes can also make a difference. If you do better with flexion exercises then I would stick with flat shoes. Heels put your back into extension.

FLEXION STRETCHES

When done as a stretch, these positions can help loosen your low back muscles (extensor muscles), open up the disc spaces in your back, reduce nerve pressure and alleviate disc pain.

BACK STRETCH

Sit in a chair and simply lean forward. If you want more of a stretch, grab the legs of the chair or your ankles and gently guide your body forward. If you are wide at the shoulders or your belly gets in the way, scoot forward on the chair and move your knees apart a little more.

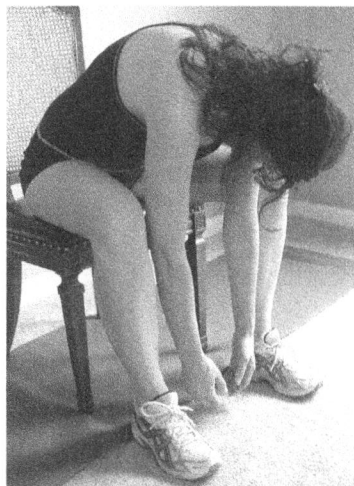

CAT STRETCH

Take a position on the floor and get on your hands and knees. Take a breath in and arch your back. Then exhale and sit back on to your heels. If you want to get lower move your legs apart so your torso can drop more. You can even push backwards with your hands to force a greater stretch in the low back.

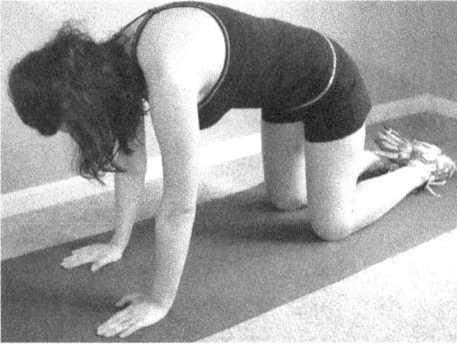

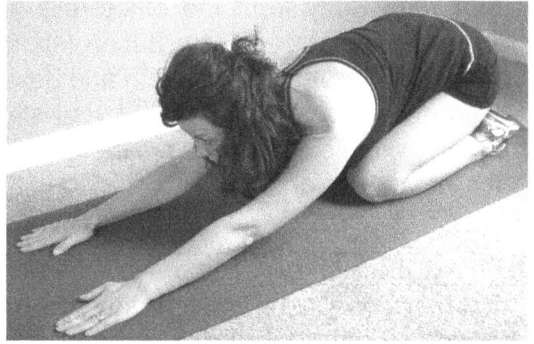

KNEE TO CHEST STRETCH

Lie on your back and with both knees and your feet on the floor. Grab one knee with your hands, pull it toward your chest and hold. Set the leg down to the starting position before repeating for the other side. If you want to bring both legs up, bring one up off the ground, then the other. Then bring them both into the chest, hold and let them down one at a time.

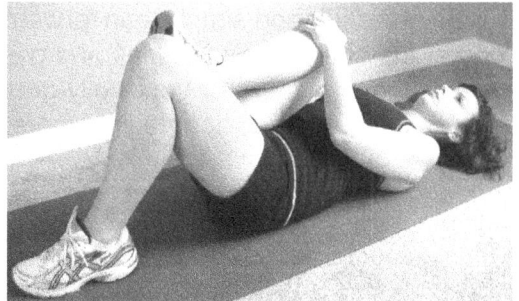

Moving both legs down simultaneously can put too much pressure for the low back, especially if you have a back problem.

If you have a bad knee, grab behind the knee joint so you don't compress the joint. If you can't reach your knees, try placing a towel behind the knee and pull the towel to move your knee to your chest, or as far as it will go.

While standing you could also put your foot on a chair, dresser or the bed and lean forward. Your knee and chest still come close together so it stretches the area just the same. Sitting in a chair you could put your heel on the chair's seat while you're watching TV and bring your knee toward your chest.

If you wanted to try to create traction to separate the joints and reduce pressure in your low back, you could stand at the back of the recliner or cushy chair at your house. Now lean over the back of the recliner by placing your stomach on the top of the backrest. Place your hands on the armrests and let your legs hang down to the ground. For added height, place a pillow in front of your beltline.

A similar position to this would be to place a bunch of pillows on the bed and place your waist on top of them so you are propped up like a tent with your backside in the air. That creates flexion in the low back. If you want to add some traction to the spine like on the chair, set the pillows up close to edge of the bed so your legs can hang toward the ground.

I found a position that alleviated pain in my inflamed back by sleeping on the couch. I wasn't on the couch because I was in the dog house. I slept with both knees bent and slid toward one arm rest so my toes touched it. This prevented my legs from straightening out and allowed me to relax because I didn't need to hold them like this. Then I put a pillow behind my knees to reduce knee stress. Next I slid toward the back of the couch so my legs didn't flop too far to one side. This kept the legs fairly straight and decreased any rotation in the hips. My back stayed flexed with open the disc spaces all night long. It really helped me out.

EXTENSION STRETCHES
Commonly referred to as McKenzie Exercises, extension exercises can be done lying down or standing and may help with disc pain. It may help push a small disc bulge back to where it belongs.

BACK EXTENSION
When you are on your stomach, do a pushup but keep your waist on the floor. As a stretch this will lengthen the abdominal region or stomach area. Rest on your elbows like a kid watching TV or go up on to your hands. Whatever level feels comfortable to you. Don't be a contortionist. Go up for 20 seconds and rest

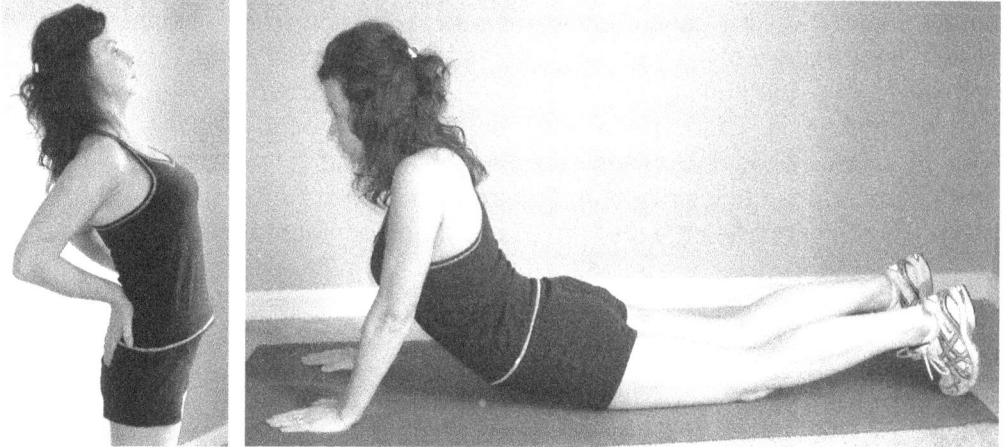

for 40 seconds.

The standing version is similar in that you put your hands on your lower back, or waist, and gently arch back. You may also put your outstretched hands against a wall like you're being arrested (no prior experience needed here), and let your waist move toward the wall.

LATERAL GLIDE
Place your hands on your hips and pretend someone is pulling your belt one way for 5 seconds and then let go. Repeat on the other side. Keep your shoulders parallel to the floor so you aren't tipping your upper body. Only your midsection moves to one side or the other.

If it is painful shifting to one side or the other, then don't do it. If both ways hurt, don't do either.

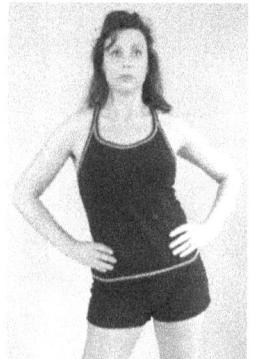

MIDBACK & UPPER BACK STRETCH

Wrap your left arm across the front of your chest. Take your right arm and grab just above the elbow. Pull the arm across the chest and turn your upper body to the right.

I also like to do this using a doorway. Put your right shoulder next to the edge of the opening of a doorway. With the same starting position as mentioned above, grab the doorway with your left hand and keep your arm parallel to the floor. You should be in the exact same position you were in when your arm was across your chest. Now just let your body weight fall away as you hold on. You are not pulling the doorway but allowing your bodyweight to distract, lengthen and stretch the muscles. Try to keep your arm close to your chest through the movement.

In a sitting position with your knees apart, try reaching your arms and shoulders through them and maybe even grab the chair base below you. Gently pull down or just reach as far as you can under the chair for an all over backstretch. Focus on arching the upper back. This stretch will also hit the lower back.

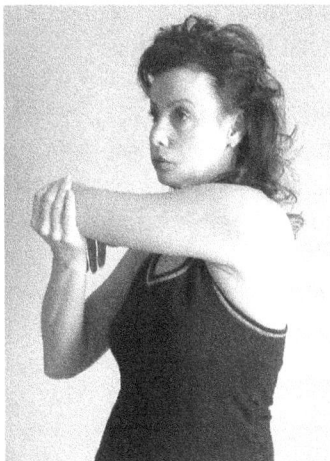

NECK & SHOULDER STRETCH

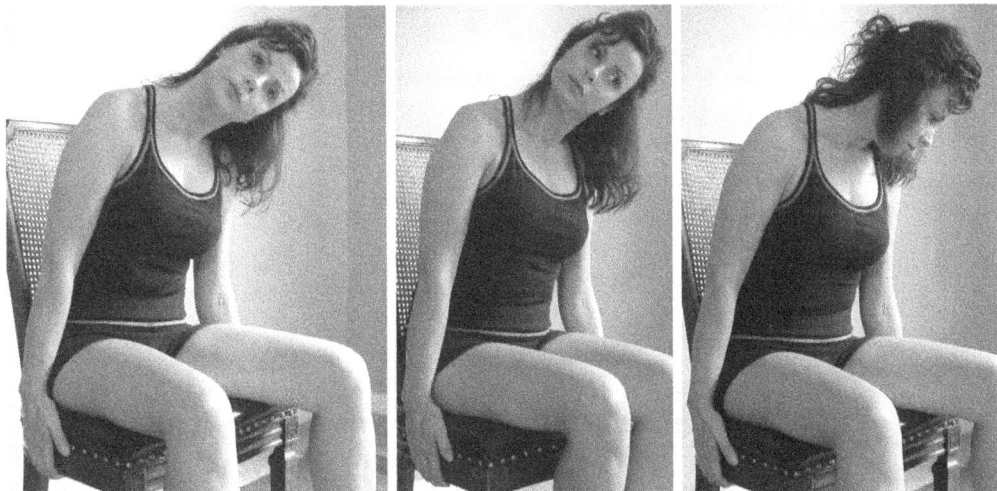

In a sitting position, place your right hand on the edge of the seat and lean away from it and toward the left. Bring your left ear toward your left shoulder. This will help lengthen the muscles from your shoulder to your neck.

You can also lean a little forward and bring your ear, and then your nose, in the direction of your armpit to stretch a little above the right shoulder blade. Do this for both sides.

If you don't have a chair, you can reach behind your back and grab your right wrist with the left hand and do these same exercises. You could also take your free hand (the left in these pictures) and push down on the right shoulder. Now tipping your head away from that side will create a better stretch. However just leaning your head in a few directions should get you to feel a mild stretch. You can always add a little stretch with your free hand by placing your hand on top of your head and gently guiding it away from the side that is being held down. Use a few fingers to limit the intensity.

A stretch and exercise you can do for forward head carriage resembles a pigeon in the city. You are sliding your head backwards like someone grabs your ears and pulls your head backwards. It is often demonstrated by putting your pointer finger on your chin and pushing your chin to glide it backwards. The head should remain even and looking forward.

To strengthen the muscles in the back of your neck, lie on your stomach and lift your head up in the same manner. Now you have to lift that *"pumpkin"* against the forces of gravity, which makes the muscles stronger in the back of the neck. This can help to correct forward head carriage or stop it from getting worse. You can also gently push the back of your head into the car's headrest for a few seconds. That's an Isometric contraction and helps strengthen the muscles.

PIRIFORMIS / HIP / BUTTOCK STRETCH

On the floor, bend and cross the left leg over the right, straight leg. Take the right elbow and place it on the outside of the left knee. Add a slight twist to the right with your upper body and push the knee with your elbow to the left in the opposite direction. You can also grab the bent knee with the hand of the opposite side and pull the knee toward it.

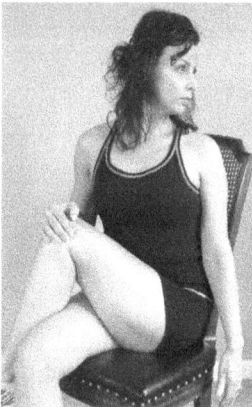

This can also be done sitting. Cross your left leg over the right knee like you are sitting at a fancy dinner. Take your right hand and grab the left knee. Carefully turn your upper body and right shoulder toward the left knee. Try to approximate your left knee and your right shoulder and bring those two together.

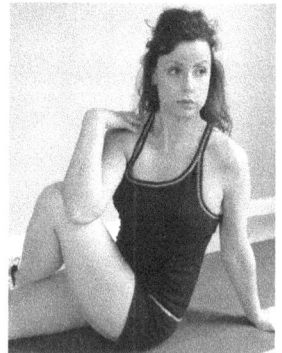

On the floor, put the left ankle on the right knee. Now raise the right knee toward your right shoulder. You can hold the ankle as you approximate the shoulder and knee of the same side.

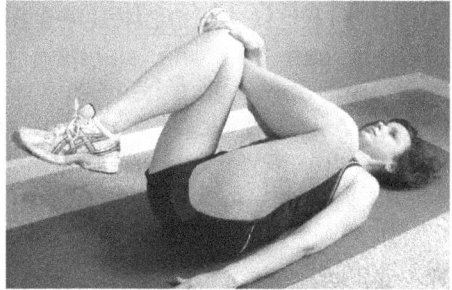

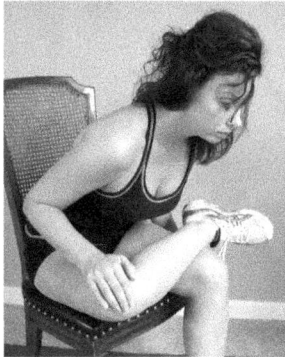

In the sitting position, cross your leg with one ankle resting on the knee of your other leg and lean forward. You should feel a stretch in the buttock region or the back of the thigh. If you have a history of hip problems and now experience pain in the hip, stop and consult your doctor.

PLANTAR STRETCH (ball of foot)

Using any of the previous positions from the calf stretch, bend your knee toward the floor and allow the heel to come up off the ground. This will force more of a stretch into the muscles that run from the ball of the foot to the heel on the bottom of your foot.

You could also put your toes up against any vertical surface, about 2 – 3 inches up, while the rest of your foot is on the floor. This too will stretch the plantar muscles.

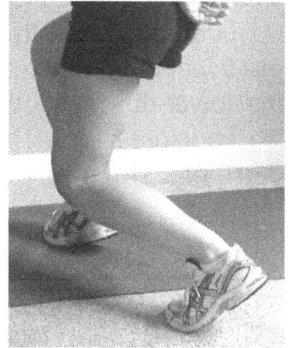

QUAD STRETCH (back of upper leg)

Stand near a wall or a vertical and sturdy object. Place your right hand on it and hold it for balance. With the left hand grab your foot furthest from the wall and bring it toward your buttock. For a little more stretch pull your foot up and back. Then you lean back over the bent knee.

Don't do the old hurdler's stretch where you sit on the floor with one leg straight and one bent. That is unless you are looking forward to destroying your knee joint sometime down the road.

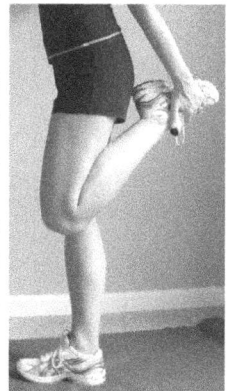

SIDE STRETCH (obliques and lats)

This can be done standing or sitting. Put your arms above your head and grab either your hands or elbows. Now lean to one side and gently pull the arm to get a greater stretch on that side. Then try it with the other side. You can even add a slight twist of the waist to change the angle of the stretch.

Sometimes I like to reach up and grab the top of a doorway and hang down. I can lift one leg and get a greater stretch on that side due the weight of my body pulling downward.

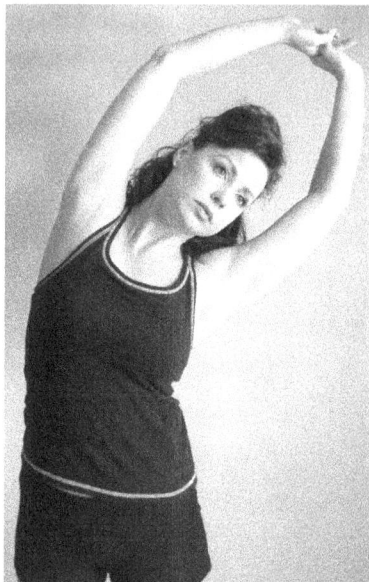

TRICEPS STRETCH (back of arm)

Grab a towel with your right hand, raise your arm above your head and let the towel hang down behind your back. Reach back with the left hand and pull the towel down. Another version is to place your elbow above your head and lean against a wall. The movement is similar to the towel stretch. You could also place one arm over your head and use the other one to push the elbow back.

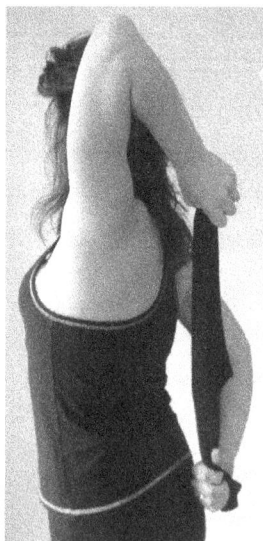

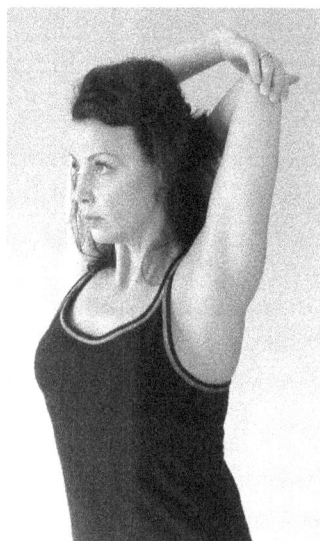

Section III

You Can Teach An Old Back New Tricks

> *"I will always use all the tools at my command, because all healing is scientific."*
> **– Bernie Seigel, M.D.**

Alternatives

You don't have to feel like someone ran you over with a truck to go see healthcare practitioners, especially when it comes to being interested in maintaining your health by using the knowledge of the body. Routine screenings, physicals and medications are all helpful to detect problems and are necessary when caring for the body. Make sure you are always under the care of a doctor to ensure your optimal health. In fact, seeing your eye doctor is a great idea. Looking into the eyes can give a clue if there is high blood pressure, heart problems, diabetes and neurological disorders.

So, I'm talking about using the body to help regulate itself. That's what it does best so let's explore some of the more *"mainstream"* alternatives to natural health, as well as some new ideas.

Some of medicine's mainstream doctors and professionals have trouble accepting new ways of thinking. They too often question how an essential oil or homeopathic substance can work, without ever fully understanding how many of the commonly used or recycled medications they prescribe every day work for their patients.

My general rule is I want every option available to me for treatment. Never leave any stone unturned and never leave a door of possibility closed. If you are being treated for something and haven't noticed any change, then why shouldn't you be allowed to explore other options? Hey, the doctor isn't the one suffering, you are. What would they do if it were their mother or father they were dealing with? Everything can affect anything and there is no reason to not explore all options of care when you or a loved one is suffering.

Door #1	Door #2	Door #3

If they are against another treatment protocol, it may be because they are uneducated, closed-minded or worried you may not come back and they lose money. Either way, find new doctors who can see beyond their prescription pads or wallets and are more interested in finding you answers and relief. Patients are grateful if a physician recognizes he/she needs to send them to another practitioner who might help. Especially if it makes a difference. That's considered doing what is best for the patients.

The mistake patients make is they think that these alternatives are instant cures. Many do not follow instructions, or think they know better, especially when it comes to scheduling. When the treatment doesn't miraculously heal

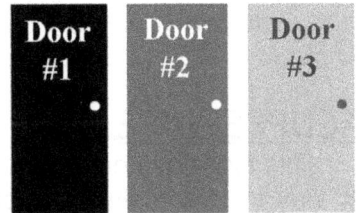

them, they stop and determine that whatever treatment they were receiving isn't good for anything. If 10 treatments are recommended and you go for three, then the failure of attaining a favorable outcome firmly rests on you.

Also just because one version of acupuncture didn't work doesn't mean it never works. If it didn't help you to quit smoking it still may help you to have less pain from a tumor. You can always try another provider if results weren't favorable. Don't paint every type of practitioner with the same brush.

If you bought groceries and the fruit was somewhat overripe, would you never go to that grocery store again? If your mechanic didn't repair your car how you expected it to be, would you never go to another mechanic? No. So why is an alternative branch of healthcare any different?

Granted, in every profession we have some people who are real weirdos. So if your doctor hasn't given you a referral to someone they might know or a provider they have been treated by personally, ask your family, friends and co-workers for a recommendation. Get a referral from someone you trust.

In general, more and more doctors have realized that no one health field is complete without the complement of their fellow health care professionals, who work together for a team approach to your health. That's what I call "Modern Medicine."

> *"Change your thoughts and you change your world."* – **Norman Vincent Peale**

ACUPRESSURE
This technique has been used for thousands of years. Only now is it making its way to other cultures, along with acupuncture. Both are based on Meridian Points, or special pathways, that are located across your entire body, and corresponding to internal organs and symptoms. There are fourteen channels, two of which are in the midline of the body. These meridians or channels contain 400 to 500 specific points along each side of the body that correspond to various organs and areas of the body.

These spots on the body control the *"Chi"* or *"Qi,"* pronounced as Chee. It is the energy force that controls blood circulation and how the body functions. It consists of many essential behaviors of life like spiritual, mental, physical and emotional activities.

It is almost like a full body form of reflexology, which will be discussed later. A practitioner applies pressure with their finger, hand, elbow or a specific device to help release these points.

It is often speculated that massage and chiropractic routinely hit many of these points during their normal treatments. This is why so many people enjoy both and feel relief afterwards.

An acupressurist may use various techniques to release these meridian points like Shiatsu, Energy Work, Reiki and Jin Shin. Each technique varies the amount of pressure, how long to apply force and how many points to hit at one time.

Schooling to become a practitioner takes 150 hours of study, while to be an Acupressure Therapist requires roughly 850 hours.

ACUPUNCTURE

Similar to acupressure, the use of needles has been around for thousands of years and focuses on the same meridian points. After a reporter with President Nixon experienced reduced pain with acupuncture in 1972, the procedure has slowly gained popularity and acceptance. The National Institute of Health (NIH) formally recognized acupuncture in 1997 as a safe and viable option for treatment of various health conditions.

Your health is believed to be affected by the energy force within you, Chi, and the balance of the forces of the universe known as Yin and Yang. These are two opposing forces. If they aren't balanced, then disease can occur in the body. Yin is believed to represent female qualities like passive, dark, cold and moist, meaning moving medially, and without any Yang.

Yang has the male attributes like always in control of the remote, never wrong and selective hearing. Okay, actually the traits are light, active, warm and dry, meaning moving lateral or sideways. Yang is void of Yin. The most prolific example is a child. They possess traits from both parents.

If you are going to experience acupuncture then you need to know about the needles that are used. There are many different needles used. There are various lengths, widths and shapes of needles, which are disposed of after each use. The sensation upon insertion is called deqi, pronounced dah-chee, and is not painful.

Practitioners can use different angles to insert the needle, as well as twirl, raise, pluck or use vibration depending on the ailment they are trying to ease or treat.

Moxibustion is a technique used where heat is applied to the points either directly or indirectly and is often complimentary to acupuncture. Cupping is a method that creates a vacuum over the point and increases the circulation to that area.

It is believed that acupuncture can increase your body's immune function, increase your endorphin levels or natural pain relievers, change the diameter of blood vessels and help control the perception of pain in the body. Several people have gone through surgery or delivered babies using only acupuncture to control pain.

Requirements to become a licensed acupuncturist varies greatly from state to state. California requires 1,350 hours of training, where as New York requires more than 4,000 hours of training. After classes, a national written and practical exam must be passed to prove proficiency.

Both acupressure and acupuncture involve taking a history as to a person's health, lifestyle and condition. A history of what providers you are seeing for the problem, what tests have been taken and what medications or supplements you may be taking are helpful in determining the best course of treatment for you.

Treatment may last anywhere between fifteen minutes and an hour. Several sessions should be experienced to see if any changes occur. Nothing changes overnight so be patient.

The acknowledged list of ailments the NIH believes acupuncture can help with includes: alcoholism, smoke addiction, digestive problems, pain, arthritis, fibromyalgia and many more.

AROMATHERAPY

This a natural treatment that cares for the body by using the scents of specific plants and other parts that make up their life force. The essential oils are removed from the plants by various means and are highly concentrated. There are more than 150 essential oils used. They are derived from many different plants, trees, bark, roots, fruits, grasses and seeds that are known for their beneficial effects.

People use the oils in baths, in massage oils, heated to infuse an entire room with an aroma, or inhaled directly. When two oils are combined it is called synergy, and is more potent than using one oil by itself. Pure oils are recommended over synthetic versions.

I tried breathing the scent of peppermint oil my first semester of school while I studied, because it was supposed to improve my memory capabilities. I forgot what happened. Haha. No … I actually made Deans list.

The oils can affect your mood, reduce stress and anxiety, promote relaxation and reduce pain, among other things. Some of these oils also have antiseptic, antiviral, antidepressant, anti-inflammatory and antifungal properties.

The father of modern medicine, Hippocrates, used aromatherapy principles to help stop the plague. In fact, for more than 6,000 years many civilizations in India, Egypt and Greece used aromatherapy.

Your nose is so powerful. Plug your nose the next time you eat one of your favorite foods. Without your sense of smell the food tastes like wet cardboard. Not that I taste tested.

We have the ability to differentiate more than 10,000 distinct smells. The nose hairs have a direct relay to the part of the brain called the limbic system that controls emotions, memory, feelings and moods. So trying to alter what we smell can really have a drastic affect on our health.

Society is already incorporating scents and sounds to make us respond predictably. Massage therapist use oils to relax you while you get a massage. Fresh baked chocolate chip cookies draw you to the bakery section of the store, or can even help sell a house because the scent reminds people of home.

Retail stores pipe in holiday music the day after Thanksgiving because it increases your buying tendencies. Vanilla candles calm and soothes men and remind them of Mom's home cooking. Next time you want to change the mood in your house, help reduce the number of colds or hide the odor of the cat box, make a trip to the health food store and do some research on scents.

CHIROPRACTIC

This profession offers patients' the opportunity to treat many conditions as well as help maintain patients' health. Some people think working on the back is a new concept, but it has been mentioned in old literature books and found on cave drawings across the world. Chiropractic is derived from the Greek word Chiropraktikos, which means done by hand.

Chiropractic is the science of treating ailments by manipulations or adjustments of articular structures (bones) of the spine, skeleton and soft tissues. The majority of cases involve musculoskeletal conditions like headaches, neck and back pain, whiplash and sciatica.

This conservative and noninvasive approach is based on the scientific fact that your brain controls the proper function of your entire body via the nervous system. For example, if the wrong messages are being sent to your organs, skin or muscles, then they will cause problems and work improperly.

Think of your brain as the fuse box to your house. Lots of wires exit and carry electrical information to many different rooms in your house (areas in your body). If you can't get a light to work in a room, it could be the switch, the outlet, the bulb, or maybe the electrical information being supplied to that area has been interrupted. That can occur in your body when there is pressure on a nerve blocking signals within the body.

I just experienced this when my can opener suddenly didn't work. I checked and decided it had served its purpose and it was time for a new one. So I purchased a new one and it didn't work either. Then I noticed nothing attached to the four outlets was working. I thought maybe a wire was bad and I might have to replace the outlet. Then I realized I had messed with the fuse box and accidentally clicked the wrong one two days earlier. One click and the old can opener still worked like a champ.

Doctors of Chiropractic, (D.C.), specialize in this form of healthcare, which focuses on maintaining the balance of your muscles and nerves, the posture of your spine, along with eating right, regular exercise, proper rest and positive thinking to keep your body functioning at its best.

With more and more patients requesting alternatives to drugs and the surmounting research proving chiropractic's effectiveness and safety, chiropractic is becoming more widely accepted. *The Annals of Internal Medicine, Spine* and *The Journal of Manipulative and Physiological Therapeutics* all reported more favorable outcomes with chiropractic treatment for chronic neck and low back pain when compared to medicines, acupuncture or exercise

Chiropractic physicians can now be found working alongside Medical Doctors of all types. They are even being introduced into the hospital setting and utilized alongside the medical staff of most professional and college sports teams.

These doctors understand that your body goes through tremendous stresses each day from things like lifting, kids, accidents, chores, falls, sports injuries and sleeping wrong. All of these factors can affect your spine and the muscles attached to it. By properly caring for the spine's health you can help decrease the wear and tear on your body, much like taking your car in for a tune up. Patients are of all ages and various health conditions.

Currently only around 10 percent of the population receives spinal care, but I'm pretty sure 98 percent of the population have spines, excluding politicians.

Maintaining the balance between your spine and the muscles is equivalent to caring for your teeth, or your car, on a regular basis to prevent major problems. The differ-ence is you can't see spinal problems like you can tartar or a chipped tooth, which are swiftly brought to your dentist's attention.

Unfortunately people usually: ignore their symptoms from their bodies signaling something is wrong; allow the problem to exist too long; cover up their pain with drugs; or continue to believe they will get better on their own. No matter what the excuse is, the spine is being neglected. It's like fixing a small spot of rust before the rust engulfs your car. Covering it with fresh paint won't solve the problem. It just masks it. The longer we let health problems exist or accumulate the harder they are to reverse or heal correctly.

There are several colleges teaching this specialty. Some colleges require a four year degrees as a prerequisite for acceptance, while others a two-year degree. The Doctorate program for Chiropractic is equivalent to five years of study. It requires completion of over 4,600 hours of class lecture, lab and patient contact with the majority of hours being concentrated in Anatomy, Diagnosis, Neurology and Radiology.[99]

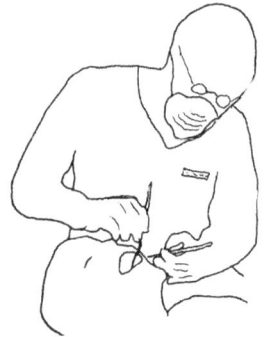

During school, students are required to pass four stringent National Board Exams to practice. Then there are Continuing Education requirements to ensure DC's continued learning and proficiency.

Upon your first chiropractic appointment you can expect to receive a thorough, physical exam, orthopedic exam, neurological tests and maybe laboratory analysis, x-rays or MRIs if needed. The Chiropractor is capable of determining if someone should be a chiropractic patient or if they should be referred to other healthcare professionals.

After careful analysis, the doctor may use modalities like heat, ice, massage or electric stimulation before he or she makes an adjustment to correct a spinal problem. Adjusting is done by placing his or her hands on the patient in a precise way and applying a gentle force to correct the specific location of vertebral joint dysfunction or subluxation. The body may make a popping noise as correction is made. The noise is merely gas escaping from the joints, like when people pop their knuckles. The body then reabsorbs these gases.

You release body tension, endorphins or your body's own natural pain reliever, and nerve information throughout your body. After treatment, some patients can experience instant relief while others may notice soreness due to the stretching of muscles and correction of mechanical dysfunction; much like wearing orthodontic braces or exercising for the first time.

Some people crack their own backs or friends' backs. This is not advised as you wouldn't have a mechanic do your taxes or have a butcher fix your teeth. *"He who adjusts his own spine has a fool for a chiropractor."* Never have an uneducated person touch your spine. You don't watch a surgery on TV and then decide to perform one on your child do you?

It might seem like a minor ache but only a doctor is able to determine the right course of action. There are many cases of simple pains like spinal misalignment or pathologies like Cancer that if an uneducated person thought *"cracking it"* would help, they would actually cause more harm or permanently injure that person. There are actually people who go to school to understand the physiology, neurology, anatomy and musculature of the body and know what is needed to be done, or not done as the case may be, so a patient will actually benefit from care. They are called Doctors.

The orthodontist can't squeeze your teeth together with braces for a week or two and expect them to stay put. When you are trying to make a permanent change in a body part that has become well-established, it will take time. Your chiropractic doctor needs time to retrain your body in terms of the bones and muscles so they function properly.

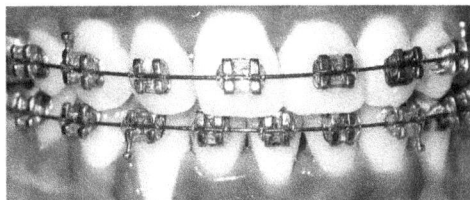

When I say well-established, I mean it is like realizing you have gained a bunch of weight and you finally have admitted there is a problem and need to do something about it. The weight gain didn't come on over night and it isn't going to be gone like that either. Now it is going to take time to lose it and retrain your body on how to eat properly.

Dieting and exercising for two weeks isn't going to do it. It takes longer than that to correct your weight problem. The first pounds come off fast but the last five take more time to complete the process and achieve your goal. Spinal correction may also take time because ligaments, tendons and the vertebrae will have firmly adapted to an improper position.

Continued care may be recommended to help your body keep proper motion and help avoid bigger problems. Weekly, monthly or every few months, visits will help you stay well just like brushing your teeth every day and having them professionally cared for once every six months or a year prevents cavities and gum disease. All the teeth do is chew food and keep your tongue in your mouth while the spine and muscles are working with your every move and action.

In the April 2001 *Journal of Occupational Medicine* reported chiropractic maintenance care of low back pain resulted in lower disability recurrences when compared to medicine and physical therapy. Similarly, the December 2011 issue of *The Journal of Chiropractic Humanities* found that facet joint degeneration, muscular atrophy, improved funtion and wellbeing and fewer episodes of injuries were achievable if receiving spinal anipulation once every two to four weeks.

If a chiropractic doctor can't help you, or after a reasonable trial period the patient's condition hasn't changed enough, he or she will refer you out. This will be to whomever they think is the next most appropriate health care professional to help you get relief, such as, an orthopedic or neurosurgeon, a physical therapist, or a massage therapist, if needed. More advanced blood tests and diagnostic films may also be requested.

Most states require insurance companies, worker's compensation, no-fault insurance and Medicare to cover chiropractic because of the positive results and the demands of the patients.

HOMEOPATHY

If you can cause a problem, then you can correct it. This is the principle that homeopathy is based on. If a remedy can cause the symptoms in a healthy person when given in large doses, then it can correct the symptoms of an illness when administered in smaller quantities.

We all have a distinct vital force or self-healing capability. If this force is disturbed then illness can occur. Homeopathy strives to boost your own body's defenses and help it heal itself.

In contrast to medicine, homeopathy believes symptoms are the body's way of expressing disease and trying to restore homeostasis, or balance, within the body. This is the same reason I explained why we sneeze to rid our bodies of germs and have a fever as a result of good cells battling bad cells that are causing illness inside us.

When treatment starts, the dose to a patient is as small as possible. Formulas are diluted enough to still cause curative effects within the body with no chance of causing illness or negative side effects. This principle follows the idea that our bodies regulate themselves by secreting small doses of hormones into our systems.

A moth can use one molecule of her own pheromone to attract suitors from miles away yet one woman who bathes in her favorite fragrance can keep guys away in general. Homeopaths slowly decrease the dose as the body adapts to it because of a concept known as potentization. This principle states that by diluting the substance further the body has a memory of it, which is built upon with each sequential dose.

Each person receives different doses and combinations for the same problem because an individual responds differently to treatment depending on their personality, demeanor and other traits.

In 1994 the World Health Organization (WHO), noted that homeopathy had been integrated within several countries health care systems. In the U.S., all of the states have different requirements for being licensed to practice homeopathy and the methods of earning a degree are just as varied. Connecticut, Nevada and Arizona only allow Medical Doctors to be licensed to use homeopathy.

The first visit includes an in-depth exam and assessment of your present and past health conditions. Let your homeopath know about any drugs, supplements or treatments you are trying. The extremely diluted remedies have no interaction with drugs, but it is safe practice to keep all providers informed of any and all treatments being tried. Successive treatments require feedback from the patient to determine what remedies are helping. Then the practitioner can adjust remedies and add others.

Although the FDA does not regulate the practice it does require bottles to list the ingredients and what conditions the contents are intended to treat. Anyone can buy homeopathic remedies at the store because the diluted formulas have been found to be extremely safe with rare side effects being reported. This isn't a license to play neighborhood homeopathy provider. To properly diagnose and treat your conditions seek the guidance of a qualified practitioner.

Research has trouble understanding the concepts of this treatment and micro doses, but there are plenty of people who have experienced beneficial results. Never rule anything out without exploring it.

HYPNOSIS

I'm not talking about the *"you're feeling sleepy"* guy, I'm talking about real men and women who help people by using the power of suggestion. It's a state of mind similar to when you are thinking about something else while someone is talking to you. So it's probably more like many spousal conversations acround the world.

Anyway, when you drift off you are totally absorbed in thought. You are not sleeping. It happens when we read, or when you try to talk to your kids when they are completely focused on cartoons that will have them wanting to collect and trade the cards or toys.

The idea behind hypnosis, which is like deep meditation, is that when your attention is focused you are more open and less critical to suggestions and can therefore, be manipulated into doing something you normally wouldn't do.

Just recall asking your husband to take out the trash, three times, while he's watching the game. He doesn't respond right away because he is distracted, I mean, focused on the game and eventually says, *"Okay, okay, I got it."* However he usually will forget he even acknowledged that suggestion later. Normally he doesn't want to take the trash out but agrees to because he is focused and less critical of the suggestion.

I remember being at Syracuse University and attending a hypnosis event. The guy talked to the whole crowd and then could tell who was hypnotized. I witnessed my friend go up on stage and eat a whole lemon, peel and all, like it was the juiciest apple and the last piece of food on the island. Oh yeah, he made students dance around like chickens and do other silly stuff too.

When you are under hypnosis you have an ability to block out all other stimulation and focus solely on a specific thought or problem. Many people have used hypnotherapy as a way to help curb eating habits, to lose weight, or to help them stop smoking. Considering the drug alternatives and their many possible side effects, this could be a real possibility for a solution to a health problem.

Sometimes therapy is used to help understand repressed events in our past that have been hidden but cause us to react certain ways. I'm sure one of the CSI shows must have used hypnosis to help solve a case. It can help someone recall faces or license plate numbers by replaying and slowing down the moments.

On a few occasions some therapists have actually asked questions in ways that caused false memories. This type of questioning should only be done by an experienced practitioner, especially when it comes to children and abuse cases.

Other common uses for hypnotherapy are to help with fears, anxiety, phobias and even to control pain during medical procedures. So if you have arachnophobia or fear spiders, hypnotherapy can help resolve that issue. Hypnosis is great to help accelerate change with regards to behavior, mental and physical well-being.

Treatment will last for 30 – 60 minutes and may take several sessions to complete your goals of therapy. When you are in the trance like phase, you have control and aren't vulnerable. The practitioner is there to help you relax and then will make suggestions or implant visual images to help you achieve your goals.

Some top athletes use hypnosis or have been taught to picture themselves making a difficult golf shot or hitting a ball out of the park. It helps them visualize and then helps them mentally put that vision into action.

Most hypnotherapists have some type of formal training; some are also a Medical Doctor or Psychologist, while others take a course and have completed more than 200 hours of study to become certified. My suggestion before selecting any healthcare providers is to get some recommendations from your doctors and friends.

MASSAGE THERAPY

We use the muscles of our body all the time with every breath and movement. In addition, most of us are moving at a ridiculous pace.

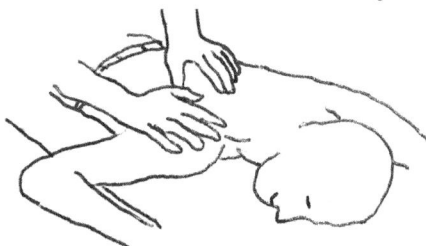

The muscles can get overworked and become tight in an instant or over time. Next they will develop knots or trigger points that can refer pain to other areas and limit your body's normal range of motion. Complaints like neck pain, stress in the muscles, headaches and back pain can be associated or caused by muscles that are in spasm or too tight.

When I think of a massage, I think of Sean Connery as James Bond trying to get a relaxing rub down and having Olga come in and work him over like she's tenderizing a steak. There are many forms of massage techniques. In fact there are more than one hundred; so, one of them has to be right for you.

They can range from superficial touch like Swedish massage, which is relaxing, to deep tissue work like Sports Massage, which is preferred by those who wish to have their muscles stripped and knots broken up, so they probably endure a little more discomfort. With whatever style of massage you go in for, you can always ask your therapist to decrease or increase the pressure to suit your tolerance.

The profession has grown from the days of ancient civilizations using massage, and rulers like Julius Caesar getting regular massages each day.

There are more than 200 accredited programs teaching the art of massage nationwide in private and community colleges. The program typically includes 500 – 750 hours of classes focusing on the sciences, nutrition, ethics and treatment. There are more than 45,000 practitioners who are credentialed and have passed national board exams.

Usually a therapist will want to know about previous massage experiences, where you are having problems and whether you have had any recent falls or injuries. Basically they need a medical history to work safely and give you the most benefit from your muscle work.

At the time of your massage you will undress in private and have a sheet covering you when the therapist re-enters the room. They are there to relax you and do a job. You can keep your undergarments on if you wish. They are going to use a lotion or oil on your skin to help their hands glide over your skin. They will uncover a body part as they work on it and keep the rest of your body covered to maintain modesty and respect for the individual.

In general you don't want to ruin your clothes and it is easier to work on the back without straps or other articles of clothing. A typical treatment will last from 30 – 60 minutes. Rooms are dimly lit with relaxing music and sometimes there may be soothing aromas from candles or incense. After your massage, drink plenty of water to help flush out any toxins that were broken up from your muscle fibers during your session. Follow up sessions may be required to work out areas that have become well-established over the years.

REFLEXOLOGY

This technique was utilized way back by early civilizations of China and then more recently recognized in the early 1930s. The theory behind reflexology is that both your hands and feet have corresponding locations throughout your body, which can indicate whether there is a problem with your internal organs.

In books you will see how all of your organs are drawn out on your hands and feet to show where attention would be focused to help the corresponding area of concern. For example, you would have work done to the ball of your left foot, behind the second, third and fourth toes, to help your lungs.

The treatment approach is to apply pressure to or massage an area. This in turn sends a signal from the peripheral nervous system, which includes nerve tracks outside of the spine, to the central nervous system, which is on the inside of the spine, like the brain and spinal cord. The brain can then make necessary adjustments to the specific area to correct any problems.

Now considering the abuse we put our feet through with standing, walking, running and different shoes, I know the tootsies could use some attention in general. How about the hands that are tired from typing on a laptop computer, holding your coffee mug or maneuvering a steering wheel? They too can benefit from some muscle work. By relaxing the stress in the hands and feet it is believed this will reduce the tension and stress throughout the rest of the body.

Using a professional is always the smarter way to go, but some of you might be a little headstrong. There are schools that have classes and there are books to learn how to perform reflexology at home. Now while watching TV, or working on the computer, you can rub the foot with a foot roller to hit specific areas. Like any treatment that involves changing muscle tension that has been building up in your body, it will need to be repeated to get lasting benefits.

At a reflexology session, the practitioner will ask for some background information before they start working on you. A treatment can last from 15 minutes to an hour. Have those nails trimmed because you need to bare your dogs, and some people use oil to help glide their hands over your skin's surface.

Sometimes in a massage treatment the therapists will massage both hands and feet but may not be as specific to a certain location if they are not educated in the art of reflexology.

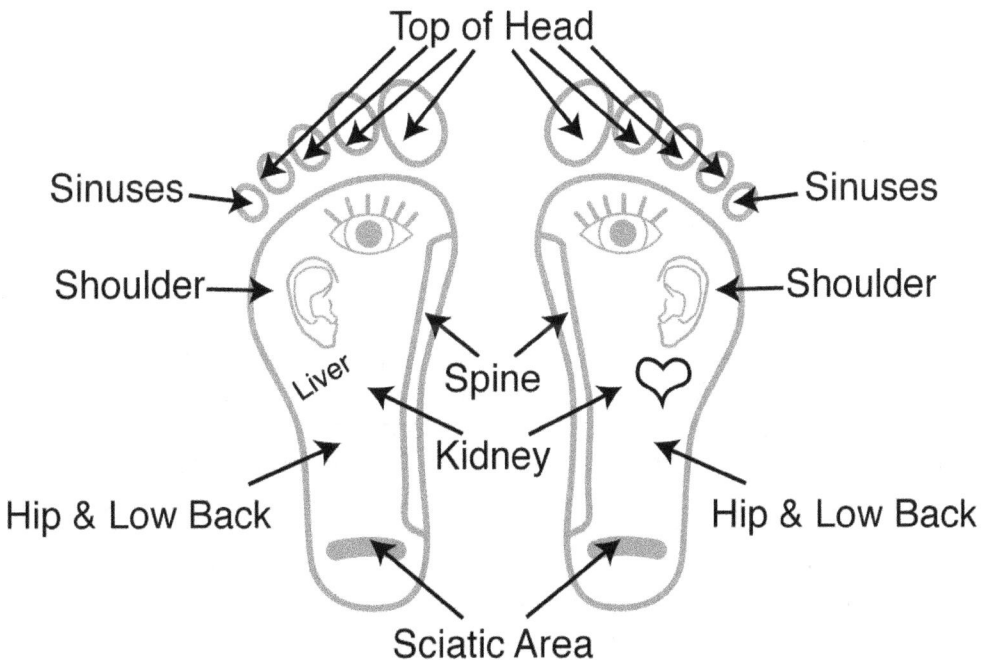

A Few Reflexology Points

"What I dream of is an art of balance." – **Henri Matisse**

Correcting Your Posture "Overnight"

Some of the demands we place on our bodies everyday will take their toll on our health if not immediately, then slowly and permanently. Think about your spine and how it was designed before you go to lift that laundry basket, workout or talk on the phone. Slight changes can help you stave off many health problems. If you could see what you were doing to your spine you would be more careful.

I am going to cover many scenarios each of us face on a daily or weekly basis. Apply the ideas to your day and live a healthier life. Bad posture will affect and modify everything from breathing to hormonal production. Some of the other conditions easily influenced by posture include: headaches, back pain, blood pressure, pulse, lung capacity and mood.[96]

"I still need more healthy rest in order to work at my best. My health is the main capital I have and I want to administer it intelligently." – **Ernest Hemingway**

SLEEPING

One of the most overlooked reasons people wake with aches and pains is that they are still sleeping on the same mattress they used in 1980. That old, lumpy sack has had its day and could be providing you with simply a surface to sleep on instead of proper support.

A 2006 study published in *The Journal of Chiropractic Medicine* found that participants in who sleep on a new mattress can immediately and significantly reduced pain in their backs.

Patients often ask me what mattress I recommend. First off it doesn't matter if you sleep at the Taj Mahal or in the barn. If you sleep in an incorrect position then the result will always be the same and your bed makes little difference. My suggestion regarding mattresses is to get what is comfortable for you.

Someone could offer me a million dollars to advertise their mattress, but if I don't use it regularly or believe in it, I won't recommend it. I have only advised the use of products that I know to have helped my family and me personally. Hopefully you will have a similar response.

We all have our own preferences. Some people need to sleep on a warm cloud, while other people, usually the spouse, like to sleep on a cold boulder. Let's discuss a few of the more common options in use today.

After about five to 10 years it may be time to re-evaluate your bed. If you have gained or lost weight then you have to take that into consideration. Maybe you have someone else staying with you and they are heavier. If you have grown or you need space, make sure you aren't sleeping on a bed that is too small. Get yourself some more space and *"spread out."*

> *"A mind, like a home, is furnished by its owner, so if one's life is cold and bare he can blame none but himself."* – **Louis L'Amour**

THE GOLDILOCKS DILEMMA

Okay, so I don't like waterbeds. If I were a fish then maybe I would change my mind. A waterbed displaces your weight and doesn't appear supportive as it conforms to your body. If your torso is the heaviest part of your body, then it sinks the most and water is displaced raising your legs and head. That can bend

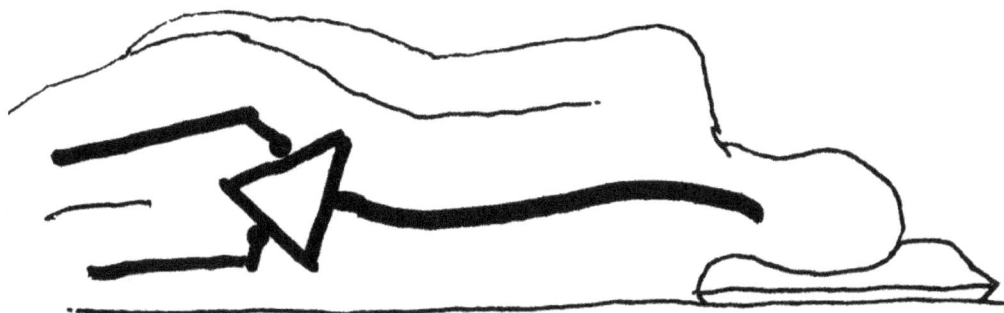

your neck to an unnatural angle or curve, with too much or too little pillow.

When you try to get out of bed your legs can move but it takes some work to get your backside back onto dry land. There is no resistance when you push to get out of bed, so if you have back pain you might have some difficulty getting up. Making sure the bed is always properly filled up with water and has available stabilizers can greatly reduce these problems and provide better support.

You also need to take other considerations into account when getting a waterbed. First, can your house or building support the weight of the bed? No need to see you on America's Funniest Home Videos. Next, if it ever springs a leak via a foreign object, you will have a mad scramble on your hands. There's no shut off valve so have a plan. You will also have a heck of a time rearranging the furniture or replacing a rug if it does leak.

There is some maintenance required with ownership. Occasionally you have to let air out of the mattress and add chemicals to keep it from becoming stinky and green. Also you should never let a child sleep on it, especially newborns. They can suffocate if they roll over because they can't raise their heads.

The biggest reason I hear for not getting rid of them is that they are warm because of the heater. Well, wear some jammies, get an electric blanket, or adopt a few cats and dogs. That should help keep you cozy. I know they have channeled and waveless waterbeds that are supposed to be better support, but you make the call. I have not tried the newer versions. People with allergies also seem to do better with these beds because they can't be infiltrated with all kinds of nasty critters, mites and pollens.

There's the space foam mattress or you can get the cheaper version and add it to your existing mattress. But, putting a foam layer over a bad mattress is like putting a new coat of paint over a rusted vehicle. It isn't a good way to judge the foam pad. You could try it on a decent mattress or the floor and see how it feels.

I think the full mattress would be the way to go but it is expensive and about as heavy as a T-Rex. Make sure you don't need a special I beam constructed box spring to support it. And if you want to put a new rug under the bed at some point you may need to call a crane operator to lift it. In fact make sure your house can handle a heavy mattress like the waterbed.

Memory foam conforms to the shape of your body while you are in it and returns to its original shape when you leave. Its goal is to support the weight of your entire body and redistribute the force on the mattress evenly so you are almost floating.

Some patients love the fact you could dance on the mattress and not disturb the other person, not that they were dancing in the dark, but because movement is not transferred through the mattress. They also like the feeling of being cradled by the foam, which also keeps them warm.

I have had other patients who hated this mattress because the embracing foam kept them too warm or made it difficult when trying to loosen themselves from its grasp. Getting out of this type of bed with back pain is a bit of a chore as well. It is also hard to sit on the mattress and put your shoes on because it slowly gives away under the weight of your buns.

I have patients who have the adjustable air mattresses so one spouse can sleep on a cement slab and the other can sleep on fluffy clouds. In addition to the benefits it may offer to keep you feeling great when you sleep, it may also help to keep your relationship strong as well.

I'm a big fan of a firm mattress with a pillow top, but that doesn't mean you will like it. This provides support while not pressing in too much on your body. Maybe we were supposed to hang from trees to sleep, but as long as I continue lying down I'm going to keep on using a mattress.

When you look at a mattress of any kind, ask to see the construction in regards to the gauge and number of springs or coils, the design, the box spring's design, padding and warranty. Compare that to others you are evaluating. Many mattresses have 10-year warranties; and some become worthless before their time. You may be able to get a pro-rated refund because it didn't last as long as the warranty stated.

It would be great if we could go to a mattress store and sleep overnight to see how a mattress feels. Even that really isn't enough time to give a new mattress a chance. If you have been sleeping on a soft mattress and switch to a firmer mattress, then of course it will feel different and may be a little uncomfortable at first. Be patient.

Check with some stores as they may have a 14 day or 30 day return policy if you are not satisfied. Some give you 90 days. These options are more convenient so at least you have an option for exchanging your bed if need be. Otherwise you will be throwing it in the spare bedroom for me to sleep on when I come over and visit. Everyone knows there's a good chance the uncomfortable one went in there. It's okay.

When you go to the mattress store, lay on the bed for 15 or 20 minutes. Get a feel for it. Make sure you have support everywhere on your body when you lie down. Have your partner join you and relax together to see how it feels. Take your time in making your decision. There is no rush. Bounce on the bed a little and test how it affects the other side of the mattress.

A solution to this conundrum is to find a few really nice hotels and plan a night away from home. Check out what mattress they use and see how you feel the next morning. If it is really good, write down what kind it is and shop for a similar version. Whatever you do, don't tear the tag off. You'll never sleep again because the mattress police will be forever chasing you down. Just kidding.

Another option is to see how another bed in the house feels. Kick one of the kids out or try the spare bedroom. I have even recommended patients throw down some blankets on the floor to soften it slightly and pretend they're camping. The whole family can have fun with this on a weekend. This can give the feel of a firm mattress with the pillow top softness. How does that feel?

You could go visit the out-laws, or in-laws, depending on how that whole relationship is going. Maybe stay at a relative's house or a friend's apartment. It doesn't matter. This is a great opportunity to see how a different mattress feels to you before buying it. If all else fails, ask everyone you know what kind of mattress they use and why they like it or dislike it. Now you have an informed place to start from as well.

Different health conditions can also dictate which mattress may be beneficial to you. Patients with acid reflux or asthma may want to raise their heads while people with circulation troubles and congestive heart failure may need to raise their legs. Elderly patients need support but not too much pressure back into their bodies. Ask your doctor for some input. The adjustable bed that raises the head or the feet may be a good choice here, but still look into what type of mattress is on it.

Regardless of what mattress you prefer, you should feel well rested, and not sore or tight when you first wake up. That is your motivation when selecting a particular mattress to sleep on.

Now that we have our mattress, let's look at the best position to sleep in. Remember the anatomical body is thought of as being in correct posture when from the side: the ears are in line with the shoulders, the waist, the knees and the ankles. From the front: the head is straight, in the midline, shoulders are parallel to the floor, arms to the side, waist parallel to the floor and knees and ankles aligned with each other. Let's discuss what you've been doing to yourself at night.

"Nice guys finish last, but we get to sleep in." – **Evan Davis**

SUNNY SIDE UP

There are essentially three positions to sleep in. The back, side or stomach. The stomach position is the worst, and it is not easy to change your habit. I know people love it more than a family member but here is what is wrong with it.

When you sleep on your stomach your head has to turn to one side and could be at 90 degrees. I joke with patients that if I introduced myself to them with my head turned all the way to the right or left, they would be thinking, *"What the heck is wrong with this guy's neck?"*

That is how many people sleep, and they wonder why their necks or shoulders start to hurt. When the cervical bones are rotated to one side for a prolonged period of time, this also affects the muscles attached to them. Over time the stretched muscles will become longer on one side while the other side, in which the attached muscles are in a closer approximation, will shorten.

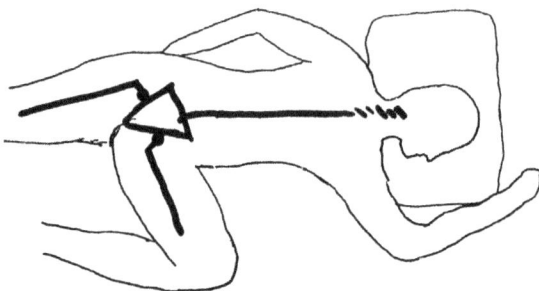

This leads to muscle tightness, knots, trigger points and misalignment of the neck. Just for starters your range of motion will decrease and then you can get headaches. Now if that isn't enough to get you off your stomach, wait, there's more.

If your face is being squished into the pillow if you are on your side, you could be increasing your chance of wrinkles. The pressure can affect your blood supply and lead to wrinkles. Now that has got to have the ladies talking.

A lot of people put their hands above their heads and under the pillow.

When I do an exercise called a shrug, I bring my shoulder towards my ear. That contracts the upper trapezius muscle, which runs from my neck toward my shoulder. It shortens, gets tighter and becomes bigger.

When you bring your arm up like that, it creates a similar situation but a different result. You are just leaving the trapezius muscle in a shortened state and in time it will shorten permanently. This can cause pain in the neck, into the arm via nerve or artery problems and give you decreased range of motion of your head to name a few conditions.

A patient named Stephanie had headaches, chronic neck and shoulder pain. I found out she was sleeping in this stomach position with her arms up. I worked on her and corrected her sleep positions and the very next day she couldn't believe how much better she felt. I told her, *"You were causing your own problems."*

In addition, consider the anatomy of the shoulder socket. It is a ball and socket joint. Sitting and with your elbows on a desk, put your right fist inside your other hand's palm. That is what the joint roughly looks like. Your right fist is making up the ball (gray area) of the upper arm bone (**B**), called the Humerus, and the open fist is the socket, called the glenoid, located in the upper right corner of the scapula (**A**).

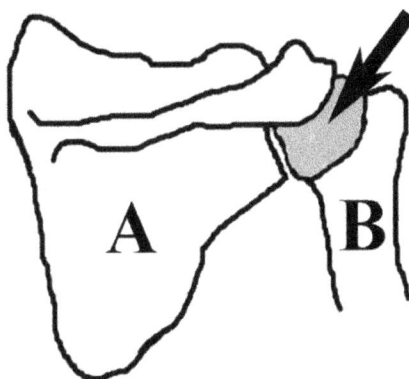

Move your right elbow up and away from the midline of your body as high as it can go. Do you see how your thumbnail is facing the ground and there is no socket to support it? Now when you lay on your shoulder with the arm up under the pillow, that is what is happening. You are encouraging the shoulder to dislocate or become unstable.

Your ribs and midback are trying to protect your internal organs; things like the heart, lungs, pancreas and liver. When you lay on your stomach you are compressing the rib cage and these vital organs. Also the thoracic curve is being reversed by time and gravity. You can end up with a flat back instead of having a spine with one of the important curves necessary to redistribute stress placed on the body.

Finally we have the low back, where only 80 million Americans have problems each year. So doing everything you could to keep it healthy and not become a statistic would make sense right?

Okay. The lumbar spine has a lordosis in which the curve moves towards your belly button. On your stomach, that curve progressively shifts inward. This causes additional stress on the discs and the posterior portions of the vertebra. Ouch. This isn't good either.

The unsung victim here is the calf muscle. When you sleep on your stomach your feet are pointed like you are tip-toeing on your toes or they may hang off the end of the bed. When the toes are pointed it shortens the calf muscles, the gastrocnemius and soleus. If they continue to stay tight, the Achilles tendon will tighten and may lead to serious problems.

How can you stop damaging your spine by sleeping like this you ask? Well I must confess. I was once a stomach sleeper. Yep it's true. But I kicked the habit. Here's how. First, put a pillow under one shoulder. That will prop your upper torso up at around 30 – 45 degrees to the mattress. Next, bring your knee of the same side up perpendicular to your body so it is in a flexed, fetal position. This helps to take pressure off the lower spine.

Place your head on the edge of your pillow. You will not be in a position that is looking perfectly straight ahead, but you might only have your head turned 30 degrees instead of 90. That's a great start. The arm of the same side will hug the pillow while the other arm will be at your side. Eventually you will adopt a side sleeping position, which is much better for your posture, spine and health.

For the stubborn sleeper, I have some ideas for you to help resolve this problem but you might throw this book out. You could try taping a tennis ball to the middle of a nightshirt so it hits you in-between the chest and against your sternum. If you roll over onto your stomach the ball will remind you. If that doesn't work try a basketball. I'm just kidding. I did have a patient who safety-pinned his shirt to the sheets when he started to go to sleep on his back and that did actually help him. No, I did not suggest that one.

You could always have your spouse, partner or friend keep an eye on you. If they see you on your stomach have them gently reposition you or wake you enough to have you do it yourself. Don't get mad. They are only trying to help.

To get that arm down I might recommend sewing the sleeves into the side of your shirt or get out the duct tape. You could also move your pillow closer to the headboard or wall. That way you will bump your hand into the wall and hopefully it will remind you to bring your arm down. You might try tucking your hands into you sleep pants pockets.

"A ruffled mind makes a restless pillow." – **Charlotte Bronte**

CHOOSING SIDES

Let's take a closer look at side sleeping. The position most often adopted is the fetal position. You would lay on either side with your knees pulled up and bent. Arms would be in front of you or at your side.

When you are on your side make sure your head is on enough pillow to keep your nose in line with the buttons of a shirt. This keeps your spine in line. Look at the wall to double check good posture or have your partner look at you to see if you've got it right. If that doesn't work, grab a small mirror and look at it while you are in your sleep position. Do your neck and torso look like they are in a straight line, or is the neck crooked?

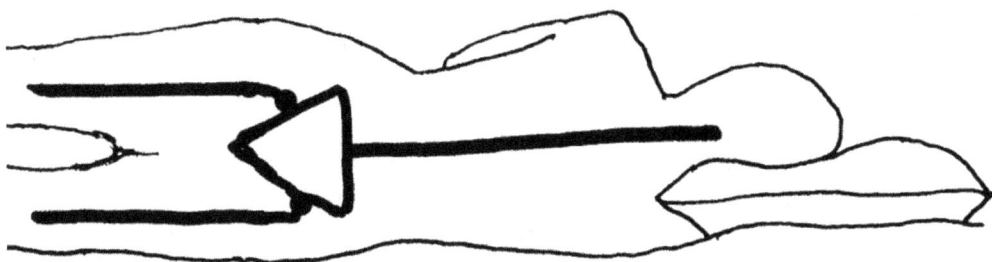

Also, don't tip your head forward like you are tucking your chin to your chest. Keep your chin up so you are looking straight ahead with your ears in line with your shoulders. Bending it forward reverses the neck curve again. It would be like walking around all day like Eeyore, always looking at the ground. This strains the muscles of the neck and can lead to tension, headaches and misalignment. All because of your poor posture.

I like to use a pillow in front of my chest, if not another body, which is basically the spoon position. It helps to keep your body perpendicular to the mattress so your waist isn't twisted. If you have a bad shoulder and it hurts to lie directly on it, place a pillow behind your back so you can lay on to it and prop your body up at around a 45 degree angle.

This will put you in between being on your side or back. Sometimes I put a pillow under my leg on the same side to completely keep my body at the same angle. I know what you're thinking, how do I ever get any sleep?

Using a pillow between the knees is a great way to keep the hips in a good alignment. Your hips and legs naturally are straight when you stand. On your side, one hip bends toward the other side and can twist the low back or stress that hip. You could use a body pillow, or any old pillow, to keep the legs straight. Hugging a pillow can also benefit the shoulders the same way.

A while back, someone came out with a curved wedge to fit between your thigh and knee to maintain proper alignment. It was shaped so it would nestle in between your legs and not slip out.The current support only supports the thigh. This allows the knee to bend laterally and stress the knee joint. I improved this design years ago and regard this statement as verification of my notarized design.

The new pillow I've thought of is still a curved wedge but it slowly decreases the width from your thighs to your ankles. A smooth transition allows proper support throughout the entire lower extremities without lateral forces on the joints. That helps the hips, knees and ankles. When on your side, try to make sure the feet aren't pointed so your calves don't tighten up too.

Last but not least, we use our hands to hold the phone, grab a mug of coffee, hold the wheel, etc. The forearm gets used and tightens constantly with no end in sight. Rarely does anyone stretch these muscles to release the tension. And, we wonder why we get carpal tunnel syndrome.

One mistake you don't want to make is to sleep with your arms curled up inward at the elbow or with your wrists bent. It restricts nerves and blood flow. If you've ever awakened with a *"dead arm"* and the pins and needles occur next, you know what I mean. The same damage can happen in the wrists. Be careful.

A few times I slept like I was in the thinker position with my fist under my chin. The next day I had to brace my wrist and immobilize it because I had no strength and it hurt to move. A few hours of rest and support helped it feel better. I guess I used to do some of my best thinking at night. Oh well.

> *"Life can only be understood backwards; but it must be lived forwards."*
> **– Soren Kierkegaard**

NO LOOKING BACK

Sleeping on your back is the most efficient way for your body to rehydrate your spine. Fluids and nutrients are free to flow to this region. Remember we can lose three inches of height as our discs get old, so every little bit helps. A healthy spine keeps you feeling fine.

Sometimes falling asleep is difficult in this position. If it isn't dark enough in the room, try shutting your eyes. Haha. I mean the curtains. If that doesn't work get a mask to block any light. I sometimes have trouble because my mind is thinking in a million directions and I can't shut it off. Of course if I relax for a second I can be asleep in under a minute.

It takes some practice to learn how to wind down and sleep in this position. Pull out a book on something really boring, hopefully not this book, and maybe that can help you nod off. It used to work wonders for me in class.

People who sleep on their backs have their nasty habits too. One of these starts fights in every bedroom and can lead to lonely nights across America. The problem is snoring. I have been in the room with two of the greatest for a weekend seminar. I thought the walls were moving in and out with each breath. I forgot my earplugs and slept on the floor, on the far side of the other bed to try to let sound pass over me. I think the building eventually crumbled to rubble.

After recertifying my CPR card I realized we are taught to tip the head back so you can ensure the tongue isn't blocking air from getting into the victim's lungs when you supply breaths. If we have our head tipped too high with a pillow, it can obstruct the mouth airway and lead to breathing through the nose and snoring. Just a thought. So change your pillow configuration and see what happens.

Sleep apnea is when a person actually stops breathing during their sleep. Typically if someone has a barrel-shaped chest or is somewhat overweight, they are likely to have some degree of this. Daily exercise and better posture may decrease the problem. The delay in breaths can be up to a minute long. This is very disruptive to the individual's quality of sleep, not to mention the worried spouse next to them.

My friends with the snoring super power have the *"Darth Vader"* mask for sleep apnea because their breathing is irregular. The mask is really called a CPAP mask, which stands for Constant Positive Airway Pressure. It continuously forces air through the nose to regulate the breathing of the individual. It can also help reduce snoring! One of my buddies lost some weight and doesn't need his machine anymore. How about that?

Another common problem I hear about is people are propping their heads and necks up with too many pillows. Remember to keep your ears in line with your shoulders. Imagine if two inches of forward head carriage causes three times the force on the neck, then propping your head up will really do some damage to your neck over months and years.[9]

Sometimes it is because we fall asleep watching TV in bed. For everyone's happiness, a TV in the bedroom is a sure way to cool off the bedroom according to some relationship experts. Now if you want to read in bed, sit up and do so. Just don't angle your neck too much so you can do it. I have seen plenty of x-rays where you could visibly see the neck changing its curve and reversing due to improper support to the neck during sleep.

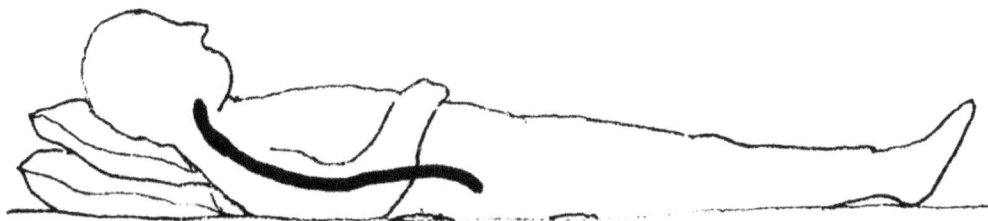

And for your own good, get your butt into bed. I don't care how tired you are, how great the game is or how mad she is. A good night's sleep rarely occurs on the couch. I have pushed the limits of tiredness sitting up. You're talking to the sleep deprivation master. My head flopped back so hard I hit the wall and gave myself whiplash, twice in the same night. When I'm tired now, I always go to sleep. The game can wait or I can hit the record button. Patients are always falling asleep on the couch only to wake up in real discomfort. Don't let this be you.

If you have a reflux problem and need to prop your head up, start at the waist. Add pillows as you get toward the head or buy a wedge. This gradual elevation of the back will cause less stress to the neck and allow you to achieve the same position.

Lying on your back puts around 55 pounds of pressure on your lower discs, yet elevating your legs with a pillow can reduce that figure to a mere 25 pounds.[3,4]

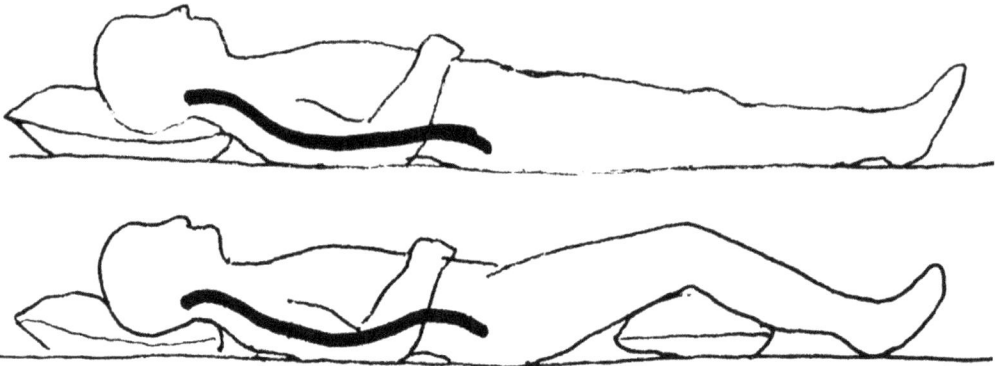

If your low back is bothering you, position an extra pillow under the back of your upper legs. This will take some stress off the low back. Bending the knees toward your chest, in flexion, helps to open the vertebra, disc and nerve roots and is helpful in some cases.

I have used a couch before to maintain this position and this is one of the only ways a couch can help your back. Lie on your back on the couch and bend your knees. Your toes should be touching the base of one of the armrests as it meets the couch. That way your legs can't straighten out. Staying close to the back cushions of the couch will keep your upper thighs straight so there is less chance of twisting your low back. Place a pillow under your leg and you will be set. Now where's that remote?

As for your arms, they can be anywhere they're comfortable, except overhead. Keep them at your side, on your chest or in any position that doesn't allow your elbows to go higher than your shoulders.

To often people come in complaining of increasing shoulder and neck tightness. One of the things they do is sleep like they are signaling a touchdown. I challenge them, and you, to walk around for 10 minutes like that and tell me how your shoulders feel. *"Oh, but it feels so comfortable when I'm in bed."*

My wife sleeps on her back with one arm up. When I pull her arm down, I feel like I'm playing slot machines all night long. Except for no payout. She was having neck and shoulder pain that was referring down into her hand and fingers. Not anymore. As long as she can get out of that habit or I stay awake and watch her all night long, she'll be fine.

I'm kind of kidding when I say this but I did say it before. You could sew your sleeves into your nightshirt so your arms can't be raised during the night. Or have your spouse check on you when they turn over or come back from a pit stop. If all else fails, I joke with patients to duct tape their hands to their waists. Seriously, you could also wear shorts and tuck your hands in your pockets.

So you are on your back, arms down, head in a correct position, except one thing. Sometimes we let our heads turn to the side when we sleep on our backs. If you can try to keep it so your nose is in line with the buttons of a shirt, you will be better off. Leaving your head rotated to one side will cause tightening of your neck muscles. If you don't have a fancy pillow or the one you're using doesn't prevent head rotation, take an extra one and place it next to your face or head. This way it can limit your motion or be something to lean up against.

Your legs can really be affected by sleep patterns. I hate the sheets tucked in at the bottom of the bed. I think most men will agree the first thing they adjust is that darn sheet. That is probably why we just pull the sheets up and consider the bed made.

Anyway, if you sleep on your back, try to keep your feet in a neutral position too. If you allow your feet to turn out you are increasing the chances of the piriformis muscle in your buttocks to tighten because you are shortening the muscle. This is the pesky little muscle that can cause sciatic pain. Sometimes I will place a pillow by the side of my thigh so it prevents the hip from rotating.

Another strategy I use is lifting my outside leg up and toward my other leg. This permits the sheets to fold up under the elevated leg.

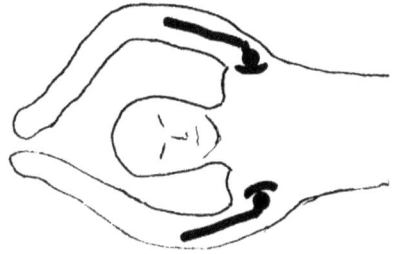

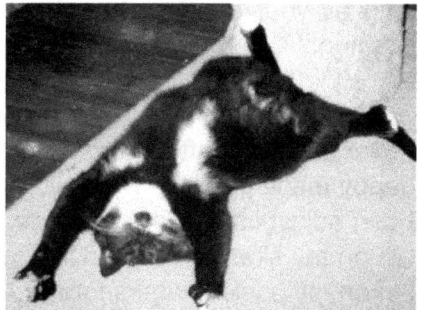

When I bring the leg down now, the sheets will be tucked in underneath my leg. The resistance of the rest of the sheets and blankets from the other side of the bed, can hold my foot straight.

I guess, if my patent attorney is ready, you could sew two tube socks together or fasten yarn from one toe region to the other. Put on the socks. Your feet can be the normal distance apart except the connecting thread keeps both feet in proper positions. Nice. And they stay warm.

I also try to keep my feet flat as if I was standing on them. If they point forward, like you are on your toes, the calf and Achilles tendon can get tight. I just had two friends who popped their Achilles tendon. One was dribbling a basketball up the court and the other attempting to play with improper warm up or stretching. Not a nice surgery or rehab.

Interestingly, my former S.U. roommate, who thought he could just run out and play at 38, used to always walk on his toes. I remember imitating his bouncy step as a joke because his heels never touched the ground. All of that walking on the toes, is like doing calf raises and never stretching for years. His wife is my editor and she just ratted him out as a stomach sleeper too. Hmm, maybe all of this had something to do with why his Achilles tendon was tight and popped.

> *"Last night I dreamed I ate a ten-pound marshmallow, and when I woke up the pillow was gone."* – **Tommy Cooper**

I'M DOWN WITH THAT

First and foremost, for good posture when you sleep you want to keep your head in a neutral position in relation to your spine. Basically if you sleep on your back you want to have your ears close to being in line with your shoulders.

It is true, pillows do come in many sizes, different levels of firmness and costs. I recommend using one pillow for your head as long as it isn't too high and fluffy, or too low. I don't care if it is lumpy, feathery soft or from when you were a kid. If it's comfortable and keeps your posture correct, use it. I don't care if it's a trashcan, as long as your head and neck are in a proper position.

One extreme case was my grandfather who never used a pillow during WWII and never used one afterwards. There is always a happy medium. I like my down pillow because I can adjust its thickness for me. Whether I need it thick and bunched up when I'm on my side, or with a fist-sized roll and a depression in the middle for when I'm on my back. It works for me.

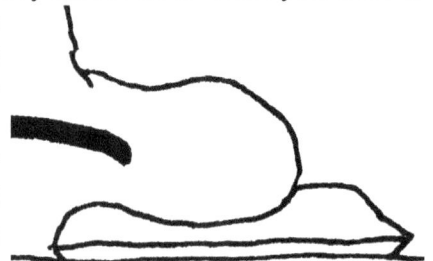

If you want to spend a bunch of money you can, because there are so many to choose from. There's everything from the space age foam, to a water pillow, to the neck curve pillows. I just had a conversation with my patient Lisa and she asked me about special pillows. She uses a down pillow now and is a recovering stomach sleeper. I told her to hit, push and maneuver the feathers so she can create a pillow similar to the ones she could buy. The difference is that hers will be fully adjustable for her height or width.

Then there are those people with 12 pillows on their beds. They tend to put too many pillows behind their heads and inevitably prop their chins toward their chests as they lie on their backs. Using two to three pillows can reverse the cervical curve causing headaches, neck and shoulder pain and muscle tension, unless they are some seriously flat pillows.

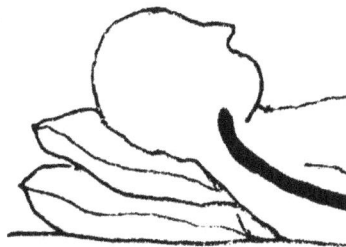

I have tried the space age foam pillow and it pushed back into my neck. It might be fine for you, but I went back to my faithful pillow. My cats love it!

Some pillows have a curve built in to them to support your neck, and a carved out section for your head to rest in. The reason this idea came to fruition was because with a normal pillow your head will hit the pillow before your neck. The head then bends forward until the neck touches the pillow. This will reverse the neck's curve, as described, in order to achieve this position.

A cut out section allows your head to drop lower than your neck, so both areas are then supported and in proper alignment.

I like the cervical curve design. It feels like hands are caressing my neck. I have a foam and fiber pool toy shaped like a cylinder that is soft and pliable. My neck feels like it is in heaven when I lay on that.

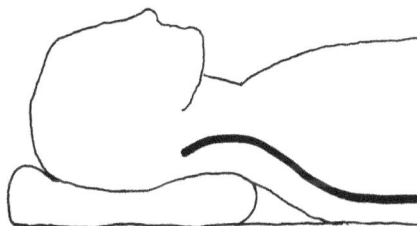

I even use a pillow with a neck curve that has a "V" angled in it. The idea is to lock your head in the "V" and your body weight then distracts and separates the disc spaces in your neck when you lay down. It does feel pretty good. You could take a small towel and roll it up like a tube, about the size of your fist, and even make the "V" to see how it feels to you.

If you have a really flattened pillow, roll one edge over to thicken it where your neck will be. Then rest your head on the single layer of pillow, while your neck is on the double layer, keeping your head and neck in a neutral position. If my head is almost on the bed and I have a fist-sized roll under my neck, I'm set.

Trying either a towel rolled up, a sock filled with pillow fibers or rolling your pillow at the edge are some great methods to try this idea before making a purchase. Pillows can be costly and filled with more fiber and science.

"Form follows function-that has been misunderstood. Form and function should be one, joined in a spiritual union." – **Frank Lloyd Wright**

The Morning Ritual

Let me tell you about a recent start to my day. This is the definition of a good start and a bad start. I was getting dressed, grabbed a pair of dress pants from my closet, and reached into my pants pocket and found seven dollars. That's a good start!

I had some time this beautiful morning, so I took my sheet, which is on top of the bed, outside to shake it violently and remove some of the fur from my cats. I raised the sheet up and brought it down quickly and popped myself right in the not so great and very tender, but funny place. I almost crumpled on my front lawn. That's a bad start! May you enjoy good starts to your days.

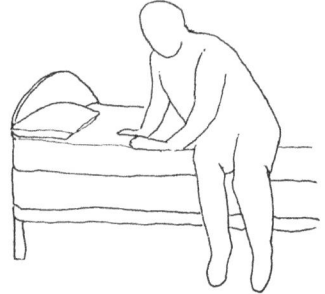

We are all guilty of rushing to get to work or off to school and sometimes we may do things that aren't in the best interest of our bodies. Unfortunately, we are more likely to injure ourselves early in the day when our bodies aren't loosened up yet and our spinal discs are filled with fluids from being inactive. Making slight modifications to the start of your day can help make the rest of it more productive and enjoyable.

"Cultivate the habit of early rising. It is unwise to keep the head long on a level with the feet." – **Henry David Thoreau**

RISE AND SHINE

The alarm clock goes off, your dog licks your face or your internal clock awakens you to a new day. Before you jump out of bed to take on the world, it is a great idea to just loosen up and stretch before you ask your rested body to start tackling your to do list.

You know the bones can be achy when you get up. They need to be lubricated, not like the Tin Man, but close. The muscles have also tightened up because they have been idle and have cooled down. Have you ever watched your cat or dog wake up from a nap? What's the first thing they do? Stretch proficiently. And we call ourselves the most intelligent species.

Because our discs rehydrate during the night, they are filled with fluids and are very susceptible to injury. Do an experiment by overfilling a Ziploc bag and under filling another one. When you place a weight, or force, on them both, the overfilled one has a greater chance of bursting. Same with discs in your back.

About 54 percent of lost disc height occurs in the first 30 minutes of our day.[100] This reinforces the importance of starting our days with some caution. Waking up without care or moving too quickly after a long drive can be dangerous, because sudden movement can create a loading stress to the fluid-filled discs of the spine. This is directly related to injuries and the loss of disc height that occurs under pressure.[101]

Research has found bending stress in the morning increases 300 percent in the disc and 80 percent more in the ligaments.[102] Changing positions or stretching before attempting to do something strenuous, can help flush fluids out of the disc and protect it. This should encourage you to take a few moments to stretch and loosen up before taking your first steps of the day.

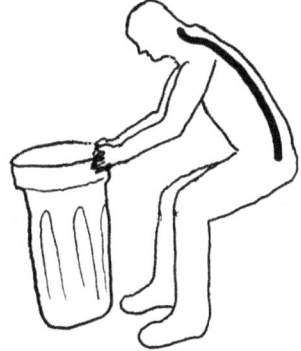

Now you understand why waking up and rushing to drag the trash out, or trying to fire up the lawn mower after you watched your game, can strain the back and put you out of commission. Stretch a little first and avoid the Sunday trip to the ER.

In fact, if you have a diagnosed back problem, lie in bed and do a few gentle extension exercises, side to side bends or knee to chest exercises, whichever was recommended to you or feels good. That way you might be able to loosen up the back a little before you start your day.

When you wake up in the morning, don't just sit up. That is a bending stress and causes increased pressure in the low back. Slide your body to the side of the bed. Next roll onto your side and use your elbow to help yourself up into the sitting position, as you let the weight of your legs drop off the mattress and toward the floor. I do this every morning.

Here are a few simple stretches you could do to start your day off right. **1.** Put your arms over head and shift your waist one-way and lean to the other side. **2.** You can pull the arm across the front of the chest at the elbow with your other hand. **3.** Lie on your back and bring your knees to your chest, one at a time or put your foot on the bed and lean into it. **4.** Place your hands on your hips and arch backwards while you are standing. **5.** Put your arms behind your back and grab your wrists and push the chest forward. **6.** With the knees slightly bent, reach for the toes and feel the muscles in the back of your legs elongate.

These are just a few moves to help grease the wheels before you start your day. No straight leg toe touches because that could damage your spine. If you want to get the blood pumping in the morning, turn on the news and do some jumping jacks or jog in place.

*"By health I mean the power to live a full, adult, living, breathing life in close contact with...
the earth and the wonders thereof - the sea - the sun."* – **Katherine Mansfield**

BREATHE DEEP, THE GATHERING GLOOM

Most of us don't breathe correctly. You mean all this time I've been doing it wrong? Yep! Usually when someone takes a deep breath they expand their chest and raise their shoulders as their lungs fill with life saving air. Wrong!

When you take a deep breath, a membrane called the diaphragm lowers allowing the lungs to fill. When this happens you should actually be expanding your stomach. Did you hear that? It's okay to push out your stomach.

As you exhale, the diaphragm rises and forces the lungs to expel the air. The benefit of this entire motion is that it also exercises the lower spine without using weights. You can practice this in your car, at home in a chair, or even in bed. Feel the stomach expand and bulge like a beer belly as you inhale, and feel your low back flatten against the seat as you exhale. And how long have you been breathing? Practice, practice, practice.

*"The best reason I can think of for not running for President of the United States is that you
have to shave twice a day."* – **Adlai E. Stevenson Jr.**

WITHOUT THE NICKS AND CUTS OF A BLADE

When you shower, you complete some of your hygiene tasks and help your body. Why not take advantage of some of that hot water. Your muscles are warmed up and you could do a few morning stretches in there. Check the six stretches just mentioned. You could probably do the whole routine but I don't want to be responsible for your water bill.

For guys, shaving your face or head in the shower is better for your back. Just like brushing your teeth. You don't want to be stuck in a position that keeps you bent forward for extended periods of time. When you stand at the sink and lean forward, your low back muscles are straining to keep you there.

The longer you stay that way the more stress you put on your muscles and spine. Remember your posture? Your body prefers to be upright. Leaning forward like that puts twice the amount of pressure on your low back versus standing straight. Install a fogless mirror in the shower so you can see what you are doing.

Ladies already have a good grasp on the ergonomics of shaving. They usually put one leg up on the side of the stall so they don't have to bend down to shave. If you can't do that maybe you can place a stool inside the shower so you can sit down or place your foot on it.

Likewise, brushing your teeth in the shower permits you to stand up straight and limits back stress. If you spill a little who cares, you're in the shower. If you need to see your teeth in the mirror and you would rather be at the sink, then just remember to stand up straight. Otherwise, you could walk around while you are brushing and return to the sink to rinse.

When you dry off, be cautious. Slowly dry yourself and bend carefully. Don't flip your head back after it's wrapped in a towel unless you want to throw your neck out. You can bring your leg up versus bending down to dry your little toes too.

"Fashion is a form of ugliness so intolerable that we have to alter it every six months."
– Oscar Wilde

IT'S ALL ABOUT FASHION

Getting dressed can be tough in the morning on a good day. The older we get the less the old bones and joints move to make it easier on us. I recall Michael J. Fox in Back to the Future getting his leg caught in his pants and falling over. I think we all can relate to that in one way or another. I've caught one foot in the wrong slot of my boxers before and had to do the Fred Astaire shuffle really quickly to save myself.

Socks are no treat either. In fact mine have worn off the hair around my ankles. I can't grow it on my feet or my head; just everywhere in between. Anyway, instead of trying to balance or hopping around like you stepped on a tack while you put your socks on, sit on the bed. Bring your knee toward your chest and look at that, you're doing a stretch for your back. It works the same when you take them off.

If you can, try putting your pants on while sitting so it is easier. One leg, then the other, stand up and fasten them. No bending or balancing act required.

When I put on my shoes, I slip my feet into them. Then I raise a foot and place it on the bed, nightstand or dresser. Bringing my foot closer to my body and allows my back to stay fairly straight as I tie the laces As discussed, less bending stress in the morning is better. So using this simple step, could keep you in step.

An important topic to discuss for women is the bra. A problem for women arises if they are medium to large breasted. The shoulder straps on these contraptions can really pull down on the shoulders and neck. I have had patients who developed pain in that area due to the constant pulling and strain. That pressure is over a delicate area called the brachial (arm) plexus. This is an area where many nerves, arteries and veins pass to provide your arms with blood or nerve information. If nerves are pinched, they can cause pain to radiate into the arms or hands.

In addition the back strap can be like a noose around your midsection. You can move the back strap so it isn't always squeezing the same spot or get bras with a wider band to spread out the pressure. I have seen some women who seem to be wearing a bra from 20 years ago. Now add a few pounds and I'm not sure how they could breathe. If it feels tight, than buy yourself some new bras. Most women don't have properly fitting bras. Ask the sales person to help find the best fit for you.

When you can, try to buy different bra styles with wider straps to help the neck, shoulder and back region. Maybe try a sports bra. They are like a supportive and stretchable shirt without the binding straps.

Sometimes, women decide they need to enhance their physiques. They may want their breasts to resemble what they once were before kids, they may decide to reward themselves after a divorce, or may have survived breast Cancer and wish to look better. There are silicon and saline and various sized implants to choose from. Before you do, understand that they also add weight and can cause stress to your back and shoulders. If you go from an A cup to a D, there will be quite a difference in the pressure those straps cause. I have had several patients complain because the weight of their new breasts was more than their body was used to carrying.

"All we demanded was our right to twinkle" – **Marilyn Monroe**

IT'S GOTTA BE THE SHOES

Ladies, this section is for you. I know. You don't want to hear this. Neither did my patients. But I have always mentioned it to them so they could try to help their posture and improve their health condition. I already mentioned how you need to make sure the shoes fit, they are cut for the shape of your feet and they are comfortable. I don't mind repeating this because most women are ignoring this part anyway.

If you go into your closet or closets and peruse the unexplored boxes or stacks of shoes, just try them on and see how they feel. Are they comfortable to wear all day? How does the foot feel the next day? All I'm asking is for you to re-evaluate them so they do not cause foot problems.

High heels on the other hand need to be discussed. They prop your body up as if you were walking on your toes or the balls of your feet. What would I know about this you ask? Halloween 2007 I had seven inch platforms on and the pressure from two outings as Gene Simmons damaged a nerve in my foot.

This may have actually caused a permanent Neuroma, or an irritation and growth around the nerve. So now I get a tingling sensation in the ball of my left foot. It feels like there is a corn kernel under my foot.

Wearing heels adds unnatural flexion on the knee and hip joint while your body weight is predominantly on the metatarsal heads, base of your toes, or the balls of your feet. This also accentuates all spinal curves, putting your back in a state of hyperextension.[103] I understand wearing them for a special event but if you feel you must wear them, maybe you could pick a lower heel for everyday use.

I actually have had patients who refused to change their footwear while they were experiencing debilitating and shooting leg or back pain. *"But the shoes are comfortable."* Not for your back and posture they're not. High heels alter the curve of your back, which can ultimately influence the rest of your spine's posture.

A few years ago, maybe six or so, the fashion world cursed young teenagers with the dumbest shoes I've ever seen. You know the ones. They have an entire sole that was like three inches high. Come to think of it they remind me of my KISS platforms. Each person shuffles on them like they are walking with stilts. Not only did it look stupid, those doofy shoes mess up your spine because of the altered gait of walking. How would you get away from someone if they were chasing you? Skip? Just because someone on TV wears it, or it is a fashion craze, doesn't mean you should jump on the bandwagon.

Good weather brings out the flip-flop. These can be so cheap and colorful, everyone is wearing them. Before you slap on a set of flops make sure you have a pair with some kind of heel and arch support. Chronic flop wearing can lead to tenderness in the heel or Achilles tendon, arch pain and could lead to back pain. If your flip-flop is a piece of *"flap,"* do your body some good by picking up a quality, supportive and stylish pair.

I am always bashing Converse shoes or any footwear that is flat inside and has no arch support whatsoever. They looked terrible for your feet when I was a kid and Larry Bird wore them. They may look cool or be in fashion but I'm about function and support.

If you notice foot pain, look to your shoes as a possible cause. Try different brands and styles. I have Fred Flintstone feet so I always buy wide shoes. Some shoes are cut differently, much like clothes. When you find your brand, stick with it.

> *"Develop interest in life as you see it; in people, things, literature, music - the world is so rich, simply throbbing with rich treasures, beautiful souls and interesting people. forget yourself."*
> **– Henry Miller**

I FEEL PRETTY, OH SO PRETTY

Ladies. When you decide to dry your hair, be careful. All that hanging your head over and whipping your head back could make you dizzy or cause a spasm in your neck. That flip could be a sure way to start your day with more than just bad hair.

The real problem is the drying and the brushing. One arm holds the dryer and moves forwards and backwards. The other hand makes long sweeping motions. The main arm I am concerned about is the hair dryer hand. That repetitive motion can cause muscles in your shoulder and on your back to get tight and become painful. The brush hand can also develop similar symptoms. Did you know the average woman spends more than two years of her entire life doing her hair?

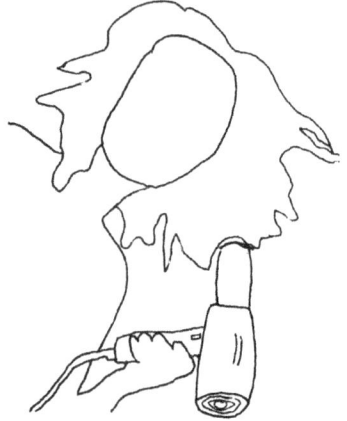

The shoulders get tight from having the arms over your head and the rotator muscles become overworked from the back and forth motion. If you can, try switching hands or mount the hair dryer to the wall. In fact a woman just patented a wall-mounted hanger for hair dryers so both hands are free to style your hair.

You could also try to switch up hairstyles. Have it down one day after all of your hard work, and up the next day. Remember, beauty comes from within, not from your hair.

Speaking of beauty, women like to put on make-up and I have nothing to say about that, believe it or not. Almost 300 pages and finally I have nothing to say. Miracles never cease. If you like how you look and it makes you feel good, do it. However, I would recommend you stand straight and not lean toward the mirror. If you are doing any eyebrow maintenance, try not to bend forward so your back isn't strained. Stand tall. My wife sits upright on the counter facing the mirror. Not because of me but it does help her back.

"Remember that nobody will ever get ahead of you as long as he is kicking you in the seat of the pants." – **Walter Winchell**

WHAT'S IN YOUR WALLET?

Guys love their wallets like women love their purses. If you've ever seen the Seinfeld episode where George has his entire life in his wallet, you know what I mean. Every picture and receipt is in there. The thing is two or three inches thick. He starts to develop pain in his back and his doctor tells him to get that wallet out of his back pocket.

I see this in my office all the time. The problem is that if you have a George Castanza wallet, when you sit down it is propping up your low back on one side. This is like putting a brick under one buttock cheek. Your pelvis gets tilted and this strains the rest of the back. This is an actual patient's wallet. It's two inches thick. In the picture, that's a vertical sugar pack to the right. I've seen worse!

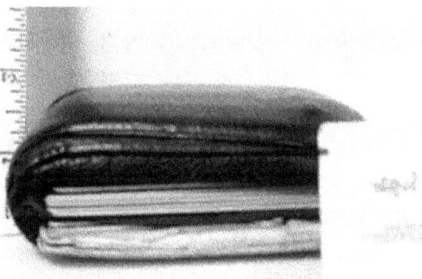

The normal posture of the lower spine is altered and becomes curved while you are sitting down. This increases the pressure on the discs and nerves unevenly, altering the muscles. The longer this occurs throughout your life the more damage you will inflict.

Often guys have sciatic pain due to the same source. The wallet in the back pocket can put pressure against the piriformis muscle in the buttock. The sciatic nerve can run through, above or below this muscle. If this muscle gets irritated it can send pain into the foot or feel like trickling water down the back of your leg.

I'm not saying don't carry your wallet, or let your wife have it. I'm not that far gone. Haha. Carry it in a different pocket. If you have to sit for an extended period of time, move it to your jacket, shirt pocket or front pants pocket. Placing it on your seat or dashboard is a sure way to forget it or get it stolen. Keep it on you.

Now you probably could also review the items you have in it. See if you can remove a few business cards, receipts, smaller bills, credit or shopping cards, etc. Seems everyone has a card you need to carry. If you shop at 13 stores you have 13 cards. Crazy. Just use you phone number when you check out or put all your cards in your smart phone if you have one.

> *"Happiness is not achieved by the conscious pursuit of happiness; it is generally the by-product of other activities."* – **Aldous Huxley**

THE PURSE-SUIT OF HAPPINESS

For years I have lifted the curse many women bear. I have raised the beast that has held them down. I have taken suitcases on trips that were smaller than their everyday purses. If you need that much stuff you should either hire staff or drag a red wagon with you.

Hilariously, I have had women confess that they have a small purse that they bring in with them. They leave their posture-distorting, heavy bag hidden in the car. They just didn't want me to see it. Some of these purses weigh 20, even 30 pounds or more! I have seen purses or carry-on bags that house everything, but the kitchen sink. Oh wait, there it is. The American Chiropractic Association states that a purse should be up to 10 percent of a woman's bodyweight but no more than 15 pounds. Shoot for that.

We talked about the shoulder neck region and the delicate brachial plexus. This strap is pressing down on that area. Women typically carry that strap on one side of the body. It feels comfortable on one side of their body and it becomes a habit. However, switching shoulders is one way to evenly distribute the stress to the spine. Do it frequently.

If you routinely carry something heavy, be it a briefcase or monster purse, you will tip your body to help adjust for the additional weight. Over time you will train your body to change and the back will curve one way. You also raise your shoulder toward your neck to keep the strap in place and support the weight. When you hold any muscle in a contracted state, or a shortened position, for a certain length of time, that muscle will become tight and painful.

What do we really need? What could be stored in the car? Are there possibly any papers, photo albums, extra makeup items, shoes or snacks that could be removed? First I would start with the six dollars in change rumbling around in the abyss of your purse. Get a change purse and keep three quarters, four dimes, nickels and pennies. That is enough to get you through any purchase.

Besides, my editor says, *"Who uses cash? Debit and forget it."* Are there books you carry but don't ever really read? I just removed a stack of papers I carried around for a year in my briefcase and never read. I'm just as guilty.

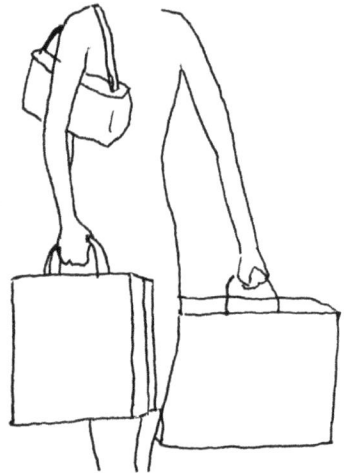

Get a smaller purse or briefcase. The smaller the container, the less junk you can put in it. With a smaller bag you will need to decide what really is essential or plan a little wiser. Whatever you can do to lighten the load, besides bootin' your spouse out, do so. It will help your posture and ease those tight shoulders.

Sometimes that big bag is in the backseat of your vehicle and there's something you've gotta have. So you twist your body to try to get it. First off, stop the car. Reaching and grabbing will contract one side of your mid back; and because you are lifting in an unfavorable position, you are likely to cause spasms in your back. Not to mention you can't see the road and you are driving!

If you need it that badly, stop, turn your whole body toward it to take some of the torque off of your lower back. At 13, my sister turned to get something out of the backseat for my mother and her legs went numb. It was pretty scary. She tweaked her disc. Yes even at a young age it is possible to injure the back.

Be careful if you need to lift a heavy bag. You might offset the balance of weight and roll the car, or knock the Earth off its axis, for that matter. The pressure on your twisted back while lifting a weight beyond your reach, can multiply the weight of the bag by over 10 – 15 times. OUCH!

Maybe you can thumb through it and find what you need. But if Dr. Lipoff's 3rd Law of Inconvenience is true, what you need will have magically disappeared, until you have almost emptied everything out to find it. Then low and behold, after hours of searching for it, there it is, practically right in front of you. If it never turned up, then the 2nd Law comes into effect, in that you must buy an exact replica in order to find the original.

Of course try to remember to move the important item to where it is accessible if you think you may need it in the near future. You could place the bag on the seat next to you or on the floor of the passenger seat if available. Maybe you can have someone else get the item or purse for you. If you must send an inexperienced adventurer into the depths of your monster purse, tie them off with rope so they can find their way back, in the event they get lost.

If you must know, my 1st Law of Inconvenience is the rule that if you drop something it will inevitably fall and roll under something; requiring you to get on the floor to find it and retrieve it, if you can. However if it involves food then sub-rule (1a) takes effect and your lid or toast will have landed face down. I don't make up the laws, I live them. So do you.

> *"We may go to the moon, but that's not very far. The greatest distance we have to cover still lies within us."* – **Charles de Gaulle**

Travel

Taking a drive or a trip can be exciting, stressful and dangerous all at the same time. Whether it is by plane, train or automobile, try to plan out your trip in advance as far as rest stops. Allow for regular breaks to walk around and grab some snacks or a meal. Ah, the joys of rushing through an airport or driving with arguing children in the back seat. It just isn't a vacation without them.

Sometimes on vacation we try new things like trapeze lessons, exploring the rain forest with rappel clips and lines or even beach volleyball. Don't try to pack too much physical activity or excitement, into your first day. Space it out a little. Give your body and mind a chance to adjust to the traveling and time zones. Kickback, relax, take two Margaritas, and a nap and call me in the morning. Not too early though.

Use caution before attempting any type of new activity, so you don't ruin the vacation all together. Doing too much could create some soreness or some excessively tired and cranky kids, or adults, which could get the trip off on the wrong foot.

I can't change the job you are driving to or the location of your next vacation, but I hope I can recommend some ideas to help prevent you from having a miserable day due to pain from your body.

> *"The best current evidence is that media are mere vehicles that deliver instruction but do not influence student achievement any more than the truck that delivers groceries causes change in our nutrition."* – **Richard Clark**

ARE WE THERE YET?

Vehicles are not made specifically for you or me. We each need to adjust features so they accommodate our personal needs. One of the first things to correct is the seat distance. There is no need to be cruising with the front seat tilted into the back of the car. The air bag might hit you in a bad spot.

When the seat isn't in an upright position, the head then curves forward so you can see where you are going. Kind of like leaning forward to look at a computer screen or TV. This reversal of the spine will lead to major problems. Move your seat forward and tilt it so your feet are flat on the floor and the knees are slightly higher than your hips.

A great way to make sure you are sitting

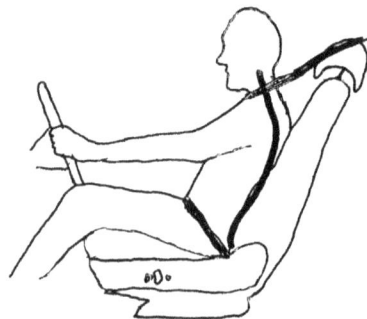

upright is to adjust the rear view mirror in the morning. When we first wake, we are at our tallest because our spine is fully hydrated. As you go to get in the car and leave, adjust the rearview mirror and don't touch it again.

After a long day of work your body will try to slouch and relax like you are sitting in a La-Z-Boy. If you can't see out of the mirror properly, then you aren't sitting up straight. This will remind you to maintain correct posture.

Cars have a big console that is next to your right leg and the accelerator pedal. If you have cruise control use it so you can return your feet to a more comfortable position than out in front of you.

If you don't have cruise control, or prefer to have control during your drive, be cognizant of that console getting in the way. In many vehicles the console can be such a nuisance that it forces you to externally rotate your hip and point your toes toward the other side of the vehicle. This is like when we lay on our backs and our feet turn outwards.

As you keep your foot on the pedal, your leg stays like that and allows the piriformis muscle to stay in a shortened state for an extended period of time. So the piriformis muscle in your buttock can tighten up and then irritate the sciatic nerve. That gives you the pain down your leg. If you feel that while you are driving, you may find yourself bending your leg, squirming around or moving your leg across to the other side, to relieve some of the tension in that muscle. I have placed an empty plastic container between my leg and the console to help keep my leg straight.

If you have to drive and you have back or leg pain there are some things you can do. If arching backward feels good, adjust your lumbar support or put a pillow behind your backside to scoot yourself forward. It will take you out of the normal flexion experienced while sitting. With some back and leg pain, tipping to one side or the other may give you some relief. Either put a towel under one buttock or slide toward the raised side of the seat because they will both shift your pelvis. If leaning right eases your pain, raising your right side will tilt your pelvis to open up the left side.

One night while driving in snowy conditions, I noticed that I had to keep my foot on the gas because cruise control might speed up the vehicle and cause a spin. My foot was pointed for a while before I realized my calf and Achilles tendon were tightening. I was basically standing on my toes. I solved this by moving my heel closer to the pedal so I no longer was flexing my foot so far forward to accelerate. That resolved the problem. You can teach an old dog new tricks.

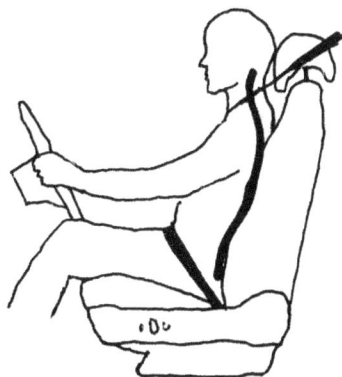

> *"When you travel, remember that a foreign country is not designed to make you comfortable. It is designed to make its own people comfortable."* – **Clifton Fadiman**

DON'T MAKE ME STOP THE CAR

A vehicle colliding with another object causes whiplash and the forces inside the vehicle are 2.5 times greater than the impact to the vehicle itself.[17]

As your head whips violently forward and backward, it causes severe damage to the spine, discs and ligaments, even at minimal speeds. As stated in the first section of the book, damage from this type of injury can last for years.

Part of the problem is due to the fact that in an accident car seatbelts restrict our upper torso and waist, or put a tremendous force on the body[104] and the head is left vulnerable, perched on a delicate neck. The head is like a 10-pound bowling ball that is set in motion.

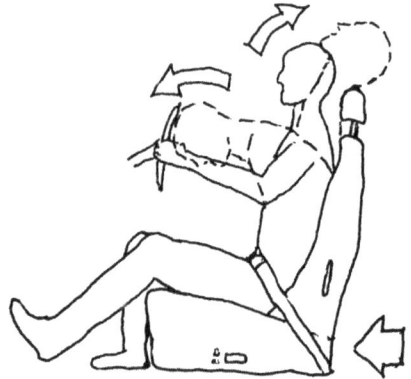

The seat belt can cause bruising to the body depending on the energy and power of an impact, as it prevents you from a worse fate. The force on the waist by the lap belt can cause internal injuries. It can even fracture your spine, which is called a belt fracture. Of course overall the seat belts save lives, so keep 'em on. *"Click it or Ticket."*

In fact I think I found an easier way to buckle up that reduces the stress to my back and the shoulder, which is what prompted me to rethink this maneuver. When you first sit in the car's seat and are facing outside, before you spin your legs into the car, grab the seatbelt so when you spin, you're in. This way, you don't have to torque your spine to grab it, or compress your shoulder to reach overhead to grab it, after you are comfortably seated.

Air bags may deploy to prevent a severe head and neck movement during an accident. They fire quickly and inflate to protect you. This helps to prevent excessive body motion, and impacting the steering wheel or dashboard itself. There is some concern that an inflating bag might hit you in the face like Muhammad Ali. It's better than glass, and can save your life. Many vehicles have them over all windows to protect passengers. Some protect your knees.

The second-generation air bags are designed to use less energy when inflating but provide the same protection. They work their best to protect you and your family when used in conjunction with your seatbelt.

One of the best ways to reduce the chance of whiplash was reported by the American Chiropractic Association that estimated more than 75 percent of drivers have their headrest at an inappropriate height. By raising the headrest so the middle of it meets the back of your head, it decreases the chance of injury during an accident by 10 percent because your head won't hyperextend.

If it is too low your neck will fulcrum over the headrest, causing severe ligament damage or worse. Just taking the time to raise it, can help you prevent major damage throughout your lifetime. You can also try to keep your head close to the padding. Around an inch away or less will reduce the force generated in an accident because of the close proximity of your head and the headrest. This may also help you sit upright and keep your neck in a more correct posture.

Some of the newer vehicles have headrests that actually move with the motion of your car during a motor vehicle accident. This limits the whiplash that can occur by preventing excessive motion in your neck and potential damage to it, by staying close to your head during the impact.

If you have any pain after an accident see a doctor to make sure you are okay. Symptoms are the window to what is really happening to your body. Think of them as an early detection system to prevent problems from getting worse.

"The sun, the moon and the stars would have disappeared long ago, had they happened to be within reach of predatory human hands." – **Havelock Ellis**

YOUR HANDS UPON THE WHEEL

Most people are taught to drive with their hands at the 10 and two o'clock positions on the steering wheel. This is the position I use when I need to be focused because conditions are bad or traffic is heavy. Try to relax. Drop your elbows so you are not holding your arms or shoulders up. If you have them up in the air you are contracting the shoulder muscles.

If over the course of weeks or months you drive a lot, this area will tighten and likely cause headaches. Try some of those neck stretches we talked about to combat this stress. The next time you have to drive at night or during bad weather, check your shoulders. I bet they are elevated due to fatigue or driving conditions.

When you take hold of the wheel, move your hands down to the four and eight o'clock positions. See if you can rest your elbows on the middle console and the armrest. To make this easier you may be able to adjust your steering wheel and lower it. That way if you have your knees bent and feet flat on the floor, you can even rest your wrists or arms on your knees and thighs. This is the position I use when I have a little more freedom to drive without worrying about the next distracted driver. It also keeps you from placing your hands and shoulders in the same old positions.

To combat the arm and shoulder tightening up, some drivers prop their left elbow on the side of the door and some may even put their right arm on top of the seat next to them. I have heard a lot of patients complain of shoulder and shoulder blade pain from this.

Although the arm is somewhat supported, there is a component of muscle contraction and stress to the joint that can cause symptoms. Remember the ball and socket design of the shoulder joint loses some of its stability as the shoulder is raised. The best recommendation would be to not leave your arm in any one position for too long.

A long drive can almost break your will, so switch up positions and throw in a few stretches here and there. When I started dating my wife, I drove six hours one-way, at least every other weekend to see her. I did this for more than two years. And I can tell you after logging some 60k miles in my car from that drive alone; stopping to take breaks is a necessity. I used to stop at a gas station, fill up, use the facilities, maybe look around the store, or play some pinball. I gave my body a chance to recirculate blood and nutrients and for muscles time to loosen up. It kept me cruisin' along.

The same thing is recommended for anyone who must take long flights where you are stuck in little seats for hours. Get up and walk the aisle. Prolonged sitting on planes has been found to cause circulatory problems like clots in your legs. Get up and shake it down the aisle so you can stay loose and keep that blood moving. Practice those leg and calves stretches and isometrics.

> *"Clothes make the man. Naked people have little or no influence on society."*
> **– Mark Twain**

LEAVING ON A JET PLANE

I know the baggage weight limit is 50 pounds but do you have to test those parameters and the stitching of your suitcase? We are definitely a country of excess. We like big cars, big houses, big meals and we like to have all of our stuff when we travel.

I know because I have a suitcase for my clothes and another for my scuba diving gear. The goal is to decide how much we actually need. Are you going to wear 10 outfits for dinner on a seven night cruise? If you can, try to figure out your wardrobe now and take into consideration your style tendencies. Maybe you can mix and match tops and bottoms and then you can lighten your load and pack less.

Remember Garanimals for kids? Match a top with a Lion on the label, to a bottom with a Lion and you will always look good. I might come out with a line of clothes with special labels like that for men so women don't cringe when we dress. You just have to match the team logo with itself or one from the division. I'll call it BeASport.

Anyway, I'm not trying to make you look like a hobo on your trip. I'm trying to save you from looking like Tom Joad from *"The Grapes of Wrath,"* dragging all of your worldly possessions through a crowded airport.

It can obviously hurt your back moving the awkward cases through a busy terminal. Then you have to consider going through a security check with all that stuff could also delay your plans. Packing simply and concisely can save your back, as well as time and aggravation.

Whenever you have to carry bags or other items, try to balance the load. If you have a suitcase on one side, put the computer strap on your other shoulder. If you have a suitcase with wheels, load that puppy up and push. You are now using your legs and pushing is easier on your body than pulling. Pushing keeps the weight in front of you centrally, giving you better control over where it moves.

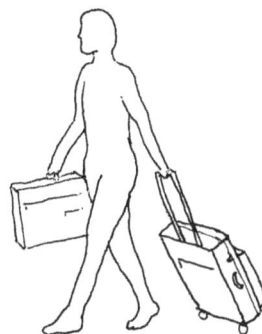

Pulling alters your walking posture and twists your spine as you reach behind you with a case that zigs and zags like it's had a few drinks too many. Always go with a suitcase you can push or improvise and turn it around. It should still roll.

If you want to live it up, rent a cart so you can wheel your stuff around like a shopping cart. Otherwise, pull to the curb, slip a couple of bucks to your airline's curbside check-in employees and they can move your bags from there. Well worth a couple of bucks to know someone else is straining their back with your gear, guaranteeing a stress free trip for yours.

"Wisdom is to the mind what health is to the body." – **Francois De La Rochefoucauld**

LOAD 'EM UP, MOVE 'EM OUT

Coach airplane seats have to be one of the most, uncomfortable types of seats known to man, and woman. I am 5' 11" and the neckpiece is tipped forward for me. I feel like I'm perpetually reading a newspaper in my lap. I either grab an extra blanket and roll it up, or bring my neck pillow, which is shaped like a tube. This helps support my neck instead of having it reversed for a six hour flight. You might try some of the travel pillows or inflatable pillows on the market, to see if they cradle your neck and prevent any tension during your next flight.

I also like a pillow behind my lower back. The seats typically cave in where your lower back rests. This reverses the lumbar spine and isn't supportive. I prefer to sit by a window so I can jump out if there's trouble. I prop my leg up on the side of the plane seat in front of me to create flexion in my spine. I do not kick the seat. Nor would I let my kids. I hate that. I look for something metal and sturdy that will not disturb the person in the seat in front of me. If your carry-on bag is with you, you could place your feet on that to raise your knees higher than your hips and reduce low back pressure by half.

If you want to read on the plane, pull out the tray or see if you can steal a pillow from a passenger. By placing the book or magazine on an elevated surface it can prevent you from looking down. That way your neck isn't flexing forward or straining the muscles and ligaments that hold your head upright. Holding your head and neck in a bent forward position will cause the muscles behind your neck to tire out and go into spasm.

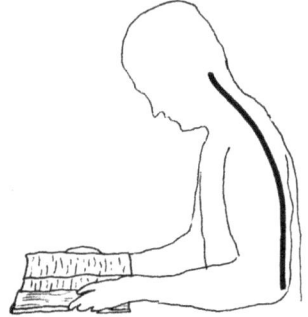

I would use this idea for reading at home or working on projects in your lap. Use a pillow or an easel to decrease your neck stress. Find a way to elevate your project so reading for prolonged periods is gentler on your neck.

If you ever wonder where all the pillows are, check if I am on the flight. It is not beyond the realm of possibilities to have one against the window too. By folding the pillow and placing it against the window you can rest your head upon it. It can bridge the distance from the window to your head. This will keep your head fairly straight so it is not tipped to one side as you rest and you don't end up with a sore neck.

Sometimes it is nice to have the fan above you blowing air on your head and neck region. If it is too cold or direct, it can cool your neck muscles down. This can lead to spasms and neck pain. Circulate the air around you but never have any fan or any other form of air conditioning blowing directly on you.

"A hotel isn't like a home, but it's better than being a house guest." – **William Feather**

LEAVE THE LIGHT ON

When you have to stay in a hotel you are at the mercy of the room's conditions. If the mattress or pillow doesn't agree with you, it can ruin your trip. Hotel pillows could be too fluffy and prop your head up beyond what you are used to or too high in general. I have treated a few patients who take their favorite pillows with them because they know they will be more comfortable. Just try not to forget them at the hotel. It happens way too much.

If you are a back sleeper and find yourself with a monster pillow, try to flatten it. You may be able to push some of the fibers around. Take some aggression out and beat that thing silly. You might be able to create a space for your head to drop into and a smaller pillow height overall. Your neck will be supported and in a better position.

Remember the pillow section from before? It is important to try to keep your head in a neutral position that is similar to when you are standing and looking straight ahead.

Another option would be to look in the closets for alternatives or call the front desk. They may have more pillows to choose from. You could also take a towel out of the bathroom and fold that to look like the cervical pillows. Just turn up the edge of the folded towel so it is double thick. If you are on your back, your head will be on the normal towel thickness and the neck would be on the folded portion of the towel.

If the towel is too thick as you pull it off the rack, open it up and do whatever is necessary to make it work for you. You could also simply roll a small towel up for behind your neck and put your head on a pillow.

> *"Household tasks are easier and quicker when they are done by somebody else."*
> **– James Thorpe**

Work and Chores

Just when you thought your workday was tough enough or you were going to get to relax, there are numerous projects and maintenance required at your home. If you own your house the list of tasks is never-ending. Even in a rental unit there is plenty of housework and cleaning. If you have a cleaning service then you may not have to worry about this section as much, so share this section with your cleaning people so they can stay well.

Some of these chores can be overwhelming to you and your spine. The repetitive movement and lifting can really take their toll. You need to be careful. Take breaks. Try to split chores amongst members of the family. Don't try to attempt too much in one day. Get help if you can. Having the right shoes and the right tools for the job is also wise. I can't tell you how many times I've used a screwdriver or a wrench as a hammer.

Here are some suggestions to make it easier on yourself to prevent an injury when you tackle a few of the more common scenarios each of us faces. If I don't mention your chore for whatever reason, like you are an underwater welder or something, try to incorporate some of the ideas that may be helpful to you.

> *"If you cannot lift the load off another's back, do not walk away.*
> *Try to lighten it." –* **Frank Tyger**

Bending or Lifting
IS YOUR BACK FOR THE FUTURE?

Most people lift incorrectly because it is easier to complete a task when you do it quickly. The problem is you increase the likeliness of causing an injury to your lower back. Every time you bend forward at the waist, your back becomes a fulcrum. This simple motion puts all of the pressure of lifting on the spinal discs, the supporting musculature, tendons and ligaments. The most common area for our discs to bulge is in the waist area, known as the L4/L5 and L5/S1 level, because of this maneuver.

Businesses that rely on workers, who lift boxes and then twist to put them in trucks at a high rate of speed, are the cause of Worker's Compensation Claims for low back pain. Even picking up your grandchild or grabbing a couple of bags of groceries can set you up for pain later.

Essentially what happens is you are loading or compressing the spinal discs. Then by twisting, you are screwing down the disc and applying shearing forces, which over time will cause a disc problem. Remember the disc is like a jelly donut. So when you place your hand on top and then twist your hand and push down, it's messy isn't it? Repeating movements like this will cause micro traumas to the spine. This is the person who has a backache that comes and goes but lasts increasingly longer. In time, they may reach to pick up a pencil and their back will *"go out."*

Many work environments encourage or require the use of back belts for their employees to help protect them and prevent work injuries from occurring. Unfortunately there is little proof that these belts actually provide any benefits.[105] Even as a reminder to the person they should not be lifting heavy things or that it would help support them if they did make a bad move, were all theories shot down for using belts. It may be better to invest a company's money in ergonomic classes and demonstrations of better body mechanics and posture.

A great idea for all of us is to loosen up first. Do a few minutes of stretching to warm the muscles up before you try to stack 200 boxes. That means you need to show up a little before your shift starts. It's like warming up your car before you drive it. If you drive just 15 minutes to work, your back can have fluids build up in the tissue and make you susceptible to injury if you just hop out and start to bend and lift.[50] Doing a few gentle extension exercises and other stretches may help to remove some of the fluid, making it safer for you to lift again.[106]

Imagine what happens to your back during a holiday. You drive about two and a half hours to see the grandkids and when you get there they jump into your arms as you lift them up to the sky. This is a classic example of how someone strains his or her back at the beginning of the visit. The best scenario is to stop close to your destination for a fill-up, remember to pick up the earplugs, and move around to loosen and prepare your back for the impending lift. A few minutes extra to loosen up could help make your entire stay more fun, not just the first five minutes of saying your hellos.

When we lift anything off of the floor we are supposed to keep our backs straight and bend with the knees. Easily said, but hard to implement in the real world and when you are working against the clock. When you do use your legs to lift you are using your body's largest and strongest muscle groups. They save your back. This type of lift is known as a squat lift.

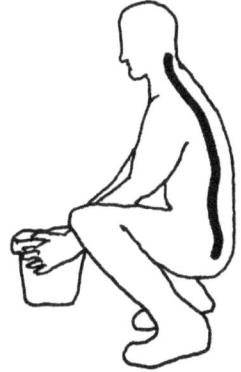

Place your feet about shoulders' width apart, bend the knees and try to bring the item in close to your body. The closer the weight is to your body the less stress it puts on your back. Before you stand back up and carry the item to wherever you need to, make sure you have no obstacles preventing you from moving easily to your destination. Nothing spells disaster like trying to step over a startled cat, crushing a board game piece into the bottom of your foot or having an electrical cord snag your leg like a booby-trap snare, all while you are carrying a television.

After picking up something that you need to place next to you, take a step with your feet so you are facing the area where you will put the item down. This keeps the spine in a stabilized and protected position. As just mentioned, twisting while carrying weight is damaging to the spine. It only takes one false move to start an episode of back pain. My patient Keith came in after bailing out a pond. He repeatedly bent over, lifting a bucket of water and twisted to throw the water behind him. He wasn't sure how he reinjured his back and I just chuckled before explaining how he sidelined himself. Again.

Another way to lift an object that is similar to the squat lift is a power lift. During this movement you don't bend the knees fully, but bend over at the waist and use a little more back and hamstring strength to hoist the weight up. You've probably seen guys do the dead lift or watched The World's Strongest Man competitions on TV, where these monsters lift the front of a Mack truck. The pivot is intended to be more centered at the hip, not the waist.

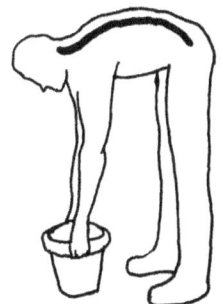

If the object is too heavy, or you get careless, you will end up rounding your back. This will create instability in the spine and the supporting muscles. The result will be an injury either immediately or down the road.

A tripod lift is when you bend down on one knee and gather your object in front of you. Then you use the other leg that doesn't have the knee touching the ground, to start your ascent to make the lift. Your legs do the lifting and your back is preserved.

A strong midsection is helpful with any lift. Keeping your core or pelvic region strong is a great help to stabilize the spine, maintain correct posture and limit damage from repetitive lifts. Studies have shown that when you maintain a lordotic curve in your low back, the erector spine muscles that run along the side of your spine, contract and stabilize the spine.[106, 107]

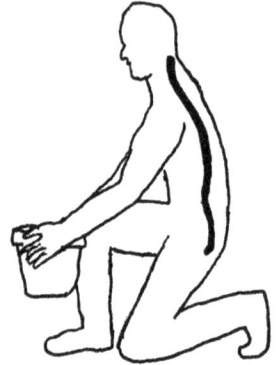

This helps to protect and guide your back through the motion. It can redistribute and balance the stress of lifting. That's why you shouldn't round your back when you lift.

I see a lot of unnecessary lifting. Women always put their purses on the floor in my office only to lug them off the ground later. If you have to frequently pick something up like a briefcase or a laundry basket, perhaps you can elevate the item. If it is already off the floor, then that is less bending you will have to do when it comes time to move that object again.

Another technique you could employ is to use one arm to brace your body as you bend to pick up something, known as a golfer's lift. One hand can make contact with the edge of a desk. Then when you bend your knees to pick something up, your arm is straight and acting like a support pole. This decreases the stress on your back and knees and can be helpful when standing back up.

A common place for this maneuver might be when cleaning the bathroom or picking something up off the floor near a table or couch. So if you are cleaning the shower, toilet or sink don't overstretch or bend over at the waist. Kneel or bring a stool in if you're going to be there for awhile. Otherwise find a brush with a longer handle.

> *"The meeting of two personalities is like the contact of two chemical substances: if there is any reaction, both are transformed."* – **Carl Jung**

WITH A LITTLE HELP FROM MY FRIENDS

One idea to make lifting easier is to have someone else do it. Do you have a friend who you always help? Then it's payback time. Maybe there's a buddy who owes you a favor for covering for him while he went to the game.

Get the project set up so it is ready to go when help arrives. Don't make someone helping you move do tedious stuff like moving smaller boxes to get to the couch. Have it cleared away so the task at hand, is in hand. Then they may say how easy it is and offer some more help. A little reverse psychology goes a long way. I knew my college degree would come in handy one day. You also never know when your help may receive that mysterious call of imaginary distress, and leave you empty-handed. Get the most work done while you can.

If the project is muy grande, then call your friends for a *"Help-me-move-some-heavy-stuff-cookout party."* Entice them with some food and drinks and make it fun. Invite a whole bunch of friends over and the job can be accomplished more quickly. Your job is to make sure everyone is well-fed and of course, that the project gets completed. Especially if you are serving beer in tandem with the day's work.

It's a great way to work, socialize and reconnect with friends during your busy life schedule. If you've got yourself some drinkers, limit the beverages, or you project may not get done or your new deck might look more like a rhomboid.

If you are at work, have co-workers help. There is no reason to go it alone. Maybe they can help you move the table and chairs into the conference room for the big meeting or event. If you need to get supplies, grab a colleague or stack them on a cart and distribute them safely.

Now I'm not advocating child labor, but, if you got 'em, use 'em. There is no reason a teenager can't help their parents around the house. Hey they live there too. What is this place a Holiday Inn? Get them off the couch and make them earn their stay. This will take some of the pressure to do it all off of you. If you want to grease the wheels and throw them some cash, then do so. Cash is always a great motivator. So are homemade treats.

Speaking of cash, if you have no friends or children, or they have an excuse that they need to re-lace their shoes in their closets, then you could call a professional. There are lots of companies that move and haul stuff. Do some research or ask neighbors and friends who they may have used. Find a reputable mover that's right for you.

When you are alone and need the job accomplished, use your brain. For instance, you can walk a dryer to the back of your vehicle by leaning it back onto two supports and then walking it forward, right in step with your feet. When you get to the vehicle, place a blanket on your car or truck to protect it and lean one edge of the dryer on the vehicle. Now if you have to lift it up, bend your knees, keep your back straight and use your legs. The vehicle will act as the fulcrum and reduce the weight of the dryer. It's Physics, baby.

> *"The future belongs to those who prepare for it today."* – **Malcolm X**

PREPARATION IS KEY
Another smart thing to do before lifting something is to make sure it isn't stuck. I had a patient Scott who went to lift an aluminum ladder but it was stuck in the mud. When he lifted what should have been 30 pounds, the resistance of the mud made it feel like 300 pounds. This caused a tremendous strain on his body because it was an unexpected force. He was out of work for months.

Likewise, I just went to lift my computer off of a chair. The strap conveniently slipped around the bottom of the chair's seat. When I lifted the expected weight and was met with a jerking force back, I could feel my shoulder and midback cringe and tighten up. Preparation is a good thing. Now where did I put the numbers for my chiropractor and massage therapist?

> *"Take a chance! All life is a chance. The man who goes furthest is generally the one who is willing to do and dare."* – **Dale Carnegie**

THE DOUBLE DOG DARE
When your kids challenge you to lift something heavy, check the weight first, like you should with anything prior to lifting it. It is always fun to win the admiration of your kids. Okay, the neighbor's kid. Oh, who am I kidding, the whole neighborhood's kids. Just be smart about your back because what you do today can have a long lasting effect on what you are able to do and how you feel tomorrow.

With any activity take breaks so you don't overdo it. Especially if you sit at a computer for a living, and then decide to chop five trees up for firewood on the weekend. That is too much for a body that isn't used to that kind of work.

"If I have seen further, it is by standing on the shoulders of giants." – **Isaac Newton**

LAST MAN STANDING

If your job involves standing most of the day, see if you can get some ergonomic mats to keep under your station or desk. Nice pads can cushion your feet and knees to keep you light on your feet all day. They also absorbs some of the impact that a concrete floor would otherwise be distributing to your low back. If you can't put the pads under you, put them in your shoes. There are many choices for shock and odor absorbing cushioned inserts.

Wearing quality shoes can help too. Good support and soles can ease some of the stress to your body. You can check different shoe companies. Some make lighter products so you don't feel like you've dragged muddy shoes around all day and tired out your legs in the process. For baseball I bought cleats that were lighter than most, to keep me running fast around the bases. At my age I needed every advantage possible.

I have advised teachers to change position while in class. They can sit or rest on the edge of their desks. Even use a chair as a footrest to put some flexion in their lower backs and reduce pressure in the spines. That was what the railing in a western saloon was for. You could put your foot up and drink longer.

Another great idea for teachers that I just mentioned during a lecture at Syracuse University for future music teachers, is to let students take turns wiping the board off. If you are responsible for erasing your board for years and years, you will develop one heck of a shoulder knot and have the tightness to prove it. Otherwise, if no one deserves the honor, at least switch arms. I realize some schools have advanced beyond the chalk dust or dry erase boards. Times are changing.

The good news is standing puts less stress on your lower back. Sitting is the worst position for your back because it compresses and squeezes the discs. Standing is better, but not as stress free as laying on your back. Most of us aren't going to get paid to work while we kick back like that. If you do, you probably will be running from the police soon.

"People who work sitting down get paid more than people who work standing up."
– Ogden Nash

SYNTAX ERROR, FORMATTING HARD DRIVE

Computers have officially taken over our lives. They are priceless for keeping things in order, helping with inventory, saving precious documents and sorting through E-mails. These little demons are also the cause of a lot of health concerns for people.

When you are sitting, you want to have good support for your back. Keep your feet flat on the floor, or slightly elevated in front of you. Remember that this position is only 55 pounds of pressure in the low back.[3, 4] Tucking them under the chair can increase extension in the back and crossing your legs puts stress on the ankles, knees and hips. If you need to sit with your legs crossed then try to limit how often you do it and switch legs frequently.

Sitting on a bent knee raises one side of your spine altering your mechanics and will put more pressure on one side of your discs. This position can also damage the delicate ligaments, tendons and meniscus of the knee. That's why athletes shouldn't do the old hurdler's stretch because it compresses the knee and can damage it over time.

If you can, position your knees slightly higher than your hips, to decrease the disc pressure in your back by one half. If that is difficult at your desk, bring a box in or a piece of wood and place your feet on that. Some chairs have legs in front of the seat that you can rest your feet on to accomplish this position.

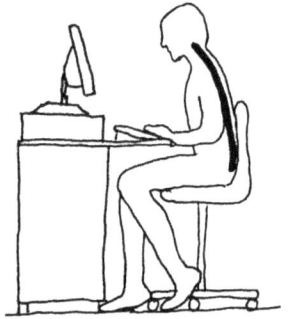

If you are short, I mean vertically challenged, to be politically correct, you definitely don't want to have your legs dangling. That will cause stress to your back. Simply bring in a box to rest your feet on, or request a different chair or desk set up.

Remember your body would prefer to stay in its neutral position, which reduces the likeliness of injury. Keeping your feet flat on the floor will help to maintain good posture throughout your back, so you will not slouch.

Regardless of your height, make sure the seat portion of your chair is not pressing into the back of your knees. It should be against the lower section of your leg a few inches above the knee. There are vulnerable nerves and blood vessels in that region.

I have a kneeling chair to keep my back straight and take some pressure off my low back by moving it to my knees. It is a good concept and does work, but if you are committed to bad posture you can persevere. It doesn't matter what chair you use, you have to nag yourself not to slouch. Put a note on your computer, your desk, your dashboard or anywhere to remind you.

"Hard work never killed anybody, but why take a chance?" – **Edgar Bergen**

ALL IN A DAY'S WORK

If you use a lumbar support or lumbar pillow it may help reduce stress on the back[108] or remind you not to hunch over so your face touches your monitor. There is a fine line for minimizing the stress we place on our spines when we sit. If we sit too far forward or lean to far backward we increase the pressure on our backs.[109,110] Sitting in a chair in the upright position at an angle of 95 – 105 degrees helps to reduce disk pressure and supporting muscle activity.[108,111] A Scottish MRI study revealed sitting at an 135 degree angle is great for the back but you then tip your neck too far forward to see, like cruisin' in the car.

All chairs are different and some have multiple options for your back to feel comfortable so try all of the supports. Good posture in this position is extremely important, considering many of us are sitting for extended periods of time.

When you routinely sit on one side of the couch, leaning on the armrest, like when you watch TV, over time you can start to curve your spine that way. Your body will adapt. Working at a desk, leaning on one side will do the same thing. I used to work from one side of the table and noticed a curve forming in my own back so now I alternate sides.

To reduce lower back stress when getting out of your chair, place your hands on the arm rests and use your arm muscles to help hoist yourself up and out. This will save your back. Use your legs too.

When you set up your station, position the height of the monitor so your eyes are looking straight ahead. The eyes should be close to level with the midline of the screen. If you are seated too high then try to raise the monitor by putting it on a stand or a phonebook.

I happen to have a stool I'm sitting on right now adjusted so my seat is lower and my lap top screen is at a better height with my arms supported on the desk. I really do try to practice what I preach.

You will also want to have the monitor screen in front of you and not off to one side. I treat patients who work with their heads turned in one direction for hours. They are working in poorly designed offices or very small spaces.

Remember the normal posture of your spine and make the necessary changes. If you are stuck looking to one side, or up or down, this will strain your neck muscles and shoulders causing them to tighten up over time. See if there are any ergonomic modifications to your workstation that you could make to reduce the strain on your body.

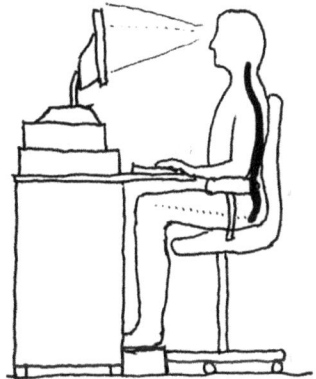

Check if you can have your arms supported while using the keyboard. You might be able to raise the arms of your chair or make some space at your desk so your arms can rest on it. Supporting the arms is vital to reducing neck and shoulder tension.

If your elbows are floating in the air then your trapezius muscles, located from your neck to the shoulder, are contracting to keep them elevated. This will keep these muscles in a continuously contracted state for a long time. They will tighten up and cause a problem. It is the same thing that happens when we drive with our arms up or at odd angles.

Avoid carpal tunnel injuries by easing stress on your wrists. Try those foam pads for the keyboard or mouse to prevent harmful bending at the wrist. You could also tilt your keyboard up toward you. I was using a laptop to type this book and realized I needed to angle the base. The keys are half way across the base of the laptop. So by raising the angle, I decreased my hand fatigue and stress by creating more of a natural position for my hands when I type.

In addition, the mouse can do a number on your wrists. If you get pains from pointing and clicking, try to keep your wrist still and use your arm to move it. Any rest from not bending your wrist back and forth will help heal the tendons and muscles.

With either the mouse or the keyboard, try not to use more force than is necessary to type or move the *"rodent"* around. Excessive energy used can result in fatigue and strain.

Like most guys, I'm a clicker. I have found my pointer finger gets sore from using the mouse. Almost like Atari thumb, for those of you who remember way back. I may try to press too hard or too often, so I occasionally switch and use my middle finger. This can be learned pretty easily. You can also use a different mouse. A vertical mouse requires your hand to rest as though you are holding a drink.

You have to remember to take breaks by getting some water or changing positions. Try to move every 30 – 45 minutes to stay loose. Studies have shown fluid creeps into tissues in just 15 minutes after you stop moving.[49] You might get fired if you reposition yourself that often, just be cognizant of your resting back before doing anything sudden or stressful.

If you go to lift something after sitting and have allowed enough time for fluids to fill into your discs and your joints, then you are more likely to cause an injury. An example employs two Ziploc bags. One you fill ¼ of the way with water and the other is filled to its maximum capacity. Lay them on the side and place a few books on them. The one that is most vulnerable is the one that is over-filled with fluid. That's what happens to your disc when you move after staying still for some time.

In addition, chronic sitting can cause your hamstrings, located in the back of your legs, to become short and tight because they are being held in a position that keeps the muscle shortened. That can lead to low back problems by creating an imbalance in your core or pelvic region. It's okay to be a hard worker but give the hamstrings a little love now and then. Stretch.

Computer users were followed during a three-year study to research what happened to their health. More than 50 percent of participants studied were likely to experience neck, shoulder, arm and wrist or hand pain.[112,113] Taking breaks reduces eye strain, can clear the mind and helps avoid developing additional problems in your body.[114,115]

Whatever you are doing, especially if you are a typing fool like me, you need to take a break. Get up and grab some water, visit the lavatory or maybe do some stretches. This gives your body a breather by lubricating your joints and gets the blood flowing again. Your eyes also need to refocus. Take a break and look outside so they can adjust to other distances. This will help keep them seeing clearly longer.

> *"The right to be heard does not automatically include the right to be taken seriously."* – **Hubert H. Humphrey**

CAN YOU HEAR ME NOW?

The phone is another one of those necessary evils we all have to deal with. Many people still cradle the phone in between their shoulder and ear so both hands are free and they can work or write notes.

That position keeps the trapezius muscle and others in a permanent state of contraction. Normally your shoulders should be parallel to the floor and your head straight. Get a headset and all will be right in the world. You will have freedom of movement and proper posture for a long healthy day at work, or talking to friends and family.

There are some simple stretches to loosen your neck that you can do at your desk. I mentioned them in the stretching section. They were the ones in which you would start by taking your right hand and grab the seat of your chair. Now just lean and tip your left ear toward the left shoulder. Feel that on the right? Having your hand on the seat keeps the right shoulder down and forces a greater stretch into the muscle.

To reach a little further back in your spine, keep your right hand on the seat and lean forward a little. Try tipping your left ear or your nose toward your left armpit. Now the stretch is a little more in the back of the neck and shoulder

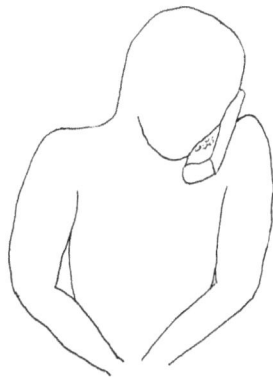

region. Hold these for 15 seconds and do them on both sides. You can do these on your couch, in the shower, or at a stop sign while in the car.

Considering everyone seems to carry much of their stress and tension in the shoulders and neck, you probably can't do these enough times during your day. One to five sets of 10 would be awesome. How about one held for 60 seconds?

> *"This country has come to feel the same when Congress is in session as when the baby gets hold of a hammer."* – **Will Rogers**

EVEN IT UP, EVEN IT OUT

Well it's time to make dinner for the family or yourself. You probably need a few things at the store. They have such great prices, you fill your cart. Now you have to bring all the bags in. The first thing I would do is, call the kids or spouse to help out. If they are hungry, they will help you bring in the food. It's not going to come inside by itself. Make it part of the weekly chores for any of the occupants of your fortress.

You could also do it yourself if you have to, but make several trips. Hey I'm the master of putting 16 plastic bags on one arm so I can work the key and hold my briefcase with the other. Extra trips? Those were for wimps. The new, older and wiser me, knows to make several trips and put the same number of bags on each side. By keeping the weight evenly distributed you can decrease the stress placed on your spine, wrists and shoulders.

> *"An income tax form is like a laundry list -- either way you lose your shirt."* – **Fred Allen**

WASH DAY, NOTHING CLEAN

The laundry basket can be heavy, especially when the kids come in wet from being outdoors. Having the basket above the floor, like on a table, would definitely make it easier to lift at this time. Have them strip down where they stand and leave the clothes near or in the washing machine. Moms and Dads also get pretty dirty.

The best solution is a laundry chute. Everyone can launch their wares to the machine without anyone gathering and collecting the mess. It's kind of like having a central vacuum system. I have a mud room with my washing machine, which is a great place to remove the wet clothes. However the clothes still have to be carried upstairs to the opposite side of the house when they are cleaned.

If there is any way to do it, put your laundry room upstairs where the sheets, towels and clothes are kept. Then you have less carrying to do to the machine and back when everything is clean. Basic rules are to never try to carry too much and keep the basket or hamper close to your body.

When the clothes are wet, a front end loading washer is the best so you don't have to bend over and lean to remove them. The weight of the damp clothes and chance of them getting caught as you lift are just the thing to start a back problem. With any type of washing unit, never try to take too much out at once.

After the clothes are dry, fold them on a shelf or into the basket as it sits on the washing machine. However you reload your basket try to keep it above your waist so you can lift it easier than hauling it up off the floor. Remember to use your knees and keep the back straight with abdominals tight.

"Cleaning anything involves making something else dirty, but anything can get dirty without something else getting clean." – **Laurence J. Peter**

IT'S A SWEEP

Nobody likes to vacuum. From the dust, to the filters and bags, it is a pain in the backside. One of the problems I have with the design of a standard vacuum is it forces you to move the machine predominantly with one side of your body. This forces your upper back to twist with the shoulder extending forward causing a stretching and torque component to the lower spine.

There should be replacement handles so they are more toward the center of your body. Even L-shaped like a portion of a shopping cart handle. A centrally located handle would balance the stress on your body and do not over develop or strain any one side. You could clean like before with the machine to the side, but your back wouldn't be strained or twisted.

Until I can put that idea into production you could try to switch hands. I know it feels weird but you will get used to it in time. I have faith your body can adapt and learn. It will help keep both sides of your back muscles strong and equally developed.

Otherwise you can place the vacuum in front of you and push it so it stays central to your spine. There will be no twist of the spine or uneven muscle use and the machine will clean just as well. Dyson created a vacuum with a swivel ball because most vacuums have fixed wheels. This reduces the stress to your body when you maneuver it.

The other problem is that people forget to move their feet. There is no reason to try to stand in one spot and strain to reach the farthest corners of a room. Walk over there. This will also reduce the stress on your back, the supporting

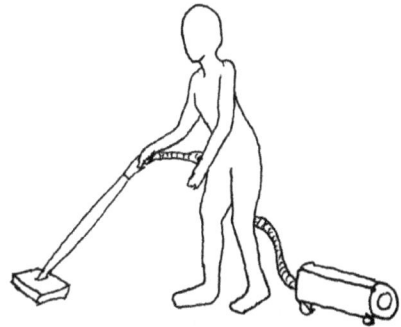

muscles and your shoulder. It can also add up to a few more calories burned.

My wife watched me vacuum and noticed I had foot marks everywhere because I walked with the machine instead of reaching forward. If you are worried about footprints, a solution for this would be to start at the farthest spot and work backwards. My argument is that company will never think you rushed through to clean the house because although the rug is clean, you would have footprints. They'd think *"Wow the floors must always look great."*

Another idea would be to do your regular vacuuming by using some of these ideas, like walking with the machine, to decrease the abuse to your body. But if there is a special occasion, than vacuum like your old self so it gets done just like you want. At least some of the cleaning will be done with less stress to your body.

There are some pretty cool inventions out like the house version of the automatic pool vacuum. These can ease the constant reaching and bending otherwise associated with vacuuming. They don't hit an exact spot on the floor but meander and scoop up what they can. I would tape a string to it and let your cat chase it for hours. Research them before you spend your money. I have heard positive and negative comments regarding their effectiveness and cost. It could decrease the time you spend waltzing with your upright.

For you steam cleaning and shop or water basin vacuum users, simply don't overfill the bucket. It is easier to lift that way. If you don't want to lift the whole unit or you have overfilled the tank, use another container to scoop water out to make it more manageable.

> *"The best time to plan a book is while you're doing the dishes."* – **Agatha Christie**

MAGIC HANDS

Any work, preparation or cleaning that needs to be done should be completed with your back as straight as it can be. Leaning hunched forward over a sink or a counter, for an extended period of time, causes the muscles of your low back to stay contracted. Remember this also doubles the stress to the disc region. The longer the muscles work while your back and neck are in these vulnerable positions, the tighter the muscles will become. This tightness can then remain long after the chore is done.

I have always been one to clean the dishes as I use them. Seems easy enough to me. For those of you who still wash 'em using your hands or are forced to because the dishwasher is clogged with mineral deposits, listen up.

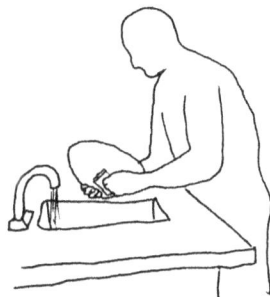

At my house I can open a cabinet door beneath the sink and put my foot on the edge to ease any stress on my lower back. This takes a little pressure off my back just like the saloon rail was designed to. If you want to keep the cowboys in the bar, make it comfortable for them and they'll keep drinking and spitting.

When I was first dating my wife she checked out my kitchen and asked me, *"Do you have a dish washer?"* I looked at her and said, *"I do now!"* It's a joke, people. I find it odd that you have to basically wash the dish or thoroughly rinse it before you put it in the dishwasher. But I never had one growing up so I do them the old-fashioned way. I hand them to my wife. Still joking. Anyway, be careful bending to load and unload the dishwasher. I did learn that if you separate your silverware when you put it in, putting it away is simpler.

To take some stress off of your low back in the kitchen try to keep large pans, or items you use frequently, in easy to reach places. Less bending for you means you are reducing the repetitive motion that can lead to problems down the road. Now you're cooking!

The same rules apply to the art of ironing, which I am not too good at. See if you can limit bending forward and maybe prop one leg on something to reduce low back stress. You could send your clothes out to be cleaned and then you won't have to worry about bending or that you are terrible with the iron.

Let's check your skills so far. *"What's wrong with this picture?"* **A.** He is bent over the ironing board and hurting his spine. **B.** There is no wire to plug the iron into the wall so he'll be there a long time. **C.** He is so clueless he forgot to put a shirt on the board. **D.** All of the above. Answer D of course. Oops, I forgot to draw in the cord and a shirt.

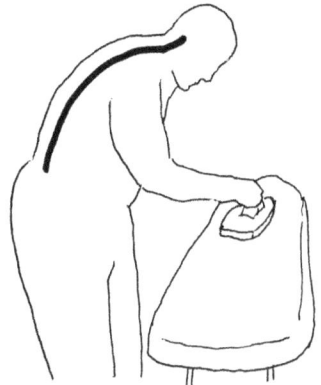

*"A painting in a museum hears more ridiculous opinions
than anything else in the world."* – **Edmond de Goncourt**

PAINT BY NUMBERS

When we move into a new place or when your spouse decides it's time to re-decorate, you will probably want to spread a new coat of paint on your walls and maybe the ceilings. I am a big fan of getting the job done with the biggest brush I can find. I would use the two-foot wide garage broom if it would hold paint.

If you have to work on the ceiling, find a roller that has an extendable handle or attach your old broom handle to it. The beauty of it is you aren't bending your head backwards for extended periods of time. You can almost keep your head in a neutral position. By simply moving your feet you can reach all surfaces of a normal ceiling without the constant reaching, pulling or neck strain. Just tip the handle at a 45 degree angle to the ceiling and move around.

I use the same technique for the walls. Instead of bending and stooping you can stand tall and hit the majority of the wall this way. You may use a roller but lately I have been using a rectangular brush with replaceable pads. It covers the wall well and may produce less splattering.

When you need to use a brush for trim work or corners and edging, do it in shifts. If you keep your arm going up and down you will strain the rotator muscles of your shoulder. You will notice when your hand is painting overhead your arm will get heavy or tired because the blood is leaving the area. Drop the arm once in a while to allow blood to flow into your muscles. You could also use a stepladder. Raise your body, keeping the area you are working on level with your eyes and arms.

"Our bodies are our gardens to which our wills are gardeners."
– **William Shakespeare**

JACK AND THE BEAN STALK

Some people like to feel the Earth between their fingers. Gardening is a great hobby; stress reliever and can provide some awesome food for the table. Hopefully you don't have to Rototill your garden first. That is like wrestling a bull by the horns.

If you have to do it yourself, do it in stages and take breaks. The vibration and jarring can irritate your back and shoulders. Otherwise check the local papers, or ask a nearby farmer so you can hire someone else to do it and really prevent any chance of back pain. There are also elevated garden beds. The plants are table-height for easy gardening and less bugs.

Who likes weeding? Good planning can go a long way. Spend a few extra dollars on landscape fabric in the fall when it's discounted, and set your seeds or plants through it. The black fabric will decrease the amount of weeds that can grow and save you hours of bending and back ache. Your plants can grow and are virtually maintenance free. Less weeds also means less competition for nutrients and the plants can grow better.

I have patients who weed or plant for hours and then wonder why their backs hurt. Too much of one position is bad. Take a break. Stand up and go get some water or lemonade. Then come back after your muscles have had a chance to relax and your joints were able to loosen up a little.

There are some cool gardening stools with all terrain wheels so you can roll from one area to another. Just don't stay seated, and then completely bend forward, straining your back. Try to alter positions from sitting on a seat, sitting on the ground or kneeling to keep your body twinge free.

"All is in the hands of man. Therefore wash them often." – **Stanislaw J. Lec**

CLEAN UP, AISLE 5

Cleaning up dust or wiping tables is a repetitive movement. Whether you are washing the car, or cleaning off the dust collectors on your shelves, it's no fun. The swirling motion can trigger shoulder pain. The Karate Kid was an anomaly. All that *"Wax on and wax off"* would have given him trigger points. That repetitive motion can lead to muscular imbalance and knots.

This motion is like the deli slicer at the food market or hairdresser brushing and drying hair. Dusting requires your rotator muscles of your shoulder to become over worked. My best advice is to do it slowly with slow strokes, versus trying to rub the finish off your woodwork. You could try to use your other hand too. As always, take breaks.

My patient Toni came in for some treatment and told me she had fallen off her ladder while she was trying to wash her windows. Now most of us have fallen off our rocker at one time or another, but she was up 15 feet, landed hard and fractured her calcaneus, or heel. My first thought was she should purchase a telescoping pole and wash the windows while safely on the ground. She confessed to me that she thought I was going to tell her she isn't supposed to do windows.

As cute as that was, her best options are to use the telescoping pole, have someone else do it, sorry Bob (her husband), move the ladder, or hire someone to come and do it. Cleaning older windows is more difficult. Newer windows tilt and open inside so you can wash them from the comfort of your room.

"I loathe people who keep dogs. They are cowards who haven't got the guts to bite people themselves." – **August Strindberg**

AND...THEY'RE OFF

Make sure when you adopt an animal, it is one you can handle because when it comes to dogs, someone should regularly take them for a walk. If you have land or a fence then you are all set. They can run around without a care. If they need to be on a leash for their exercise then plan smart. If you are 5' 4" and 128 pounds, getting a Great Dane might be too much for you to handle. Choose a dog that is not going to overwhelm or overpower you.

Some places have dog and pet sitters. They can help with the exercising and may help to get your pet accustomed to other animals. Eventually when you take a stroll you will encounter another dog, or a squirrel. Be prepared so your pet doesn't jerk you out of your shoes. Be alert to your surroundings. If you are going to the park, then you will probably see squirrels and birds. Will you be able to control Phydeaux?

You could send your best buddy to obedience class so he/she will know how to walk with you whether on a leash or loose. I have this same problem with my sons, haha. Dogs also will need to learn to obey commands in case there is a threat. And if you know the mail person comes at a certain time don't take the dog out then. That's just asking for a leash-yanked shoulder or neck. Trust me, I've seen the resulting injuries in my office and much worse.

Actually a friend was walking her little Jack Russell and a labrador retriever broke its leash, attacked the little dog, dropping its owner, who was recovering from recent back surgery, to the ground. My friend's dog is okay, but the woman fractured her hip during the incident. I'm sure her back was sore too.

I enjoy my morning litter scoop for my cats. I try to walk around a bit before having to bend over to scoop poop. Especially first thing in the morning when my back is vulnerable. If you're a cat owner, bend your knees. If you can, compile their *"piles"* in a bag or container you can take out to the trash before it becomes completely full and heavy. Several light loads are smarter than one heavy one.

When I buy cat litter containers I always buy two so I remain balanced bringing them in the house. This reduces back strain by 50 percent. Of course they come out heavier, haha. That's why taking out smaller quantities is smart.

Some people have taught their cats to use the toilet. I don't know about you but I think I'm going to have a hard enough time getting my sons to hit the target.

With any big animal, like horses, there is always a chance of getting pulled, kicked or thrown. I had them when I grew up and had plenty of nicks and bruises. Clean up is also a lot harder. Just take everything into consideration before making a decision about your next pet. Remember, the kids will plead how they will take care of the animal but inevitably, you will be the one doing the work.

"Live each season as it passes; breathe the air, drink the drink, taste the fruit, and resign yourself to the influences of each." – **Henry David Thoreau**

SEASONS CHANGE

When fall comes the leaves in the northeast change and are beautiful. All those wonderful colors are so vibrant and magical, until they are wet, brown and covering your lawn like a blanket. I'm not sure what happens to the wind pattern around my house, but my neighbors' leaves blow up my driveway toward the garage and behind my house.

Inevitably the wind brings more leaves from all over the region and keeps dumping and blowing them into my driveway. Needless to say I have come to despise raking. What stinks is my neighbor across the street boasted to me he has never raked because the wind blows them off his yard. That's the same magical wind that does a 180 and blows them up my driveway.

This chore is a lot like vacuuming in that it tends to be a one-sided chore. If you have to rake try to do it in stages. I have a nice yard, almost an acre. It contains a lot of leaves. If you are planning on raking everything up in a day make sure you take breaks. The body needs time to rest and recover.

Try to use both sides of your body when you are making the motion. That will give you a little more time to complete your task and the stress on the body will be distributed evenly to both sides. The handle on a rake forces you to turn to your side and predominantly use one arm. Using one side over years will cause it to over develop, leading to muscular imbalance, and distortion to your spine and posture.

Like anything else, walk to where you need to be. There is no reason to reach and pull. This will cause more contraction and stress to the muscles. If you are right there you can move the leaves more easily.

Some people have trash pickup for leaves. You can bag them in convenient and semi-light bags and take them to the curb. Some people take them to a pit and burn them with the neighbors.

You could also lay out a tarp and pile the leaves on top of that. Then tie it up to your eight-year-old for him to drag, (I was just checking to see if you were paying attention). Or use a tractor or four-wheeler and drag them to a field or an annoying neighbor's yard. Hmm, maybe that's how all those leaves made it into my driveway. Anyway, with this method there is no lifting or carrying.

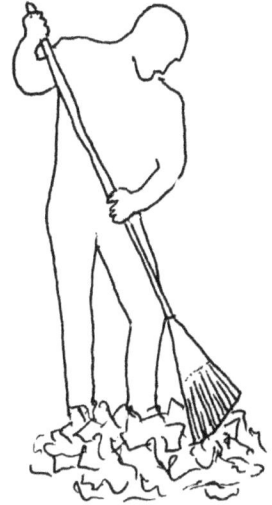

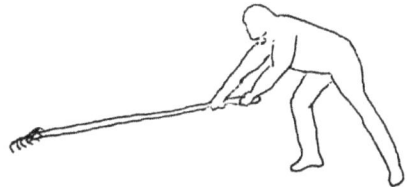

The best version of leaf removal I know is the mulching mower. For those of you who have a non-mulching mower like me, you can do the following. You can just round up them critters and keep mowing over them by starting wide and closing the circle inward. Eventually you can chop the leaves into such small particles they can provide nutrition for your lawn or blow away in the wind.

We just had a hurricane here and lots of trees came down so there's tons of yard work. Yeah. This reminded me of the way I move brush and fallen trees. Like the leaves, you can use a tarp or a big, full branch. With a branch, I might put a rope underneath it and then pile tree debris up on top of the leafy end. I can then wrap the rope around the bundle and tie it tight. Now take part of that rope, or use another one, and tie it to the thicker end of your bottom branch. Tie this to the truck or tractor and haul it away. Less trips. Less work.

> *"The older I get, the greater power I seem to have to help the world; I am like a snowball - the further I am rolled, the more I gain."* – **Susan B. Anthony**

SNOW, SNOW, GO AWAY

Well when it snows, it snows. Each year many Americans deal with this white nuisance for a couple months. Everyone has heard about north Central NY when they accumulated more than 10 feet of snow in less than a week. What do you do with that?

I think the home flamethrower makes sense here. My idea is you will never have a fight over who will clear out the driveway. Who wouldn't want to fire up that bad boy and melt some snow? It will take stress away from the low back and heck, you can cook up dinner in a pinch if you need food ready fast.

If you can find a guy to plow your driveway and not destroy your lawn then the only place you will experience pain during the winter will be in your wallet. If you are convinced snow blowing the driveway is the best solution, then you have to do it wisely.

Yep, I enjoy a nice romantic walk with my girl, the snow blower, every evening, and some mornings, because nothing says love like gasoline fumes and engine noise, with cold and dangerous equipment. Speaking of loud, to decrease the ringing in my ears I have been using ear plugs when using the mower, snow blower, and saws. It just makes sense.

For any piece of gear you have, I am a big fan of an electric starter. I don't care if it's your Harley or your leaf blower. Stepping outside and yanking a cord, which involves one side of your body, is just asking for trouble. This is the classic move that debilitates even the healthiest individual. They come off the couch cold and try to fire up the equipment. Remember the discs are fully hydrated when you are immobile for a period of time making them more vulnerable.

If you have to pull the cord, loosen and warm up your body and see if it will start with ease before you start to tip the machine with your forceful pulls. If it still doesn't start, make sure the key is in the ON position. Oops. Yep … long story.

When I am using the snow blower I try not to wrestle with it. I walk behind it and let it do its thing for about 20 – 30 minutes. It is easy enough to stand behind and turn around making several passes.

When the snow is clumped, heavy or mostly ice, is when you are most likely to strain your back. Those conditions cause the machine to work less efficiently. I have had those nights when it seemed like the blower was headed in every direction I didn't want it to go. Your shoulders and back are all subject to injury if you manhandle the snow blower. Take your time. And if something ever gets stuck in the blades, turn it off, use a stick, not your hands, to free it.

If you haven't been able to con a neighborhood kid or one of your own to shovel the snow for you, then it is up to you. It is better to make sure you are loose, so don't shovel first thing in the morning. Allow your back to warm up properly. Also when it is cold your blood vessels are constricted so use caution if you have any heart problems. That instant stress could cause a heart emergency.

Check the height of your shovel before you begin. If the shovel handle is too short you will bend forward more than you need to and may injure your back. The constant leaning forward causes the low back muscles to stay contracted. Stand up straight and stretch a few times to relieve some of this tightness.

If the handle is too long then the weight of the snow is farther from your body and can seem heavier than it is. This is a lot like a seesaw when a child and adult can balance depending on where they are in relation to the fulcrum point, or middle of the seesaw. When shoveling, slide your hands up so they are comfortable and it causes less stress to your back.

Make sure you aren't overloading the shovel if the snow is wet and heavy. Move less snow and go slow. If the snow is light and fluffy then it shouldn't be too bad if you load the shovel, unless you shovel with a trash can. I used to use one at my mom's house. Gets the job done quickly but isn't great for the back.

Now if you are moving all this snow, you then need to put it or throw it somewhere. Of course the proper way to lift a shovel piled high with snow is to bend your knees and keep your back straight. *"Who does that?"* I mean, try to lift with your legs with knees bent, move your feet and dump the stuff where you need it. Otherwise you could step forward in the direction you are throwing it so there is momentum and it is easier on your body.

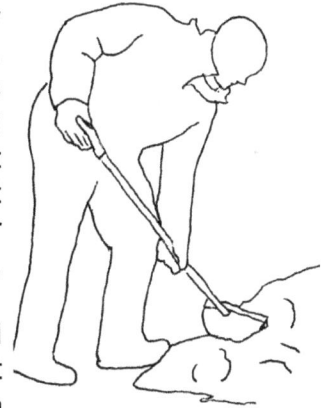

Another option depending on the landscape is to push the shovel to the edge of your driveway or sidewalk. Then take a leg and use your foot to lift and fling the snow or push it over the edge. Then there is no bending of the back.

After all of our talks I know you would never twist and throw the snow. That would be foolish because you are loading the spine and then twisting or shearing the compressed disc. And that may lead to a really serious problem.

Due to all of the snow we had in NY I had to shovel off my roof. This is a 60' long 40' wide roof with two to four feet of snow on it. My patients were shocked I did it all in one day and wasn't sore. I took my time, started at the roof peak and tried to let gravity do some of the work.

When I had to fling snow I bent my knees, lifting and using a little momentum to flip the snow forward. Sometimes it would roll off with the snow below. Other times it needed a little encouragement. I also could just step forward and throw it using the motion of filling the shovel and then flicking the end.

I first attempted to move some four foot high snow from the peak of the roof, down onto the three foot snow height below it, so it could roll off together. Wouldn't you know it, the shovel popped out of my hand! It slid on the snow and went right over the roof. I had to trudge back to the ladder from the farthest point on the roof, walk through the deep snow on the roof and the ground and retrieve the shovel so I could try it all over again. It is funny now, but not when I did it. I'll bring a wrist strap if there's ever a next time.

The other technique I used was to basically perform a row exercise from either side. I took a wide stance and plunged the shovel into the snow beside me. Then I tried not to twist my back as I threw the snow off like I was rowing a boat. I alternated sides of my body, as I worked my way up and down the roof. Sure I may have looked like a drunken sailor but it didn't hurt my back.

I just realized while I was building a new walkway that I shovel in an interesting way. I had to move gravel for part of this project. One way to shovel is to step into the pile and let your body weight fill much of the shovel. You could also angle the shovel upward and ram it into the upper portion of the pile so when you thrust it into the pile, the gravel, dirt or mulch, will fall onto the shovel. The other option is to scoop it from the bottom of the pile, but that involves a little more lifting. Of course try to alternate sides.

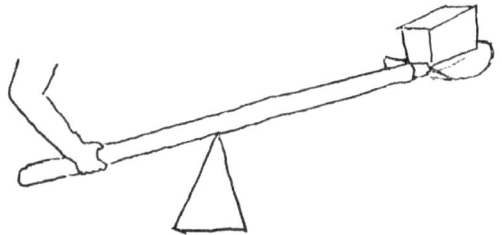

What I thought was neat was when I started to move the shovel like a fulcrum. I place my right hand at the end of the shovel handle. Once the shovel's loaded, the middle to ¾ of the handle actually rests on my right thigh. I can then press down with my right hand and use my thigh as the fulcrum.

The shovel comes up, the left hand guides the direction and you never lift the weight. Like a seesaw on my leg, I can move lots of stuff without over-straining. I was able to fill my wheelbarrow very easily.

It doesn't matter what the project is, these techniques can be implemented for anything like shoveling dirt, gravel or mulch. The key is to protect your back and realize it is a vulnerable part of your body that needs special care and attention.

"Natural abilities are like natural plants; they need pruning by study." – **Sir Francis Bacon**

MOW MORE, MOW LESS

Yep. It's almost as good as *"Hakuna Matata."* That's my motto when it comes to mowing lawns. If you drop the mower deck right down to the dirt and give the lawn a brush cut, you won't have to mow the lawn again for a while. That will free up your time to do something else more constructive.

Sure, the grass may look terrible but it just means you don't have to mow. That's one of the things I like about Arizona. You place your rocks and there they are. They don't move, drop leaves or collect snow.

Of course not everyone wants to scalp their lawn, but there are other ideas to make mowing less painful and time consuming. If you have an opportunity to do some landscaping or would rather hire someone, you can beautify the lawn while reducing the amount of mowing and edging. Do a little research, see what you like, what grows well in your area and then tackle the project.

A good mower can make the job easy. So can a lawn service. With any household chore, you can always look for a neighborhood kid who is looking to make some extra cash mowing, shoveling or raking for instance, and this can reduce the stress to your back. A couple of bucks, to save your back, are worth it. Otherwise grab one of your own kids and put them to work, or at least make them help you. They can learn responsibility and the need to earn their keep, or at least make some money.

I just used a mulching mower and will never mow with anything else again. What a fantastic job it did. No clumps of grass even if I may have been slightly delinquent in my mowing schedule. It also chops up the grass so I may never have to rake again. Yeah!

A good riding mower also should have a comfortable seat. If you are going to be bouncing around on this piece of equipment you better have a comfortable cushion to reduce the impact to your back.

If your lawn is like a cornfield and you are bouncing on the seat like a pogo stick, it can compress your discs and cause muscle tightening. If you don't want to buy a new lawn mower or tractor because the seat isn't like your La-Z-Boy, maybe see if they have other seats you can replace your existing one with. If you need to you could put an old boat cushion or pillow on it to soften the ride.

You could also slow the mower down so it isn't racing across an uneven lawn like a go-kart. Slowing down can diminish any unevenness in the terrain, will probably do a better job cutting the lawn and might even save gas. You wouldn't want your hair stylist racing either.

If you have a smaller lawn, your mower just broke, or you don't want to buy a mower, you may be using the old standby push mower. Some of these have motorized wheels to help move the little beast up hills and across your lawn. This reduces the effort you have to put into it.

Now if part of your exercise routine is pushing an ornery mower, then don't let me stop you. Don't use the motorized wheels.

As a friendly reminder, it is a push mower, not a pull mower. Pushing is always easier than pulling, so limit the back and forth yanking of the mower. Walk with the mower so you do not reach from one end of the lawn to the other. Move your feet. Just like vacuuming, make sure the handle is at a good height for your body and move to the area you are working on instead of over-reaching. That is asking for trouble.

With strategic stonewalls, flower gardens and mulching you can reduce the amount of trimming needed. Trimmers in general are terribly designed machines. So if you have big, smooth, landscaped curves, then you can probably get close enough with just the mower and avoid using this contraption.

A weed whacker or trimmer is a real cumbersome devil, which requires us to hold it in front of our body while leaning forward. Some have straps for your shoulders to reduce the back strain.

It's like using a 20-pound chain saw while leaning forward. Remember that a weight in front of you can be multiplied by 10 – 15 times to equal the actual weight and stress it causes to the back. Just leaning forward creates 200 pounds of pressure per square inch on the discs. Add the saw, which equals about 300 pounds of low back stress, due to the leaning forward with a weight in front of the body. Now this becomes 500 pounds of pressure on the low back discs as you carry the weed whacker all around your yard for long periods of time.

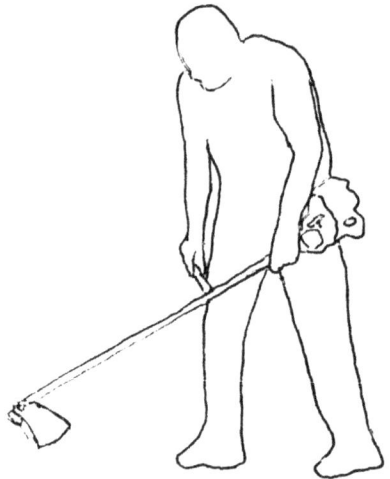

> *"One man practicing sportsmanship is better than a hundred teaching it."*
> **– Knute Rockne**

Play Time

Call them weekend warriors; call them boys and girls who can't let go of their youth. I resemble this remark. Exercise is good no matter what age or level. I'm more concerned with the preparation, than the participation.

As kids we could get away just diving in. Remember during recess time we would all just start running or kicking a ball around. If we try to do either as adults, we have a high probability of injuring ourselves or being incredibly sore the next day. With any sport or activity it is advisable to take some shots or throws and then loosen up after your body has warmed up a bit.

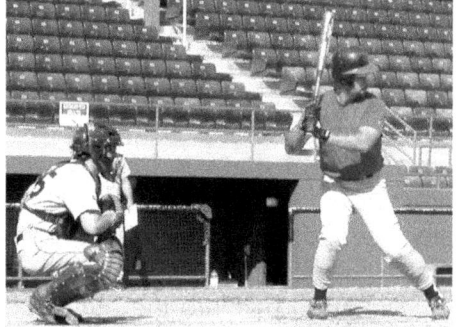

The weekend warrior may decide to play a sport or take part in an activity after not training during the week. Sometimes there are no pregame stretches either. Just show up and start swinging. Actually my friend Pat did show up late for a game once when he was next to bat. He barely had his uniform on or his shoes tied, and one sock was still down when stepped to the plate. He took the first pitch and knocked it over the fence. Now in his defense, we both practiced throughout the week to prepare and not shock our bodies come game time. However, I still recommend loosening up the old joints first.

For your health and weekend activities it is best to try to stay in good shape year round. Then when you compete or partake in activities over the weekend you will feel great afterwards. Try to pace yourself. Play one round of golf instead of two Saturday, and then try again Sunday if you are itching for another round. Don't come into the season and play 36-holes. Play a couple of 9-hole courses or 18s, with time to recover in between outings.

If you walk the course, then push the cart. Don't pull it. We push a grocery cart because it is easier and will cause less stress on the body to simply move forward then to drag something behind you. Also your torso won't end up twisted and asking for trouble. They have three-wheel carts that make pushing your cart really easy. They even call them *"pushcarts."* The two-wheel version is called a pull cart but oddly enough you can turn them around and push them on the course. Who'd a thunk it?!

Before you show off how far you can smack the ball with your new driver that is the size of a pumpkin, loosen up first. Avoid twisting and fast movements until you have warmed up your muscles and tendons. Or pay the consequences.

Most golf courses have putting greens to help you warm up but only a few of them have driving nets to loosen you up before you show the gang how you drive like a pro. If they have a driving net take advantage of it. Taking a few swings can help you prevent an injury and help your game. If they don't, stop by and hit some balls at a nearby driving range first.

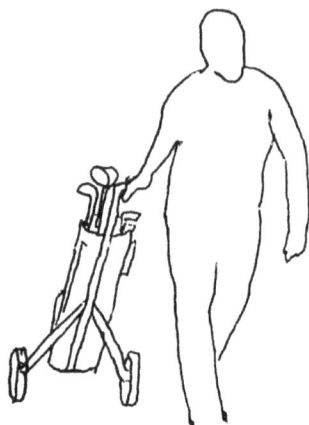

Drive the ball into the net to perfect your swing and warm up, collect your golf balls, walk to the tee and show them where you live. That means crank up a monster drive. They didn't pay money to see Babe Ruth walk.

When I am rushed and have to start before I am really ready, I know that after the fourth hole is when my game really shines because then I am completely loose. Okay, shine may not be the operative word here, but it is better. Could it get worse, is the question. In a pinch you can always swing and knock off a few dandelion tops to help get the old bones moving.

If you carry your bag or wheel it around I have the solution to help your back and your game. I have no even clubs in my bag. I use my driver, a fairway wood, chip, putter, a 7 iron and a 9 iron. I do carry a rarely used 5 iron but I eliminated half of the clubs. I can't learn how to use all of those clubs. So I decreased the poundage and have forced my game to get better with fewer clubs. Ten yards extra or less with one club really won't make or break my game but the weight could break my back. More clubs equals more decisions and mistakes.

Focus on the ones you use most. If you want to add the other clubs, do so slowly, as you get better and have a need for them. As much as I like playing guitar, I don't carry one with me at all times on the off chance someone might decide to break into song and I may need it. I do carry a pick though. Just in case.

You could add some of the other clubs on a practice day or when you're out with your friends. Of course if you are cruising in style in a cart with a golf buddy, you can take the whole set plus a cooler with water to stay hydrated. Now you're livin' the dream.

> *"Good ideas are not adopted automatically. They must be driven into practice with coura-geous patience."* – **Hyman Rickover**

WE'RE TALKING 'BOUT PRACTICE

That's right Allen Iverson, because practice makes perfect. You only get better with practice. Practice hard, play hard. Anyway, I know of a ball player who has thrown right-handed for years and is now in the big leagues. He was never instructed to train both sides of his body so he is completely over developed and imbalanced. Now he has to train hard to try to get the less used side to catch up with the rest of his body.

These imbalances have distorted his spine and may lead to posture changes and problems. By keeping both sides equally strong he will have greater ability, velocity and strength overall. You are only as strong as your weakest link.

Kids may practice for hours when playing a sport to get better. We also have them enrolled in so many activities they run around constantly. For the sake of developing a better athlete, try to have your child swing the bat from the other side of the plate or dribble with their left hand once in awhile.

If they can switch hit or kick a soccer ball accurately using either leg, they will be in great demand and be more successful. Might even mean a scholarship. This is a subtle way to develop and strengthen the less dominant side, aside from weights or resistance training.

> *"Didn't I ever tell you? Bumbles Bounce!"* – **Yukon Cornelius**

BOING! BOING! BOING!

I'm not talking about Tigger. I'm referring to what happens to your spine when you bounce up and down with certain sports. When there is too much pressure to the disc it can cause it to push through the vertebra above it or below it.

When it does penetrate the endplate, or the top and bottom surfaces of the vertebra in contact with the disc, it is known as Schmorl's Nodes on an x-ray film. That continuous and sometimes severe force on the vertebra can eventually lead to disc problems later in life.

When the integrity and the biomechanics of the spine have been altered by the endplate damage, it has been shown to alter the distribution of future compressive forces in the disc. This will result in displacing that stress into the outer annular fibers of the disc.[115] It even causes

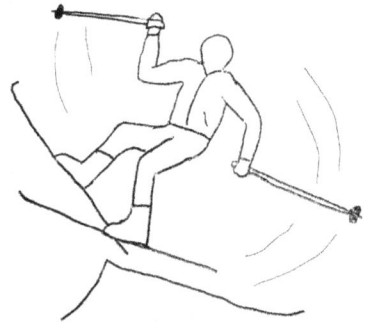

changes in the adjacent discs.[31,48,115] This is a perfect example of how when one area functions improperly it can cause increased stress to the segments associated with it.

I have evaluated many patients' x-rays at my office before reviewing their histories. I have commented that their conditions could have started back when they were riding horses, cruising on a jet ski, hitting moguls on a ski slope, riding a snowmobile, bouncing on the ATV or water skiing. They just look at me like, *"How did he know that?"* Usually there is some type of repetitive pounding that pushes the disc into the vertebrae.

Another source to cause this condition would be a major fall onto your backside. Falling out of a tree, off your bike or slipping on ice and hitting your butt are prime examples of how this could happen to any of us.

I love to go scuba diving but the boat ride can be murder because sitting is the worst position for your low back and the discs. When the weather or waves are rough I stand up for the ride as much as I can. This way I can use my knees and legs to absorb some of the shock and impact. If you have back pain, stand up for the boat ride on your next trip.

If you like to Jet Ski or snowmobile, don't just sit. Get your legs involved with the ride. It will eliminate some of the pounding on your spine and enable you to make the fun last. Some of the newer seats are angled to force more weight toward your legs, which helps solve the increased stress to the low back.

The same thing could be said for your Caddyshack outing. Try to have a calm and sober individual driving the cart so you aren't four wheeling and losing your clubs on the way to find your ball. The bouncing around could injure you or at least hinder your performance due to an aching back.

"To become an able and successful man in any profession, three things are necessary, nature, study and practice." – **Henry Ward Beecher**

LET THERE BE MUSIC

The halls are alive with the sound of mistakes. I can only imagine what my mom went through when I was growing up. I loved to play guitar, sing and crank it up. Didn't matter if it was to the radio, CDs or solo. To this day I'm not sure how I managed to salvage my hearing after all of the concerts I played and practice sessions. However I would suspect my hearing will continue to fail the longer I am married. Haha.

I can remember playing guitar for hours. It's the only way to improve. At college I played at least 24-hours a week. Alright, so maybe some college classes were missed in the process.

Practice makes perfect so if your child is practicing a lot, take a look at their positioning. Here are a few ideas and examples of postures required for playing some of the more popular instruments.

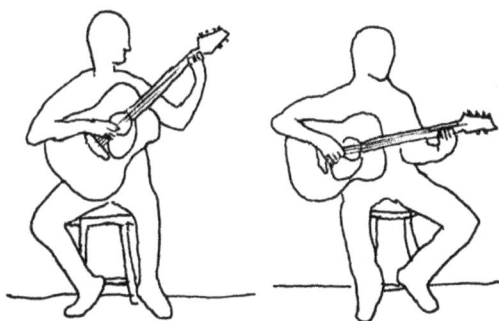

Sure lugging the tuba isn't every kid's dream, but it is difficult. I think a little talk from the child's parents can convince them they really don't want to be hauling an instrument the size of the family car. However if that is what they wish, try to do it safely or compromise to pick up that instrument when they get older … and bigger. Help them select a smaller wind or string instrument, but these too can do some real damage. Instruments like guitars, violin or cello can really strain your body.

Musicians often have their heads turned to one side, but with violin they have to pinch the instrument between their ears and shoulders. I have had some patients who play violin complaining about trapezius pain because they are tipping their heads to one side to hold the body of the violin in between their shoulders and chins. That's like holding the phone and we know that is a no-no.

This contracts the trapezius muscle and if you are playing for hours, and over several years, the area will become a problem. The shoulder will become tight and may even become over-developed. Constant stretching may help a little. So will taking breaks.

Many piano players have to support the weight of their arms by holding them up, as they tickle the ivories. In addition, they may slouch or hunch over the piano as they play which will increase the curve of their midbacks. Some keyboards can be angled, like a computer's keyboard, to reduce the stress on the wrists and back. Pianists also lean with their heads tipped forward as they learn to play. Although the sheet music is angled on the stand, copy it and blow it up so it might be easier to read. Then maybe they won't lean and strain their necks.

Having the strap of a guitar always putting pressure into your shoulder can cause muscle tightness in the trapezius muscle just like a big, heavy purse. Try different positions like sitting to alter your posture and mix it up. As usual stretch the shoulder region regularly.

Like piano, you may be bending your head forward to look down at the strings or music sheets and that can strain your neck. Many musicians read music. The best method is of course to use an easel or stand to hold the music upright. It keeps it at an angle so it is easier to read and puts less stress on the neck.

With a bigger string instrument like a cello you have to hold your arm up and out to move a bow back and forth. Holding your arm up will tire out the muscles. Moving your arm back and forth will tighten the muscles. This is similar to the stress someone puts on their shoulder while driving with one hand on the top of the wheel, or a postal worker who sorts mail back and forth, respectively.

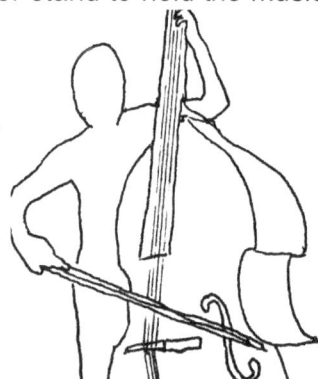

You also have to stand to play these the bass so bring something to prop one foot up to decrease low back strain. Grab a stool to rest part of your weight on; not to sit, but to lean against and reduce the stress or offer a change of positions.

I was just watching a music DVD and noticed the bassist had an instrument that had the frets angled. The bass has a long neck and is a stretch as you play near its end, or head of the instrument. It can strain the wrists and fingers. So as he played with his fingers closer to the body of the instrument, the frets angled in at the top, like this (\ ). As he moved his hand down and away from the body the frets at the tops were angled outward like this (/). This reduces the stress off the shoulders and wrists as it required less contortioning of the body. Very smart.

See if your young, dedicated musician can learn a few stretches to loosen any muscles that are being overworked to avoid pain when they want to jam in the Holiday play. Of course, taking short breaks is always helpful, but so is moving their heads and looking away for a while, taking a quick walk and performing a few stretches as if they were waking up in the morning. This will help to get the blood flowing and keep their muscles loose.

Another thing to do would be to strengthen the body. Hit the gym to strengthen your body and to add some endurance to all of the muscles that will be used during practice sessions.

If you sign yourself or your child up for lessons, see if the instructor can give you advice on how to play the instrument without stressing your posture. They may be able to advise you on adopting an upright posture with consideration for your head positioning, shoulder level, or proper arm and leg placement to help reduce spinal fatigue. Otherwise it will be up to you kid.

> *"Behold the turtle. He makes progress only when he sticks his neck out."*
> **– James B. Conant**

FIRST ONE IN, FIRST ONE EATEN

I was diving in Cozumel one vacation and noticed I had unbelievable pain in the back of my neck at the base of my skull. It became more and more intense and was causing a monster of a headache. It was almost enough to prevent me from making my next dive. I said almost. Nothing stops a dive.

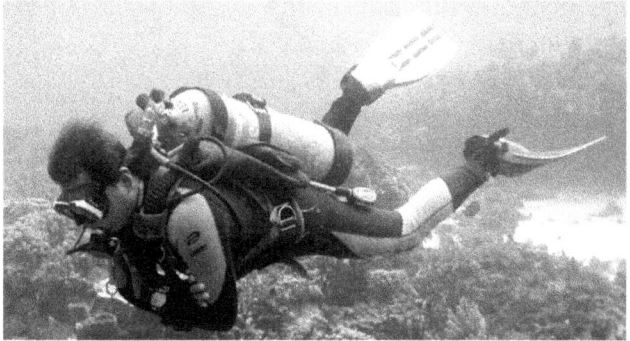

Anyway, when you are diving and floating horizontally you have a tendency to look where you are going and around at all of the neat sea life and coral formations. My muscles that extend to hold my head in this position were getting too tight. Try tilting your head all the way back. Now if you lay on your stomach try to keep it there for an hour. This is what I was doing to my neck.

After going through this a few times I recognized that massaging the muscles at the base of my skull, the suboccipitals, would help relieve the tension and my symptomatic headaches. So without giving up diving, which isn't an option, I figured out this was a typical case of having the body stuck in one position too long that created my problem.

Now while diving I tip my head forward periodically to stretch the muscles and help improve the circulation to that area. Works like a charm. I helped a fellow diver continue enjoying her dives after she too complained of this problem. A few minutes later she was back in the Liquid Blue.

Considering my low back is vulnerable as well, there are times that diving aggravates that region and it tightens up. Diving is like lying on your stomach and raising your legs to gently kick. With the gear and tank around your torso this adds a lot of weight and extension to the low back. To combat the strain and to alleviate the muscle tightness I occasionally pull my finned legs towards my chest and perform flexion exercises.

Some motorcycles require the rider to pose in the same position. Similar to riding low on a bicycle to cut wind resistance, some youthful people ride the crotch-rockets. You know the bike you have to lay down on to ride. They go like a gazillion-miles-an-hour, and riders zip dangerously in between the cars. The head of one of these riders is in the same situation as a scuba diver's.

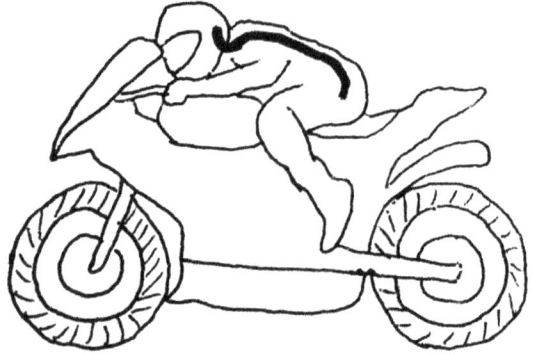

Because your body lies against the gas tank of the motorcycle you have to tip your head up and back to see where you are going. After a long ride this can cause a painful arrival.

Motorcycle riders are also susceptible to having their shoulders tighten up if they ride too long with their arms up and unsupported. You know the ones that Orange County Choppers make with the handlebars way up and out to the side so your arms are straight and elevated to control your ride.

As we age most of us feel more comfortable on an upright motorcycle such as a Harley Davidson. Then some enthusiasts ride the fancy bikes with the handle bars way up high. You may want to rethink this if you have a neck, arm or shoulder problem. It doesn't look too comfortable to me considering my shoulders, knowledge of human anatomy and steering. Whatever you ride, take breaks and find a way to relax the muscles. Get your motor running and head out on the highway, safely.

> *"When I was a kid my parents moved a lot, but I always found them."*
> – **Rodney Dangerfield**

Children
A LABOR OF LOVE

First off, no man could do it. I witnessed my wife deliver our two 10-pound sons naturally without drugs. That was like nothing I've ever seen. I would have cried uncle. She did it twice! Ladies, I tip my cap. For starters you have to endure up to a 30 pound belly, or more, that grows and puts a tremendous strain on your back. Granted it is slow growing so your muscles can strengthen and adapt; but the awkwardness and stress is undeniable. It changes every movement from the position you can relax in, to how you sleep and walk.

After checking with your OBGYN, see if you can strengthen your core muscles well before your delivery date. Training your body before getting pregnant is the best idea. It will help you deal with the additional stress on your body as the child grows within, and will help with your recovery and protect your back for years to come.

I'm not sure how parents contort their bodies to carry and feed their bundles of joy. They hold their babies and shift their upper torso to one side like someone cut them in half and shifted their waist two inches to one side. It reminds me of patients with a painful disc. Sometimes this is done for convenience of feeding and other times it is to keep one hand free for chores. They should be in Cirque du Soleil.

A good idea would be to switch arms so you can abuse both sides evenly. For instance, try not to always bottle feed with the right arm. Basically, you are curving the spine and straining your back and your muscles. Also try not to place too much pressure on one hip. You should attempt to stand straight instead of bent forward when you hold your little munchkin. Over long periods of time, like years of raising several kids, either of these positions may change your spine's natural curves and posture permanently.

I like the idea of the chest wrap, or backpacks and slings, to hold your child while you are running errands. Your hands are free and the little tyke gets to come along for the ride. Like any backpack you want to make sure the weight is close to the body and these carriers do the trick.

Picking up your child's bodyweight by reaching over the top of the crib will get old and painful. Cribs that allow the front to drop are great to minimize this stress, but some children have become trapped between this type of crib front and the mattress. Try to bend your knees if you can, but you will have to spread

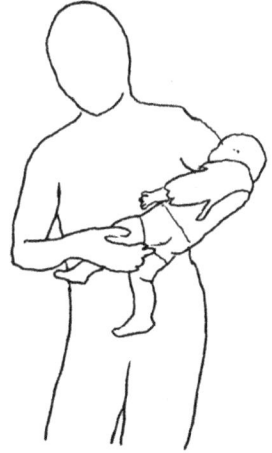

your knees to get close enough to the crib for it to be of any benefit. Hopefully they will stand up and come closer to you as well. I know how challenging it is raising kids. There into everything and require a ton of work and attention.

Sure we love our children, but they can put us through the ringer. Right, Mom? For the next five to 18 years, or more, you are responsible for a lot more work. When you need to go out and bring your child, forget the heavy purse and ever being on time. You have more weighty issues to deal with now. You have the snack and activity bag, the stroller or possibly the carrier to be your companions whenever you go somewhere. Help would be great.

When it comes time to load your kid into the car, get ready for lifting the 30-plus-pounds out in front of you, lifting far from your core muscles and in small confines, which can very difficult. Bend your knees the best you can to protect your back. Sometimes I even step into the car or kneel to take some of the twisting and bending motion out of the equation. Better yet, encourage them to climb up, with guidance, so you don't have to lift them into their car seats.

When you pick up a baby you have to carry their chunky thighs. They may only be 10 pounds now, but eventually they are going to grow. It would be wise to try to balance any weight you carry. For instance, put the snack bag on one shoulder and carry the child on the other side.

Some of the handles for the carriers are in a terrible spot. I've seen too many parents hobble in all contorted, lugging the source of their bodily pains on each arm. Currently the handles for carriers are in the middle of the portable seats. This forces parents to adjust by leaning sideways when carrying the weight. This awkward negotiation of balance and flexibility can strain the low back, your upper back and shoulders. That's a combination for bad posture and injury.

My colleague and I tried to change this design too. The handle would be on the side of the carrier and not in the middle. If you have the carrier in your right hand, the handle's side bracket should come up in a straight line so it is next to your leg. The bracket on the other side would be curved, to meet the bracket against your leg, and form a handle sort of like an "n." Sometimes the child would face forward; and, other times you would turn the carrier around so the handle could be next to your left leg. In that case, the child would face backwards. Otherwise the handle could be removed and snapped in again or slid to the opposite side, to reverse the grip, so the child would face forward on that side too.

This would allow the carrier to rest at your side and the handle would be turned 90 degrees. It would now be in the position that your hand would naturally fall if you put your arm at your side. This would reduce stress to the shoulder, neck and entire back. Any idea like this is now protected by this book.

I have also observed that some strollers have handles that make you lean forward because they are not long enough. Make sure you get one with adjustable handles so you are not hunched over and can walk upright. Otherwise you may look like Cro-Magnon man with his offspring.

Now after reading several sections in this book, people may think I want kids so they can do all of the chores around the house while I relax. That is simply not entirely true. Eventually, children should be able to clean their rooms. You don't need that responsibility too. See if you can make it a game or a contest. That way it becomes more fun than work. Yep, the old reverse psychology routine. Maybe give awards, points to redeem later for something cool or special snacks. Yes without flax seeds, tofu or soy.

The same discipline should go with the toys. Teach the kids to put away their toys when they are done using them, or before they go to sleep. That way you aren't bending to pick them up or tripping over them while venturing to the kitchen for a late night snack. Offer them an allowance if you feel like it. I never got one. I had a roof over my head and plenty of food. Helping with the chores was my duty as a member of the family because I was taken care of and had shelter. Good enough for me.

"Men are only clever at shifting blame from their own shoulders to those of others." – **Titus Livius**

A WEIGHT ON YOUR SHOULDERS

Well the kids are back in school and there are many relieved parents out there. Sorry "teach." But as the kids return to class there is one burden almost all of them will bear. It's not preparation for the state exam; it's the monster book bags they all carry.

A poll of the American Academy of Orthopedic Surgeons reported the continued exposure to such weight loads would impose postural problems and lead to damage to children's backs.

Pick up your kid's book bag sometime. Does it seem like it is too heavy? Watch them walk to the bus. Are they hunched or twisted? Now is the time to re-evaluate their book bag and what's in it to try to prevent them from developing back and neck pain.

I remember lugging my blue duffle bag filled with my sports gear and my books back and forth. Of course if I spent a little more time focused on school work in study hall, that could have minimized the work I needed to bring home, but I was also majoring in procrastination at the time.

The Consumer Product Safety Commission has estimated that more than 12,700 children ages five – 14 had to be treated for injuries caused by their book bags. They also reported 7,277 visits to the Emergency Room as a result of carrying book bags. They found back injuries related to back packs was up 330 percent since 1996.

This is extremely serious considering these stresses are applied to children who are growing. This is the most important time in spinal health and could be the start of life-long back or neck problems. An NIH study found students who use backpacks had an increase of back pain as they got older. Less than 10 percent of preteens had pain which then elevated to 50 percent in 15-16 year-olds

Damage to a growing spine, much like getting hit in sports like football or being involved in a motor vehicle accident, can have a negative affect for years to come. That's why I try to educate the public on how chiropractic can help resolve these issues early and prevent problems later in life.

An improperly loaded spine will cause stress and wear to be distributed to the back unevenly. A 2010 study published in the SPINE medical journal took MRI films of children with various weighted book bags. They found a direct relation between heavy book bags and changes in lumbar curvature and disc height.

It is easier to solve a spinal problem in the early stages rather than when your body has adapted and handled that stress for years. Fix the alignment of your car before you need to replace the brakes, rotors, calipers, etc, due to the continued uneven forces caused by driving your poorly aligned vehicle.

Just look at your children as they haul their back packs and are tipped forward, backwards or to the side. They aren't supposed to walk like Cro-Magnon man or Atlas with the world on his shoulders.

A study published in Ergonomics on how carrying book bags affects gait and posture in kids reported a clear alteration in posture and gait due to the daily stress of carrying book bags and athletic bags. They also found using one strap was far worse than when using two.

The American Academy of Physical Medicine and Rehabilitation brought to light a finding they observed in that carrying a heavy backpack can increase students' likelihood of falling. If the book bag weighs more than 25 percent of the students' body weight the researchers observed them experiencing difficulty opening doors and climbing stairs, which resulted in a greater potential for a risk of falls.

If the students managed a lower ratio of book bag to bodyweight they were much more stable and able to complete normal school tasks without difficulty. As the book bag climbed from weighing 5 percent of the students' bodyweight to 15 percent, their balance reduced. However they were far better off than those procrastinators bringing home all of their books and sports gear each night. Whoops!

We have all experienced this when we carry groceries in. How many of us load up one arm or both and then fumble with the keys and wobble; leaving marks on the walls or breaking bags open from swaying due to the unevenness of the weight? If you haven't, stop by. I sure could use some help the next time I bring groceries in.

One NIH study evaluated children ages 10 – 13 as they started by standing on a platform with and without their book bag and then stepped up to a high step and stepped back down. The first time the subject had no book bag. After that they carried a bag weighing 15 percent of the subject's bodyweight and then 20 percent.

They found that the greater forces apply to the students who carried the heaviest bags while stepping up and back down. But the stress wasn't only felt with each impact force; it was also compensated for in the spine.

The supervising researcher, Dr. Mary Ellen Franklin was quoted as reporting the following: *"Your body tries to keep the center of mass between the feet, so with a backpack, the trunk is in a more forward position, placing abnormal forces on the spine. This requires shifting the head forward ... but this would mean looking down. You compensate by bringing the head up, which makes part of the neck curve to a greater extent. It's very stressful on the neck."*

Parents usually only think that a heavy book bag can cause lower back pain but studies prove it can also affect the neck. The Associations between Adolescent Head-On-Neck Posture, Backpack Weight, and Anthropometric Features from *SPINE* reported a definite change in head and neck angle that was greatest in younger children while carrying book bags.

The School of Exercise and Sports Science in Australia noted an increased postural change in the neck and shoulder not solely due to the weight of the book bag but also the time it was carried.

Here is a summary of what the research and some common sense tells us about book bags.

Backpack/Book Bag Rules:
• Don't over pack. It shouldn't weigh more than 15 percent of his/her body-weight. A 50-pound child should carry no more than 7-8 pounds in their book bag, 75-pound child – 11-12 pound book bag, 100 pound child – 15 pound book bag, etc.
• Try to plan better so everything doesn't have to come home. Parents may be able to help determine what is needed or not.
• When you pack the bag use some thought to avoid heavy items on top or prevent shifting of items.

• Pick an appropriately sized bag for the size of your child so it isn't swinging around. The bigger the purse or house the more we pack into them.
• Get a pack with two shoulder straps to reduce shoulder pressure.
• Keep the majority of the weight around waist level. The higher the load is carried, like between the shoulder blades, the more likely it is to lead to more postural stress.
• Speak with your child about why it's important to use both straps.
• Instruct your child to lift the bag to put it on with their legs and to use two hands and face the bag.
• Using only one strap is similar to carrying a heavy purse. It can lead to the body shifting to one side, resulting in an elevated shoulder, neck pain, postural problems and back pain.
• Some backpacks have a waist strap to ensure that the weight stays low and close to the body.
• Look for red marks on your child's shoulder to determine if the book bag is positioned correctly or too heavy.
• If the weight is too high it will force your child to lean forward or it could pull him/her backwards and damage his/her lower back. I know they're not as cool as flinging a pack over one shoulder but I'm more about function and protecting the body versus what looks hot.
• Is it possible to get a ride or be picked up to decrease the amount of time the book bag is worn?
• Roller bags don't look cool and they can be really heavy without books. They can also be difficult to maneuver. As they get overloaded, who wants to pick that up and put it on the bus?
• Can they get some of their work done in a study hall and bring home less?
• Does the school have a program that offers books online, enabling students to complete their assignments at home with a computer?
• Can you borrow an extra book from school, or the library, to have at home so your student doesn't need to keep bringing their book back and forth each day?

So if the research states that not only is the weight of the book bag a factor, but also the position of it and the time it is carried, isn't it time we rethink this entire situation? Maybe there's a solution to protect your children's backs. See if you can make some changes to keep your children healthy and pain-free while they keep growing. Now is the time to make a difference.

> *"I am entirely certain that twenty years from now we will look back at education as it is practiced in most schools today and wonder that we could have tolerated anything so primitive."*
> **– John W. Gardner**

GOT NO CLASS

In classes across the world, every kid goes through this. The class is boring and they slouch in their seat. First, if you have a big kid, make sure the chair fits him/her. I have a patient who is 6' 8" and he has adjustable seats at his school. Otherwise he might never fit in a standard seat. The same goes for a small child. If there aren't smaller chairs, provide a box so he/she can put his/her feet on it.

When children slouch in their chairs it is like the driver of a car with the seat too far backwards. Their lower backs lose the normal lordotic curve and become reversed and rounded. Anytime you change the curve, you change your posture for the worse. The bad part of this change for children is that this is the most vulnerable time in their lives because they are growing and their bodies are changing. Slouching in class followed by a few tackles in recess can start a problem that grows with your child.

The midback region will increase its curve because the body is bent forward and is necessary to keep the head upright. Otherwise they would be reclining. The head will also move forward and start to reverse the neck curve. This is the position that brings the ears in front of the shoulders. Kids already have the computer monitor and game consoles doing that to them.

> *"Anybody who watches three games of football in a row should be declared brain dead."*
> **– Erma Bombeck**

PLAY IT AGAIN SAM

Again the TV set and computer screen are on my *"Use in Limited Quantities and Be Careful"* list. Too many hours on the couch in front of the TV, or playing a computer game, can lead to forward head carriage, headaches, neck and eye strain. In addition to that, too much sitting can cause hemorrhoids. Think about that for a minute.

Even though we can see the video screen we still tend to bring our heads forward and lean our bodies toward the game. I know, I catch myself doing it when I am typing. It's really not much different from Internet surfers and chronic E-mailers. Over time your body will acclimate to this position and remain there. Kids and many adult males like to play games on the computer. Thanks to the World Wide Web, you can play against friends at your house, friends who live across town and even strangers across the Internet.

I have played a few games with and against complete strangers where you run around and shoot at each other. It is a riot. You can have conversations and cheer on your teammates and before you know it, four hours have passed. The back, neck and eyes get real sore. So does the trigger finger. So I am familiar with the aches and pains that come with playing a game for hours.

In addition to the temptation of gaming with a computer, kids, and many adults, want a PS3 or Xbox 360 so they can play games with their friends. There are hundreds of games to choose from, and many hours and days of creativity, imagination and exercise can be lost in the technology vacuum.

When I was a kid I was gone at daylight and returned, with some prodding, for dinner. We ran around, explored and played outdoor games all day, every day. That is why I was thin and able to consume a 5-pound tub of peanut butter each week in the form of inch and a half thick fluffernutter sandwiches. In addition to that, during those growing phases my weekend diet included almost the entire box of Cheerios or a loaf of whole wheat, French toast (made with 8 or so eggs, milk and full calorie syrup) for an approximate total of 3,000 – 4,000 calories for breakfast alone. I was an eating machine.

I know the eating habits of a growing child remain the same. It's a challenge to keep the refrigerator stocked. The fact that too many kids now only exercise their fingers on a keyboard is part of the reason so many children are over-weight. Allow a certain number of hours they can play computer games each week. All kids go through the, *"engulf-the-refrigerator"* stage, in their teenage years. Parents need to make sure they are working it off.

One of the funniest disciplinary actions I heard from a relative was that when a child in the family was bored or misbehaved, he/she had to move a pile of rocks from one area of the property to another. Now this could help build muscle, change a kid's habits and incorporate some needed exercise. I'm not saying to buy a pallet of stones and make your kid work, it was just a funny story about exercise and discipline.

"If winning isn't everything, why do they keep score?" – **Vince Lombardi**

SCORE ONE FOR THE GIPPER

There are some great computer games to get your kids off the couch now and these should be welcomed, as long as their schoolwork comes first. I mentioned the boxing game before but another great one is Dance, Dance Revolution (DDR). It has kids and adults sweating as they try to keep up with the programmed dance steps. It's tough and fun for the whole family. It might even get more boys to dance when they go to dances or later when they get married.

There was just a recent DDR competition in a mall in my town. Lots of kids danced the night away in the event. The *"winner,"* and I use this word gingerly, was a 30-year-old who lives at home with his Mom. Okay … just playing games can create other issues to be aware of, but I won't get into them any further in this book.

There are also computer games like the Nintendo Wii that require you to hold a controller from the game console or Microsoft's Kinect, that doesn't. Each registers your movement and simulates the movement using characters in the game. You could be boxing against Sugar Ray or trying to hit a Nolan Ryan fastball, as you swing your arms. At least this gets kids moving, is less mindless and burns calories. In the old days, we had things like that too. It was called getting our butts outside and playing with the neighbors. It's good for social interaction skills as well.

When a child plays a hand-held game and it is in their lap. He/she is reversing the curve of his/her growing neck by looking down constantly. If children must play, try to get them to elevate the game. Put it on a pillow, on a table or have them rest their elbows on the chair and hold the game in front of them. It can reduce shoulder stress to the muscles of the upper back and neck as well. Make sure they sit back in their chair too so they don't round their backs.

This idea has other great uses in our daily lives. It is an excellent position for reading books, working on crossroad puzzles or knitting. There are even book easels so your eyes can focus more directly and there is less strain and neck bending.

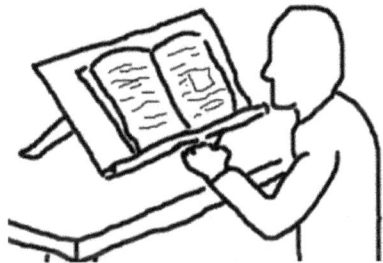

My patient Dorothy had been sewing for years and she had permanently curved her neck like a candy cane. She could not lift her chin up high and was always lifting her eyebrows and lids to see in front of her. This is why it is important to raise the projects, or things you are doing, causing minimal stress and long-term postural changes to your spine.

"Children are the only form of immortality that we can be sure of." – **Peter Ustinov**

THE WAY OF THE FUTURE

When I was a child my sleep was a bit restless. A few times I fell out of the bed and never woke up. It was not uncommon to find me on the floor in the morning or with my feet on my pillow. Kids move all around when they sleep and the habits they establish now may carry over into adulthood. Many men wind up sleeping on the couch, or in the doghouse, as they get older.

There are some dangers for kids when they sleep improperly. We have already covered the benefits to sleeping on your back and side for your health and posture. The same applies to our kids. Check on them at night. See if they have made their way to the floor or if they are contorted at the base of the mattress. Make sure they don't sleep on their stomachs, or with their arms over their heads.

I have young patients who complain of the same ailments adults do. Parents should check the quality of support their children's mattresses provide them. They also need a good surface to sleep on. Please don't just give them the old one. A soft mattress can deform their spines and is harmful as they grow.

Children also fall asleep in car carriers and strollers. For the sake of their necks, try to prevent their heads from flopping over. You could put a blanket up against the head to bring it back to the midline. Some seats have some kind of neck support. There are a lot of options in the form of pillow/supports to help protect your child's neck.

If you ever notice something unusual about the way your child is standing, leaning or holding a shoulder up, take him/her to a qualified professional who understands the body and its mechanics. Addressing the problem early can help eliminate a problem that could last a lifetime.

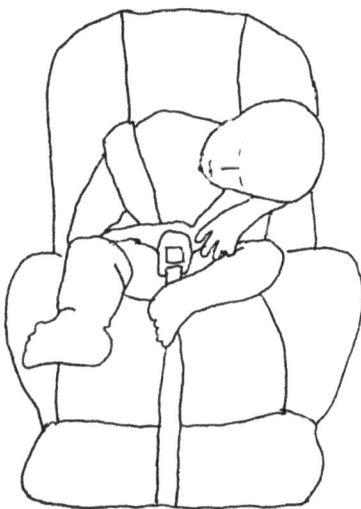

> *"Nothing in all the world is more dangerous than sincere ignorance and conscientious stupidity."* – **Martin Luther King, Jr.**

Activities I don't like.

Over the years I have seen hundreds of people working out incorrectly. I never know if it is rude to try to tell them how to do something safely; or that they are going to hurt themselves over time. I have seen people exhibit terrible form, attempt to lift too much weight and demonstrate inexperience at its worst. I made most of these mistakes myself.

When I was in high school I did biceps curls with a straight bar. Now they recommend against this because it keeps your shoulder in a vulnerable position. I never read the research on the proper techniques of safe lifting because I thought I knew it all at 15.

In college I was a prime example of someone using dreadful form. I used 62-pound dumbbells for curls and everything else. I was strong, but I was stupid and probably added to the shoulder injuries I feel now. Learn from my mistakes and lift wisely. It is better to know what you are doing than to injure yourself with inexperience.

> *"We live in a time when the words impossible and unsolvable are no longer part of the scientific community's vocabulary. Each day we move closer to trials that will not just minimize the symptoms of disease and injury but eliminate them."*
> **- Christopher Reeve**

THAT'S GONNA LEAVE A MARK

Hey, who doesn't like to go to an amusement park? I love the roller coasters. Spending some quality time outdoors getting the crap scared out of me on a ride and eating food I typically don't consume on a regular basis is a great way to pass time together with family and friends. It's okay to take a break and indulge a little. I tried a deep-fried Oreo once. It was nothing great but I wanted to feel what 500 calories felt like as it slid toward my stomach.

Anyway, some of the activities at the park, although enjoyable, may wreak havoc on our spines today and our posture later. I'm not going to ruin all of your fun I just want to mention a few of the nastiest ones to help keep your family trip pleasurable and uneventful.

I want you to come home in one piece without any new aches or pains. I was just at Universal Studios for my first time and was ecstatic about some of the rides. They are awesome! From my earlier visits to other parks I learned a valuable lesson. Keep your head against the headrest before the ride starts and bolts away. Even with that precaution, the one type of coaster I avoid at all costs is the old wooden kind. I know because I was on one once and had a stiff neck for a few days after.

That basket of wood and Elmer's glue is the most rickety and jarring ride ever created. I'm all for history and how it all started, but not when you need to bring bags of cotton candy to support your neck. These coasters bang you side-to-side, making you feel like you went a few rounds with Muhammad Ali. That's whiplash. The muscles and bones of your neck get strained. You don't need that problem when you are trying to keep two kids happy at the park.

Another popular ride at amusement parks lurks in the confines of dimly lit shadows just waiting to injure unsuspecting riders. If you really want to add to your neck problems, just jump on the chiro-practic nightmare known as the bumper cars. When isn't it a great idea for the whole family to enjoy ramming motorized cars into unsuspecting strangers and each other from all angles? *"Hey I really got little Tori. She looks like she might be crying. Wow that was fun, Dad. Can we do it again?"*

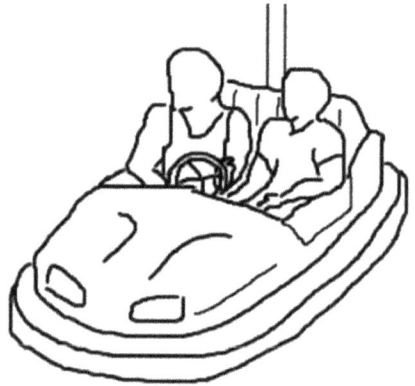

This ride mimics a motor vehicle accident and remember the human body sustains damage with an impact of just 2.5 mph.[18] It is a prime cause for headaches and neck problems in kids. If you decide to ride this torture device, make sure you and your child are okay afterwards. I'm not sure who invented this ride but he or she was probably related to the guy who invented the inflatable dartboard or waterproof towel.

> *"Experience is that marvelous thing that enables you to recognize a mistake when you make it again."* – **Franklin P. Jones**

I WOULDN'T DO THAT IF I WERE YOU

More and more families like to tempt fate and purchase trampolines for their children. First, you need a protective net so you don't appear on America's Funniest Home Videos falling off, banging your head into a tree or getting stuck inside the rim as you try to dunk a basketball. Seen 'em all.

Second, don't invite the whole family on board. This isn't a dance floor. When you jump you are expecting the trampoline to be at a certain level. If someone else is bouncing in a different rhythm, the trampoline may be lower from what you would normally expect when you are jumping alone. When you do land it can jam your body or send you flying into the bushes.

Make sure the unit is assembled correctly and in a secure, level location.

Check and recheck hooks, springs and pads regularly. Never jump on to the trampoline from a higher surface and don't jump off to dismount. If you don't have someone videotaping this agony of de-feet, neck and back, stop and climb off. You don't jump out of a moving car do you? There is no need to try crazy flips and somersaults. That is best done with professional help and supervision. Flipping is asking for trouble.

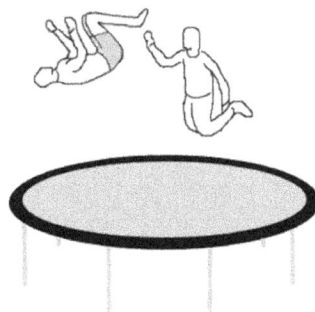

I have two friends who used to jump on trampolines. Both flipped and landed on their necks because they didn't follow some of the recommendations from above. One is a doctor and the other is a CEO of her own business. Both were lucky to not have killed themselves or damaged their spinal cords. They had only fractured their necks and had to have surgery to correct the problem. They were millimeters away from paralysis.

I have had kids of all ages complain of aches and tightness after bouncing and distorting their bodies on trampolines. As with any activity, talk to your children and the neighborhood kids about the dangers and set specific house rules. If you can, keep an eye on them, just like when they're swimming. Make sure they let you know if anything happens or someone gets hurt.

A few months ago we visited our neighbors who wer out playing and yes, they have a small trampoline. My oldest wanted to get on it and reluctantly I let him and gave him some instructions. The parent listened and then told me they just let the kids all jump at the same time so I pointed out the white warning on the safety net.

Soon after my youngest wanted a turn. He went up and the neighbors' youngest daughter wanted to go too. Somehow I let them go for it. In a minute my son was on his back and the girl was jumping violently watching my son flop like a fish out of water crying. In another moment of weakness both boys wanted to get on together and within two minutes they collided heads. Now I'm done.

Hey remember jumping off the swing set? How about trying to go as high as you could? Now who tried to jump off when the swing was pretty high? I did. I forget what my excuse was for tearing up and dirtying my school clothes. I know I almost landed in the monkey bars. Even though you may have dabbled in *"Evil Knievelism,"* take the time to convince your kids not to do the silly things you did when you were young. Unless, perhaps you like driving and waiting in the Emergency Rooms.

I was a kid. I listened about 60 percent of the time and followed through about 30 percent, on a good day. The way I saw it, that was like hitting .300 in baseball. And that was enough to get you into the Hall of Fame in Cooperstown.

> *"The object of all health education is to change the conduct of individual men, women, and children by teaching them to care for their bodies well, and this instruction should be given throughout the entire period of their educational life."* – **Charles H. Mayo, M.D.**

Final Thoughts

Well I have thoroughly enjoyed writing this book with all my ranting and raving. I truly hope you found it enlightening, inspiring and fun. Life is about family, love, great experiences, health and friends. It is impossible to change everything we do because most of us are set in our ways, but changing a few things here or there can really make a difference in your health. This old dog has learned a few new tricks. So can you.

Think about some of the ideas and information I have written about. Each topic can potentially prevent you from experiencing debilitating pains from your back, muscles and everywhere in between. By gaining a better understanding of your body and how it works, you can make any number of changes that could radically affect your present and future health.

If I can help inspire and teach one person to take better care of his or her posture; and the importance of proper exercise and nutrition and everything associated with it, I will be satisfied. Great health is yours for the taking.

> *"I find that a great part of the information I have was acquired by looking up something and finding something else on the way."* – **Franklin P. Adams**

THE BROADER SPECTRUM

Some people mistakenly believe that having money is the key to all happiness, but we have learned there is something more valuable. A large house or fancy cars won't help your health if you haven't cared for it. How many rich and famous stars are in rehab, divorced in four months, or abuse drugs to deal with their fame? They just get a prettier coffin and more paparazzi. They've got too many problems.

Look around you and be appreciative of what you have, and do not be upset about what you don't. We all have more than most.

When you have a child, you hope for a healthy baby. Boy or girl is a second consideration. Without your health, life is complicated and trying. Every time you think things are bad or you just can't get ahead, take a look around you. So many people have greater battles and health challenges than we do. Do your problems equal theirs? Put things into perspective.

Stop looking in and start looking out. If you have your health you have everything. So many people take their health for granted; some abuse their bodies with bad habits, while others simply realize its importance too late. Some were never given the opportunity to experience it at all, or lost their health for an extended period of time, like kids suffering from debilitating diseases. A child should never know pain like that without getting a chance to experience the world.

Take time to enjoy life and your health. *"All work and no play makes Jack a dull boy."* We have to take the opportunity to seek out life's great experiences. There are so many magical places to go alone, or with family. Make time. It is therapeutic for you and can really help a family bond. I had to learn this too. A brief change from the norm can rejuvenate you and recharge your system. It can enhance work, play, your relationships and of course, your health.

The Framingham Heart Study reported that men with cardiovascular conditions, who took more vacations, lived longer. We all know how great it is to get away but often that feeling vanishes when we return to normal life. This study proves there is still a benefit to escaping for a break no matter how long or how frequently.

Go explore some of the fantastic parks, the wonders of the world, museums, mountains, deserts, waterfalls, sporting events, or go camping. Life is waiting. It doesn't matter what age you are. Get out there and enjoy it. And, it's exercise.

While you're out adventuring, try to smile a little more and treat others like you wish to be treated. One study was able to predict from yearbook photos which women would live longer, solely based on their smiles.

I love having conversations with everyone from the CEO to the janitor, the baggage checker to the policeman. They are all human. People just want to be recognized and acknowledged.

They have important lives and are people just like you. They deserve some respect. I just thanked a security guard for watching the vehicles at an all-night store. Yeah he gets paid to do it but it's a terribly boring job. He was appreciative of the gesture and we had a pleasant two-minute conversation.

Saying hello or being light-hearted can brighten someone's day. My wife and I just returned a *"clear glass"* potpourri-looking thing to a store. When the guy asked why we were returning it I told him, *"She didn't like the color."* He got a kick out of the comment, and we all smiled and laughed.

Recently I listened as a clerk at a video store was telling an older gentleman to watch *"Balboa"* with the alternative ending because it gives a different feel to the movie. The clerk was basically critiquing the movie for him and the gentleman was slightly puzzled.

I had to chime in regarding my rental of *"Lady in the Water."* I told the gentleman that if you watch *"this movie"* with the alternate beginning, it's actually a man in the water. I thought that was hilarious. Like Jerry Seinfeld, I never run out of wise cracks. Studies have shown there are real health benefits to positive thinking and laughter. Maybe you should get crackin'.

> *"Have no fear of perfection - you'll never reach it."* – **Salvador Dali**

EMBRACING OUR IMPERFECTIONS

Be thankful for the loved ones around you. Do not take them, or anything else, for granted. It can be ripped from you in an instant. Cherish each moment. Life is precious. We all have been blessed with a great group of friends who have been there to help us through the good times and more importantly the bad times. Who are your friends and what do they mean to you? Have you told them? Maybe it's time.

Sometimes we don't get to talk to them as often as we would like or don't see each other as regularly, because life draws us in all directions. But you know that there is a cardinal rule: they will be there for you and you will be there for them if you ever need one another. Let them know they are treasured and don't forget to say *"thank you."* Make it a point to say thank you for all the years of their support. Sadly most of us only find the time for friendly gatherings when there's either a wedding or a funeral.

Those two words could probably be repeated to a lot of people we know. Take the time to let others know how you feel about them and what their love and friendship means to you. Let them know they are appreciated. Sincere gratitude can improve your positive thinking, energy and even improve your health.

I just listened to a story about a great guitarist named Steve Lukather who lost one of his best friends suddenly. They were in the band Toto together and Jeff was their unbelievable drummer. The last thing they said to each other on the phone one day earlier was, *"I love you man."*

In the precious words of Leo Buscaglia, *"There is nothing greater in life than loving another and being loved in return, for loving is the ultimate of experiences."* That applies to lovers and great friends.

Many spouses could look at their relationships and realize they are critical of stupid things when they are ignoring the fact that someone has granted them their heart. What greater honor or privilege is there then to offer someone your love and commitment? Relations are never easy and they are far from perfect.

Sometimes when you think the grass might be greener, you only find a cow pasture. The CDC has found people in happy relations were healthier across the board, regardless of race, sex or age. So take your sweetie out for a nice healthy walk and hold hands.

We all have idiosyncrasies or quirks. Someone else might seem really great because they give you attention, but I would bet you in a matter of time you will be in a similar situation. Guys have their sports and inability-to-communicate genes, while women have shoe needs and want-to-talk genes. It's almost a lock. I'm over-generalizing and kidding.

Maybe if you put a little more focus into your relationship with that someone special, the one with your ring on their finger, you would find there is no room for anyone else to even step into that space. Howard Stern once said something like, *"In every situation always act like your significant other is with you."* Think about it. That is a great concept. Become a team again and support each other's aspirations and dreams.

Have they changed over the years? If you wish your spouse was in better shape, go workout together and start eating healthier. Maybe you have grown apart by enjoying different hobbies. That's fine. Find one or two you can share. Everybody needs a little time for themselves. Remember the common goal. It will be a better ride. Whether together or alone, research is proving when we are happy, we are healthier individuals.

If you have kids, the relationship road is even more difficult. Those little monkeys limit the quality time you share together and you will need a maximal effort to stay on track. Remember those beautiful moments, intimacy and memories, which originally made you inseparable? I hope so, because now you will need to schedule a date night to escape and rediscover each other?

Sometimes we wake up at 4am and have wonderful discussions, without any interruptions, but those kids are still our greatest creation.

And when the kids leave for college you better have salvaged some type of bond because the house will be empty with only the two of you. That is until they move back in, live in your basement and eat you out of house and home, again. Ah ... good times. It's a crazy ride.

Take some of these ideas throughout this book and try to implement them in your life in any way you see fit. If I can change one bad habit, get one person off the couch, or make someone realize their health is the most important gift they do have control over; then the fact that my butt hurts from sitting down for so many years writing this book, is worth it. Stay well my friends. Stay happy. Don't forget to smile and sit up straight. **Isn't it time you were Back At Your Best!**

"Tomorrow is the most important thing in life. Comes into us at midnight very clean. It's perfect when it arrives and it puts itself in our hands. It hopes we've learned something from yesterday." – **John Wayne**

Quick Reference Words

Abduction – Moving away from your body's midline. Like raising your arm out to the side.

Adduction – Moving toward the body. You are **add**ing to it. Like bringing your arm back down.

Anterior – The front of the human body. *"See **ants** in front of me."*

Biomechanics – Understanding the laws of motion and applying them to the motion of the human body.

Cervical – The 7 vertebral bones that make up the spine in the neck.

Concentric Movement – Shortening or contracting a muscle, like making a muscle with your upper arm.

Disc – Shocking absorbing space in between your vertebrae that is filled with fluid.

Eccentric Movement – Elongating a muscle as you lower the weight before your next repetition.

Extension – Bending backwards. *"When you bend over **backwards** for someone you over-**extend** yourself."* A movement increasing the angle between two body parts, like straightening the arm to point.

Flexion – Bending forward. Bringing the knees to chest. *"**F**orward **F**lexion."* A movement that decreases the angle between two body parts, like making a muscle with your arm.

Hypertonicity – Extremely tight muscle, whereas, Hypotonicity is too relaxed.

Inferior – Below the middle. *"An **inferior** product is of **less** quality."*

Kyphosis – The rounding curve of your mid back. It bows away from you. **Hyper**-too much curve. **Hypo**-too little.

Lateral – Bending or moving to one side or the other. Also moving further away from your midline and moving to the right or left.

Ligament – The structure attaching bone to bone, like the ACL in the knee.

Lordosis – The curve of your neck and low back that curves into your body.

Lumbar – The 5 vertebral bones that make up the spine in the low back.

Metabolism – The rate at which your body processes, utilizes and transports food through the body.

Midline – An imaginary line from the nose through your belly button that divides your body into right and left.

Musculoskeletal System – The combination of the muscular system, which incorporates the muscles that provide motion to the joints and the skeletal system, which are the bones, ligaments and tendons of the body.

Posterior – The back of the human body. *"The **posts** are in the back."*

Posture – The normal positioning of your body that affects the health of your body, how it functions and how stress is distributed throughout the spine.

Pronation – Turning the hand or foot outward.

Radiculopathy – Pain radiating or travelling down your legs or arms

----

Sciatica – Pressure on a large group of nerves bringing information to your lower body.

Spine – The 24 moveable bones that move together to provide motion and still protect the spinal cord.

Superior – Above the middle. *"If it is **super** then it is **above** the rest."*

Supination – Turning the hand or foot inward. Hands turn in and *"cup"* as if to hold soup.

Tendon – The structure attaching muscle to bone, like the Achilles tendon.

The ME Principle – You can eat whatever you want, in **Moderation**, with a steady diet of **Exercise**.

Thoracic – The 12 vertebral bones that make up the spine in the mid back.

Trigger Points – Knots that form in the muscles and can cause pain.

Vertebra – Referring to the individual bones making up the spine. Plural version is vertebrae.

References

1. Konno Y. *The effects of relaxation and postural training on external perception: Improvement of visual acuity, visual field, and hearing acuity.* Abstract - Japanese Psychological Research 1997; 119.

2. Lennon J, Shealy CN, Cady RK, Matta W, Cox W, Simpson WF. *Postural and Respiratory Modulation of Autonomic Function, Pain, and Health.* Amer J Pain Man 1994; 4(1): 32-35.

3. White AH, Anderson R: *Conservative Care of Low Back Pain.* Baltimore, Williams & Wilkins, pp. 427-434, 1991.

4. Nachemson A. *Disc pressure measurements.* Spine 1981; 6:93-7.

5. Mayo Clinic; November 3, 2000.

6. Taptagaporn S. *Occupational Back Pain.* Occupational Health 1999; Volume 2 (9).

7. Bullock-Saxton J: *Postural alignment in standing: a repeatability study.* Austr J Physiother 1993; 39:25-9.

8. Cailliet R: *Soft Tissue Pain and Disability*, 2nd ed. Philadelphia: FA Davis, 1988:13.

9. Curl D: *Chiropractic Approach to Head Pain.* Baltimore, Williams & Wilkins, 1994.

10. Mannix LK. *Epidemiology and impact of primary headache disorders.* Medical Clinics of North America 2001; 85(4):887-95.

11. Sternbach RA. *Pain and "hassles" in the United States: findings of the Nuprin pain report.* Pain 1986; 27:69-80.

12. Hu XH, Markson LE, Lipton RB, Stewart WF, Berger ML. *Burden of migraine in the United States: disability and economic costs.* Arch Intern Med 1999; 159:813-8.

13. Schwartz et al. *Epidemiology of tension-type headache.* JAMA 1998; 279:381-3.

14. Lipton et al. *Prevalence and burden of migraine in the United States. Data from the American Migraine Study II.* Headache 2001; 41:646-57.

15. Slipman et al. *Therapeutic zygapophyseal joint injections for headaches emanating from the C2-C3 joint.* Am J Phys Med Rehabil 2001; 80(3):182-8.

16. Foreman SM, Croft AC. *Whiplash Injuries: The Cervical Acceleration / Deceleration Syndrome.* Baltimore, Williams and Wilkins, 1988.

17. Severy DM, Mathewson JH, Bechtol, CO. *Controlled automobile rear-end collisions, an investigation of related engineering and mechanical phenomenon.* Can Services Med J 1955.11:727-58.

18. Davis CG. *Low Speed Rear End Impacts: Vehicle and Occupant Response.* J Manipulative Physiol Ther 1998; 21(1):629–639

19. Troyanovich, J Manip Physio Ther 1998.

20. Frank C, Amiel D, Woo SL-Y. *Normal ligament properties and ligament healing.* Clin Orthop 1985; 196:15-25.

21. Kaneoka et al. *Motion analysis of cervical vertebrae during whiplash loading.* Spine 1999; 24(8): 763-70.

22. Bogduk N, Yoganandan N. *Biomechanics of the cervical spine Part 3: minor injuries.* Clinical Biomechanics 2001; 16(4):267-75.

23. Carette S. *Whiplash Injury and Chronic Neck Pain (editorial).* New Engl J Med 1994; 330:1083-4.

24. Radanov BP, Sturzenegger M, DiStefano G. *Long-term outcome after whiplash injury.* Medicine 1995; 74:281-97.

25. Barnsley L, Lord S, Bogduk N. *The pathophysiology of whiplash 1993.*

26. Kaneoka et al. *Motion analysis of cervical vertebrae during whiplash loading.* Spine 1999; 24(8): 763-70.

27. Grauer et al. *Whiplash produces an S-shaped curvature of the neck with hyperextension at lower levels.* Spine 1977; 22(21): 2489-94.

28. Bogduk N. *Point of View.* Spine 1999; 24(8):771

29. Hohl M. *Soft tissue injuries of the neck in automobile accidents: factors influencing prognosis.* J Bone Joint Surg 1974; 56A(8):1675-82.

30. Adams MA, Hutton WC. *The Effect of Posture on the Fluid Content of Lumbar Intervertebral Discs.* Spine 1983; 8:665-671.

31. Shiraz-Adl. *Finite-Element Stimulation of Changes in the fluid Content of Human Lumbar Discs – Mechanical and Clinical Implications.* Spine 1992; 17:206-12.

32. Moore et al. *Osteoarthrosis of the Facet Joints Resulting From Annular Rim Lesions in Sheep Lumbar Discs.* Spine 1999; 24(6):519-25.

33. Kirkaldy-Willis WH. *Managing Low Back Pain.* New York: Churchill Livingstone, 1993.

34. Dvorak J, Dvorak V. Manual Medicine. *Diagnostics.* New York: Thieme Medical Publishers Inc., 1990.

35. Whita AA, Panjabi MM. *Clinical Biomechanics of the Spine.* 2nd ed. Philadelphia: JB Lippincott Co 1990.

36. Bogduk N, Amevo B, Pearcy M. *A biological basis for instantaneous centers of rotation of the vertebral column.* Proc Inst Mech Eng 1995; 209:177-83.

37. Taptagaporn S. *Occupational Back Pain.* Occupational Health 1999; Volume 2 (9).

38. Wilke H-J, Neef P, Caimi M, Hoogland T, and Claes LE, *Intradiscal Pressure Values for Different Positions and Exercises.* Spine 24, 1999; 8:755-762.

39. McNally DS, Adams MA. *Internal Intervertebral Disc Mechanics as Revealed by Stress Profilometry.* Spine 1992; 17:66-73.

40. McNally DS, Shackleford IM, Goodship AE, Mulholland RC. *In vivo stress measurement can predict pain on discography.* Spine 1996; 21:2580-7.

41. Kraemer J, Kolditz D, Gowin R. *Water and Electrolyte Content of Human Intervertebral Discs Under Variable Load.* Spine 1985; 10:69-71.

42. Adams MA, Dolan P. *Recent advances in lumbar spinal mechanics and their clinical significance.* Clin Biomech 1995; 10:3-19.

43. Handa T et al. *Effects of hydrostatic pressure on matrix synthesis and matrix metalloproteinase production in the human lumbar IVD.* Spine 1997; 22:1085-91.

44. Virri et al. *Prevalence, morphology, topography of blood vessels in herniated disc tissue. A comparative immunocytochemical study.* Spine 1996; 21(16):1856-63.

45. Kauppila L. *Ingrowth of Blood Vessels in Disc Degeneration.* Bone Joint Surg 1995; 77A:26-31.

46. Carreon et al. *Histologic changes in the disc after cervical spine trauma: evidence of disc absorption.* J Spinal Disord 1996; 9(4):313-6.

47. Horst M, Brinckman P. *Measurement of the distribution of axial stress on the end plate of the vertebral body.* Spine 1981; 6:217-31.

48. Shiraz-Adl. *Finite-Element Stimulation of Changes in the fluid Content of Human Lumbar Discs – Mechanical and Clinical Implications.* Spine 1992; 17:206-12.

49. Bogduk N, Twomey LT. *Clinical Anatomy of the Lumbar Spine.* 2nd ed. Melbourne: Churchill Livingstone 1991.

50. Kendall FP, McCreary EK. *Muscles, Testing and Function.* 3rd ed. Baltimore: Williams and Wilkins 1983.

51. Travell JG, Simons DG. *Myofascial Pain and Dysfunction. The Trigger Point Manual.* Baltimore: Williams and Wilkins 1983.

52. U.S. Department of Health and Human Services, Centers for Disease Control and Prevention, Coordinating Center for Health Promotion, National Center for Chronic Disease Prevention and Health Promotion, Office on Smoking and Health. *The Health Consequences of Involuntary Exposure to Tobacco Smoke: A Report of the Surgeon General.* Atlanta, Georgia 2006.

53. Centers for Disease Control and Prevention. *Cigarette Smoking-Attributable Mortality and Years of Potential Life Lost—United States, 1990. Morbidity and Mortality Weekly Report [serial online].* 1993;42(33):645–649 [cited 2006 Sep 23].

54. Glantz, S. Tobacco: *Biology and Politics.* Health Edco, Waco TX. 1992

55. EPA Report. *Respiratory Health Effects of Passive Smoking.* 1992.

56. CDC. *Smoking-attributable mortality, years of potential life lost, and economic costs---United States, 1995--1999.* MMWR 2002; 51:300--3.

57. Mokdad AH, Marks JS, Stroup DF, Gerberding JL. *Actual Causes of Death in the United States, 2000.* JAMA 2004; 291:1238-1245.

58. Aligne CA, Stoddard JJ. *Tobacco and children. An economic evaluation of the medical effects of parental smoking.* Archives of Pediatrics and Adolescent Medicine 1997; 151: 648 - 653.

59. American Cancer Society

60. American Lung Association

61. Whitaker RC, Wright JA, Pepe MS, Seidel KD, Dietz WH. *Predicting obesity in young adulthood from childhood and parental obesity.* N Engl J Med 1997;337:869-73.

62. Finkelstein EA, Fiebelkorn IC, Wang G. *National Medical Spending Attributable To Overweight And Obesity: How Much, And Who's Paying? Health Affairs.* The Policy Journal of the Health Sphere 2003; 23(3): 219-26.

63. Mokdad AH, Marks JS, Stroup DF, Gerberding JL. *Actual Causes of Death in the United States, 2000.* JAMA 2004; 291:1238-1245.

64. Mokdad AH, Ford ES, Bowman BA, et al. *Prevalence of obesity, diabetes, and obesity-related health risk factors, 2001.* J Amer Med Assoc 2003; 289(1):76-79.

65. Sturm R. *The Effects of Obesity, Smoking, and Problem Drinking on Chronic Medical Problems and Health Care Costs.* Health Affairs 2002; 21(2):245-253.

66. Sturm R, Wells KB. *Does Obesity Contribute As Much to Morbidity As Poverty or Smoking?* Public Health. 2001; 115:229-295.

67. Wattigney WA, Harsha DW, Srinivasan SR, Webber LS, Berenson GS. *Increasing impact of obesity on serum lipids and lipoproteins in young adults. The Bogalusa Heart Study.* Arch Intern Med 1991;151: 2017-22.

68. McMurray RG, Harrel JS, Levine AA, Gansky SA. *Childhood obesity elevates blood pressure and total cholesterol independent of physical activity.* Int J Obes Relat Metab Disord 1995;19:881-6.

69. Berenson GS, Srinivasan SR, Wattigney WA, Harsha DW. *Obesity and cardiovascular risk in children.* Ann N Y Acad Sci 1993;699:93-103.

70. Rosenbloom AL, Joe JR, Young RS, Winter WE. *Emerging epidemic of type 2 diabetes in youth.* Diabetes Care 1999; 22(2):345-354.

71. Venkat Narayan KM, Boyle JP, Thompson TJ, Sorensen SW, Williamson DF. *Lifetime risk for diabetes mellitus in the United States.* Journal of the American Medical Association 2003; 290(14): 1884-1890.

72. The Center for Disease Control and Prevention (CDC)

73. Ferraro KF, Thorpe RJ Jr, Wilkinson JA. *The life course of severe obesity: Does childhood overweight matter?* Journal of Gerontology 2003; 58B(2):S110-S119.

74. Freedman DS, Khan LK, Dietz WH, Srinivasan SR, Berenson GS. *Relationship of childhood obesity to coronary heart disease risk factors in adulthood: the Bogalusa Heart Study.* Pediatrics 2001; 108(3):712-18.

75. Epstein LH, Wing RR, Valoski A. *Childhood obesity.* Pediatr Clin North Am 1985;32:363-79.

76. Malina RM. *Ethnic variation in the prevalence of obesity in North American children and youth.* Crit Rev Food Sci Nutr 1993;33:389-96.

77. Kavey RW, Daniels SR, Lauer RM, Atkins DL, Hayman LL, Taubert K. *American Heart Association guidelines for primary prevention of atherosclerotic cardiovascular disease beginning in childhood.* Journal of Pediatrics 2003; 142(4):368-372.

78. U.S. Department of Health and Human Services. *Bone Health and Osteo porosis: A Report of the Surgeon General.* Rockville, MD: Department of Health and Humans Services, Office of the Surgeon General, 2004.

79. Wyshak G. *Teenage girls, carbonated beverage consumption, and bone fractures.* Arch Pediatr Adolesc Med. 2000; 154 (6):610-613.

80. Jacobson M. *Liquid Candy.* The Center for Science in the Public Interest 2005.

81. Schulze MB, Manson JE, Ludwig DS, et al. *Sugar-sweetened beverages, weight gain, and incidence of type 2 diabetes in young and middle-aged women.* JAMA 2004; 292:927-934.

82. Strauss, RS. *Childhood Obesity and Self-Esteem.* Pediatrics 2001; 105(1): 15.

83. Moshfegh A, et al. *What We Eat in America; Usual Nutrient Intake from Food Compared to Dietary Reference Intakes.* U.S. Department of Agriculture, Agricultural Research Service. 2005; NHANES 2001-2002.

84. DiMeglio DP, Mattes RD. *Liquid versus solid carbohydrate: effects on food intake and body weight.* Int J Obes Relat Metab Disord 2000; 24:794–800.

85. Bray GA, Nielsen SJ, and Popkin BM. *Consumption of high-fructose corn syrup in beverages may play a role in the epidemic of obesity.* From the Pennington Biomedical Research Center, Louisiana State University, Baton Rouge, LA and the Department of Nutrition, University of North Carolina, Chapel Hill, NC.

86. Putnam JJ, Allshouse JE. *Food consumption, prices and expenditures, 1970–97.* US Department of Agriculture Economic Research Service statistical bulletin no. 965, April 1999. Washington, DC: US Government Printing Office, 1999

87. Schwartz MW, Woods SC, Porte D Jr, Seeley RJ, Baskin DG. *Central nervous system control of food intake.* Nature2000; 404:661–71.

88. Saad MF, Khan A, Sharma A, et al. *Physiological insulinemia acutely modulated plasma leptin.* Diabetes1998; 47:544–9.

89. Farooqi IS, Keogh JM, Kamath S, et al. *Partial leptin deficiency and human adiposity.* Nature 2001; 414:34–5.

90. Farooqi IS, Matarese G, Lord GM, et al. *Beneficial effects of leptin on obesity, T cell hyporesponsiveness, and neuroendocrine/metabolic dysfunc tion of human congenital leptin deficiency.* J Clin Invest2002; 110:1093–1103.

91. Colditz G, *"Economic Costs of Obesity and Inactivity,"* Medicine & Science in Sports & Exercise 1999; 31(11 Suppl.): 663–667.

92. Pratt M, Macera CA, and Wang G, *"Higher Direct Medical Costs Associated with Physical Inactivity,"* The Physician and Sports Medicine 2000; 28(10)

93. Fiatarone MA, Marks EC, Ryan ND, Meredith CN, Lipsitz LA, Evans WJ. *High-intensity strength training in nonagenarians. Effects on skeletal muscle.* Journal of the American Medical Association 1990; 263(22): 3029 – 3034.

94. Fiatarone MA, O'Neill EF, Ryan ND, Clements KM, Solares GR, Nelson ME, Roberts SB, Kehayias JJ, Lipsitz LA, Evans WJ. *Exercise Training and Nutritional Supplementation for Physical Frailty in Very Elderly People.* New England Journal of Medicine 1994; 330(25): 1769-1775.

95. Lee IM, Paffenbarger RS. *Physical Activity and Stroke Incidence, The Harvard Alumni Health Study.* Stroke 1998; 29:2049-2054.

96. Fentem PH. *ABC of Sports Medicine: Benefits of exercise in health and disease.* British Medical Journal 1994; 308:1291-1295.

97. Wong, SL, Katzmarzyk, PT, Nichaman, MZ, Church, TS, Blair, SN, Ross, R. *Cardiorespiratory Fitness is Associated with Lower Abdominal Fat Independent of Body Mass Index.* Med Sci Sports Exercise 2004; 36:286-291.

98. Janssen, I, Katzmarzyk, PT, Ross, R, Leon, AS, Skinner, JS, Rao, DC, Wilmore, JH, Rankinen, T, Bouchard, C. *Fitness Alters the Associations of BMI and Waist Circumference with Total and Abdominal Fat.* Obesity Research 2004; 12:525-537.

99. New York Chiropractic College, NYCC Admissions Handbook. 2007.

100. Reilly T, Tynell A, Troup JDG. *Circadian variation in the human stature.* Chronobiology It. 1984; 1:121.

101. Eklund, JA, Corlett, EN. (1984) *Shrinkage as a measure of the effect of load on the spine,* Spine, 9,2,189-94.

102. Adams MA, Dolan P, Hutton WC. *Diurnal variations in the stresses on the lumbar spine.* Spine 1987; 12:130.

103. Mennell, JM. Joint Pain. *Diagnosis and Treatment using Manipulative Techniques.* 1st ed. Boston, Little, Brown and Company. 1964.

104. Larder DR, Twiss MK, Mackay GM. *Neck Injury to car occupants using seat belts.* BMJ 1985; 298:153-68.

105. National Institute for Occupational Safety and Health (NIOSH) is part of the Centers for Disease Control and Prevention (CDC) within the Department of Health and Human Services. *BACK BELTS; Do They Prevent Injury?* Publication No. 94-127; 1996.

106. McGill SM, Norman RW. *Low back biomechanics in industry: The prevention of injury through safer lifting.* In Grabiner M (ed): Current Issues in Bio mechanics. Champaign, Il, Human Kinetics, 1993.

107. White A. *The Back School of the Future.* In White L (ed): Back School. Philadelphia, Hanley and Belfus. 1992.

108. Schuldt K, Ekholm J, Harms-Ringdahl K, et al. *Effects of changes in sitting work posture on static neck and shoulder activity.* Ergonomics 1986; 29:1525.

109. Anderson GB, Murphy RW, Ortengren R, et al. *The influence of back rest inclination and lumbar support on lumbar lordosis.* Spine 1979; 4:52.

110. Anderson GB, Jonsson B, Ortengren R. *Myoelectric activity in individual lumbar erector spinae muscles in sitting. A study with surface and wire electrodes.* Scand J Rehabil Med 1974: 3(suppl):19.

111. Anderson GB, Ortengren R, Nachemson AL, et al. *The sitting posture: An electromyographic and discometric study.* Ortho Clin North Am 1975; 6:105.

112. Szeto, GPY, Straker, L and Raine, S. *A field comparison of neck and shoulder postures in symptomatic and asymptomatic office workers.* Abstract- Science Direct 2001.

113. Hanson, M, Graveling, R, Donnan, P. *Investigation into the Factors Associated with Symptoms of ULDs in Keyboard Users.* UK Institute of Occupational Medicine 1996.

114. Galinsky TL, Swanson NG, Sauter SL, Hurrel JJ, Schleifer LM. *"A Field Study of Supplementary Rest Breaks for Data-entry Operators,"* Journal of Ergonomics 2000; 43(5): 622-638.

115. Mclean, L, Tingley, M, Scott, RN, Rickards, J. *"Computer Terminal Work and the Benefit of Micro-breaks",* Applied Ergonomics 2001; 32(3): 225-37.

116. Adams et al. *Mechanical initiation of intervertebral disc degeneration.* Spine 2000; 25(13): 1625-36.

> "Most human beings have an almost infinite capacity for taking things for granted" – Aldous Huxley

Small Sampling of Recommended Reading

BOOKS

Andres Stoll, M.D. – *The Omega 3 Connection: The Groundbreaking Anti-depression Diet and Brain Program*

Andrew Weil, M.D. – *8 Weeks To Optimum Health, Healthy Aging, Why Our Health Matters, Spontaneous Healing*

Arnold Schwarzenegger – *The New Encyclopedia of Modern Bodybuilding*

Bernie S. Seigel, M.D. – *Love, Medicine & Miracles, 101 Exercises For The Soul, Faith, Hope & Healing*

Betty Perkins-Carpenter, Ph.D – *How To Prevent Falls*

Bill Pearl – *Getting In Shape*

Bob Delmonteque – *Lifelong Fitness*

Byron J. Richards, CNN – *The Leptin Diet; How Fit Is Your Fat?*

Deepak Chopra – *Ageless Body Timeless Mind, Perfect Health, Grow Younger, Live Longer*

David Zinczenko – *Eat This, Not That*

James F. Balch, M.D. & Phyllis A. Balch, C.N.C. – *Prescription For Nutritional Healing*

Jillian Michaels – *Master Your Metabolism*

Joyce Vedral – *Bone Building Body Shaping Workout!, Bottoms Up*

Kenneth Cooper, M.D. – *Antioxidant Revolution*

Lauren Cordain, Ph.D and Joe Friel, M.S. – *The Paleo Diet For Athletes*

Lee Haney – *Ultimate Bodybuilding Book*

Michael Roizen, M.D. & Mehmet Oz, M.D. – *YOU: On A Diet, YOU: The Owner's Manual*

Morgan Sperlock – *Don't Eat This Book*

Nicholas A. DiNubile, M.D. – *Framework*

T. Colin Campbell, M.D. and Thomas M. Campbell II. – *The China Study*

William Bortz, M.D. – *We Live Too Short and Die Too Young, Dare to be 100, Living Longer for Dummies*

Index

Back

At Your

Best

Balancing the Demands of Life With the Needs of Your Body

Dr. Jay M. Lipoff, C.F.T.

www.ingramcontent.com/pod-product-compliance
Lightning Source LLC
Chambersburg PA
CBHW081143270326
41930CB00014B/3019